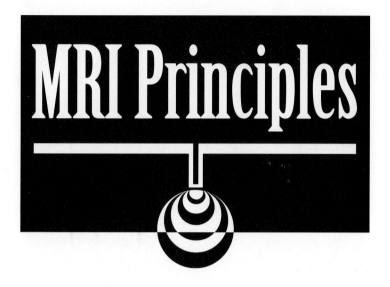

MRI Principles

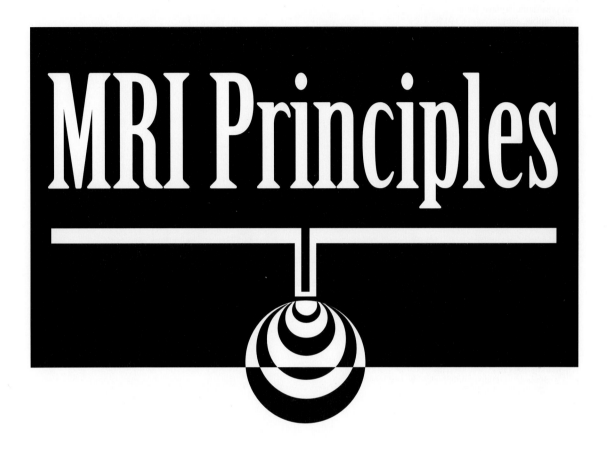

DONALD G. MITCHELL, MD

Professor of Radiology
Director
Division of Magnetic Resonance Imaging
Thomas Jefferson University Hospital
Philadelphia, Pennsylvania

W.B. SAUNDERS COMPANY

A Harcourt Health Sciences Company

Philadelphia   London   New York   St. Louis   Sydney   Toronto

W.B. SAUNDERS COMPANY
A *Harcourt Health Sciences Company*

The Curtis Center
Independence Square West
Philadelphia, Pennsylvania 19106

Library of Congress Cataloging-in-Publication Data

MRI principles / Donald G. Mitchell.

p.   cm.

ISBN 0–7216–6759–7

1. Magnetic resonance imaging.   I. Title.   [DNLM: 1. Magnetic
   Resonance Imaging—methods.   2. Mathematics.
   WN 185 M681m 1999]

RC78.7.N83M55   1999   616.07'548—dc21

DNLM/DLC   98–12902

MRI PRINCIPLES   ISBN 0-7216-6759-7

Printed in the United States of America.

Last digit is the print number: 9   8   7   6   5   4   3

To Debbie, Rebecca, and Liz, for your love and support

PREFACE

From the initial observation that dense materials attenuate x-rays, the complex field of medical imaging has blossomed. Armed with a knowledge of anatomy, pathophysiology, and the relative densities of various tissues, radiologists and other physicians have used radiography to diagnose disease in every body part and organ system.

Less than two decades old, clinical magnetic resonance imaging (MRI) offers diagnostic power far beyond that of radiographic density or any other single principle of imaging. Unlike any other imaging method, MRI utilizes *several* different principles, alone or in combination, to address a medical question. More than any other method, a solid understanding of the principles underlying MRI is essential for its effective use.

My intent with this book is to provide a framework to continue learning practical MRI principles as they evolve. Memorizing protocols is not sufficient, because these protocols are too complex and numerous and they change too rapidly. However, by understanding their basic underlying principles, new MRI advances can be learned easily and applied appropriately to clinical practice.

Like most physicians, my decision to pursue medical training was associated with a choice not to pursue advanced training in mathematics and physics. This left me unprepared for the mathematic equations and expressions offered as explanations for the MRI principles I was determined to learn. "Why can't any of these physicists explain anything in English?" I lamented to Simon Vinitski, PhD, who has helped extend my MRI knowledge over the years. Surprised at my question, he replied: "Because the simplest and clearest way to express something is through an equation!" Indeed, an equation is a simple and unambiguous method of expression, *unless the reader skips over the equations!*

This book is not "MRI Principles for Dummies." The MRI principles are described more comprehensively here than in most other texts.

In my experience, all physicians, MRI technologists, and other individuals involved with MRI are intelligent. Rather, many of us have not maintained our mathematic skills and vocabulary, so that we are not able to benefit from the clarity provided by "simple" equations.

This book is the culmination of more than a decade of my continuing efforts to teach MRI principles to others the way I learned, through plain English, copious illustrations and examples, a moderate amount of repetition, and a near total avoidance of mathematic expressions. Even basic principles in the early chapters are reinforced by examples of MR images.

Chapter 1 is an overview of the first seven chapters, describing briefly how proton signals give rise to images. Chapter 2 describes proton environments and introduces the concepts of T1 and T2 relaxation. In Chapters 3 and 4, T1 and T2 contrast, respectively, are discussed independently, along with the parameters that affect each. They are discussed independently to decrease confusion between these two important components of MR image contrast. Chapters 5 through 7 introduce the principles and processes by which MR signals are used to form images. Chapters 8 through 10 concern various trade-offs regarding image quality and characteristics. Understanding these chapters will help readers make adjustments to image protocols and pulse sequences to achieve the desired image quality and acquisition time. Chapters 11 and 12 describe the elements of pulse sequences, making use of the basic principles introduced earlier. Chapters 13 through 18 discuss how these pulse sequence elements, as well as the use of standard and new contrast agents, are combined to impart the desired image contrast. Chapter 19 reviews MR image artifacts.

I am grateful to the miracle of modern computing that empowered me to act as technical illustrator. The computer drawing tools at my disposal allowed me to create precise line drawings, obviating the need to explain my desired teaching points to a professional illustrator.

Even the mathematically sophisticated should benefit from these visually based explanations.

The lack of an advanced mathematics background should not prevent one from learning how to harness the continually increasing diagnostic power of MRI.

DONALD G. MITCHELL

ACKNOWLEDGMENTS

This manuscript has benefited from review of earlier versions by the following MR experts: Daisy Chien, PhD; Eric K. Outwater, MD; Yi Sun, PhD; and Simon Vinitski, PhD. Adam E. Flanders was particularly helpful regarding new techniques for neuroimaging. Patrick L. O'Kane, MD, copy-edited a later draft. The following individuals, most of whom were residents and fellows at the time, reviewed one or more drafts of this manuscript, contributing invaluable feedback that has significantly increased the clarity and educational value of this final product: Thomas Aretz, MD; Manoj Bhatia, MD; Granville Batte, MD; Bradford Botger, MD; Kevin Cregan, MD; Matthew C. Difazio, MD; Deborah Fein, MD; Andrea Fisher, MD; Vincent Giuliano, MD; Ralf P. Grasel, MD; Abbott Huong, MD; Shahid M. Hussain, MD; Pamela T. Johnson, MD; Ravi Kasat, MD; Robert Larson, MD; Phillip Lim, MD; Sanjay Maheshwari, MD; Burton Marks, DO; John Matzko, MD; Steven Moss, MD; Rita Patel, MD; Michael Ruhoy, MD; Ahmed Sa-dek, MD; Janio Sklaruk, MD, PhD; and Kim Wilson, MD. I am also grateful to David C. Levin, MD, Chairman of Radiology, Thomas Jefferson University Hospital, for providing resources and an environment conducive to research, education, and projects such as this.

Most MR images were obtained by or under the guidance of Peter Natale, RT. Additional images, credited in the figure legends, were provided by David A. Feinberg, MD, PhD; Michael Moseley, PhD; Neil M. Rofsky, MD; Lawrence Tannenbaum, MD; and Keith R. Thulborn, MD, PhD.

All illustrations were created by me, primarily using the following software for Apple Macintosh®: NIH *Image* and Adobe Photoshop® 3.0 and 4.0 for preparation of MR images and bitmap illustrations, Adobe Illustrator® 6.0 and 7.0 for line drawings and other vector illustrations, arrows, and figure annotations, and Adobe Dimensions® 2.0 for three-dimensional arrows and spheres.

DONALD G. MITCHELL

CONTENTS

1

From Protons to Images

Magnetic resonance imaging (MRI) is based on the phenomenon of *nuclear magnetic resonance* (NMR); that is, the resonance of atomic nuclei. *Resonance* is defined as an amplified response to a stimulus that has the same natural frequency. Nuclear magnetic resonance, in particular, involves measurement of signals coming from nuclei in response to radio waves that have the same natural frequency (resonant frequency) as the nuclei themselves.

Hydrogen is the simplest and most abundant element in the human body. Every water molecule contains two hydrogen atoms, and larger biological molecules, such as lipids and proteins, contain many hydrogen atoms. A hydrogen atom consists of a proton nucleus and a single electron. Electrons, while important for understanding radiography and critical to a different method called *electron spin resonance,* can safely be ignored for the remainder of this book, as we concentrate on *nuclear* MR. Hydrogen nuclei, which do not contain neutrons, are often referred to simply as *protons.*

An overview of the entire process by which images are created from protons is introduced in this chapter. The remaining chapters of the book are devoted to expanding on different components of this process.

SPINNING PROTONS

All current MRI techniques in routine clinical use are based on receiving and processing signals from protons. The exact molecular environment where these protons are located has a profound effect on the nature of the MR signals created, and thus gives rise to the remarkable power and versatility of clinical MRI and MR spectroscopy. The behavior of biological protons in the presence of a magnetic field is considered in greater detail in Chapter 2.

Protons have a magnetic axis. In nature, the orientation of these axes is random. In the presence of a magnetic field, however, protons spin around an axis that is aligned with the main magnetic field. This spinning of protons within a magnetic field is referred to as *precession.* The dominant axis of these spinning protons is oriented parallel to the axis of the *main magnetic field*; slightly fewer spins are oriented in a 180° opposite direction (antiparallel). For the purposes of understanding clinical MRI, we will consider the *average* alignment of protons rather than dwelling on the behavior of each individual proton (Fig. 1-1).

The precessing of protons gives rise to small secondary magnetic fields, or magnetization. The average magnetization of protons at a given time is referred to as *net magnetization.* At equilibrium, protons precess with their net magnetization aligned longitudinally, along the axis of the main magnetic field. This is referred to as *net longitudinal magnetization.*

This equilibrium longitudinal magnetization can be considered potential energy. When the equilibrium longitudinal magnetization is disturbed, as by an appropriate radio pulse, MR signals are generated. These signals can be measured and used to construct images.

MAGNETIC FIELDS

At the core of all MRI instruments is a homogeneous magnetic field. The purpose of the magnetic field is to establish net longitudinal magnetization of protons within it. Some MRI instruments utilize *permanent* magnets, which inherently contain magnetic materials that directly create magnetic fields. A permanent mag-

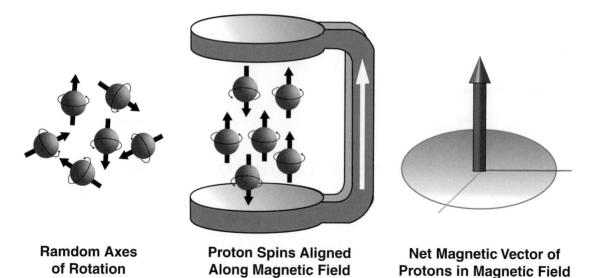

Ramdom Axes of Rotation   **Proton Spins Aligned Along Magnetic Field**   **Net Magnetic Vector of Protons in Magnetic Field**

FIGURE 1-1. Proton rotational axis in the absence of a magnetic field *(left)* is random. In the presence of a magnetic field *(middle)*, protons tend to align themselves so that the net axis of their rotation *(right)* corresponds with the direction of the main magnetic field.

netic field is oriented along an axis that extends between the two poles of the magnet. Usually, an MRI system that utilizes a permanent magnet contains a magnetic field that is perpendicular to the long axis of the magnet bore and scanner table (Fig. 1–2). Alternatively, *resistive* electro-

magnets generate magnetic fields perpendicular to an electric current flowing along a cylindrical coil (Fig. 1–3).

The strength of the magnetic field created by a permanent or resistive magnet is limited to approximately 5000 gauss (5000 times the

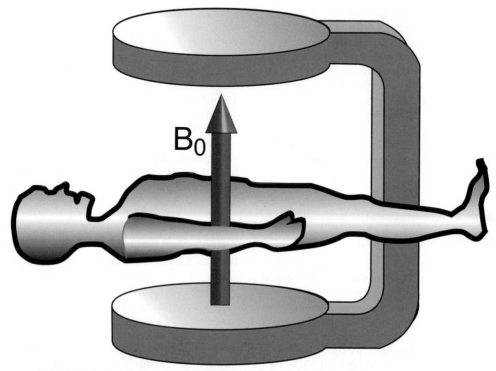

FIGURE 1-2. Main magnetic field (B_0) oriented along the axis of a permanent magnetic field.

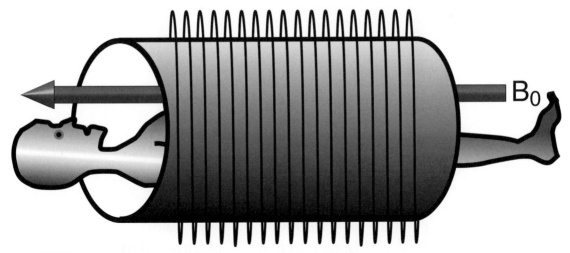

FIGURE 1–3. Main magnetic field (B_0) oriented along the axis of a resistive or superconducting magnetic bore.

strength of the earth's magnetic field), or 0.5 tesla (T). Stronger magnetic fields can be created by *superconducting magnets,* wherein resistance to the flow of electric current can be nearly eliminated by using appropriate materials and sufficiently low temperature.

The frequency with which protons precess is directly proportional to the strength of the main magnetic field. This frequency is often referred to as the *resonant frequency* because it is equal to the frequency of a radio pulse that induces resonance (echoes, reverberations) in the protons. One of the few equations used in this book, the well-known Larmor equation, expresses this relationship between precessional (resonant) frequency and magnetic field strength.

$$\mu = \delta \times B$$

where μ is the resonant frequency, δ is the *gyromagnetic constant,* and B is magnetic field strength.

The Larmor equation states that the resonant frequency is equal to the product of the magnetic field strength and the gyromagnetic constant. The gyromagnetic constant is a number without units that describes an intrinsic characteristic of a nucleus in a given environment. For water protons, the gyromagnetic constant is 42, which, when multiplied by magnetic field strength (in units of megaHertz [MHz]), leads to resonant frequencies of 21 MHz at 0.5 T and 63 MHz at 1.5 T. The gyromagnetic constant of protons within lipids and other "nonwater" molecules is somewhat different, the result being resonant frequencies that are close, but not identical, to that of water protons. The difference in resonant frequency between lipid and water protons, referred to as *chemical shift,* is covered in greater detail in Chapter 2.

RADIO PULSES AND TRANSVERSE MAGNETIZATION

When the net magnetization of tissue protons is aligned longitudinally, its strength is dwarfed by that of the main magnetic field. This severely limits possibilities for detecting net tissue magnetization at equilibrium (Fig. 1–4). To detect net tissue magnetization for the purpose of forming MR images, it is necessary to disturb equilibrium. Equilibrium is disturbed by exciting protons by exposing them to a radio pulse. This excitation pulse causes the protons to resonate.

The frequency, amplitude (strength), and duration of an excitation radio pulse determine its effects on the tissue. To excite a proton precessing within a magnetic field, the frequency of an excitation radio pulse must match the frequency at which the proton is precessing. Because the resonant frequency of water protons is close enough to that of lipid protons, most radio pulses can be tuned to excite both water and lipid protons. The amount of proton excitation is a product of both the amplitude and duration of the radio pulse.

We can think of this excitation in terms of rotation of the axis around which the protons precess. At equilibrium, net magnetization is aligned with the main magnetic field in the

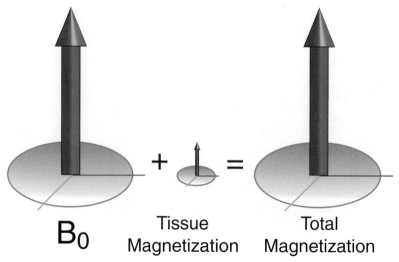

FIGURE 1–4. In comparison with the main magnetic field (B_0), tissue longitudinal magnetization is dwarfed. Therefore, its impact on total magnetization is negligible. This prevents it from being measured directly.

longitudinal plane. A radio pulse of appropriate frequency rotates this magnetization away from equilibrium into the transverse plane, producing transverse magnetization. Transverse magnetization can be detected and measured, since it is not obscured by the longitudinal magnetization of the main magnetic field.

At the appropriate amplitude and/or duration, a radio pulse may rotate all of the net magnetization of a group of protons from the longitudinal plane into the transverse plane. Rotation from the longitudinal to the transverse plane is 90° of rotation. A radio pulse that completely converts longitudinal into transverse magnetization is therefore referred to as a *90° pulse* (Fig. 1–5).

Excitation by a radio pulse produces a signal that is an *echo* of the excitation pulse. The amplitude of this signal is greatest when it is first created. The signal decays rapidly owing to nonuniformity of the magnetic field. This initial rapidly decaying signal is called a *free induction decay* (*FID*; Fig. 1–6). Because of its rapid decay, it is not suitable as a basis for spatial location. The timing of radio pulses and their effects on the information content of MR signals are considered in greater detail in Chapters 3 and 4. Methods of restoring MR signal after the FID are discussed in Chapter 5.

SPATIAL LOCALIZATION

All forms of imaging require methods of resolving tissues at different locations and de-

picting their correct positions. Therefore, a reliable method of locating the source of MR signals is needed. This is not a simple process, since the MR signal itself, like other radio waves, does not possess any directional information. (When we listen to a radio, we cannot determine from which direction the radio station is broadcasting.) Therefore, a variety of clever techniques are employed in combination to allow us to resolve the complex collection of radio signals in three dimensions, to produce useful MR images.

The fundamental process used to determine the location of sources of MR signals is the application of supplemental magnetic field gradients, referred to as *imaging gradients*. In a homogeneous magnetic field, water protons resonate at the same frequency, regardless of location. If we superimpose a second magnetic field upon the main magnetic field, we cause a predictable variation in the magnetic field along a predetermined axis. The resulting total magnetic field (the sum of the main and gradient magnetic fields) is highest at one end and lowest at the other; between are intermediate values along the axis of the gradient. Since the resonant frequency of a proton is directly proportional to the magnetic field around it, the magnetic field gradient produces a predictable variation in resonant frequency along this axis. Thus, application of the magnetic field gradient causes protons at one end of the gradient to spin slower and protons at the other end to spin faster. In this text, an imaging gradient is depicted in Figure 1–7.

Magnetic field gradients are usually produced by gradient coils within the bore of the main

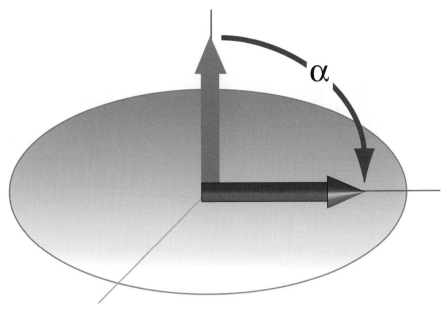

FIGURE 1-5. A 90° excitation pulse (α) rotates longitudinal magnetization into the transverse plane, allowing it to be measured.

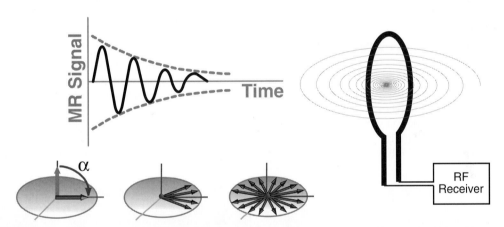

FIGURE 1-6. Free induction decay. Following its creation, transverse magnetization produces a signal that decays rapidly. It is therefore not a suitable basis for most MRI techniques. RF, radiofrequency.

FIGURE 1-7. Magnetic field gradient applied in addition to the homogeneous main magnetic field. The magnetic field increases to the right along the axis of this gradient, increasing the resonant frequencies of the affected protons.

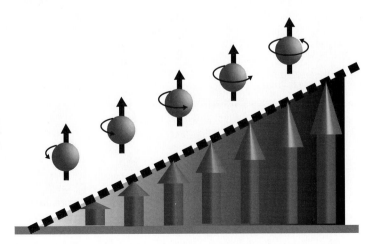

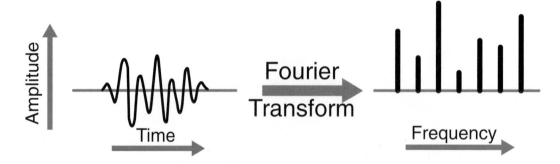

FIGURE 1–8. Fourier transform analysis involves converting the frequency data in a complex wave into a map of amplitudes for each frequency.

magnet. Magnetic field gradients are applied in three orthogonal axes, at different times, allowing three-dimensional localization of the signals' origins. The application of these gradients, and the methods by which the signals are used to construct images, are discussed in greater detail in Chapter 5.

MRI INSTRUMENT OVERVIEW

The MRI instrument includes one or more computers, a radio transmitter and receiver, one or more radio transceiver coils, magnetic field gradient coils, and the main magnet. The timing and strength of magnetic field gradients and radio pulses are controlled through an acquisi-

tion computer that uses parameters chosen by the MRI operator. The commands from the computer are sent to gradient and radiofrequency (RF) amplifiers, which generate, respectively, gradient and radio pulses. The impulses for radio pulses are sent from the RF power amplifier to the transmit-receive driver, which triggers the generation of the radio pulses. The resulting radio pulses are transmitted from an antenna, or coil, to excite the protons in the body part of interest.

In some instances, the same coil is used both to send and receive MR signals. In other instances, as for imaging superficial structures, a separate coil, referred to as a *receive-only coil,* is used to receive the MR signals. The signals from the body part of interest are sent from the receiving coil back through the transmit-receive

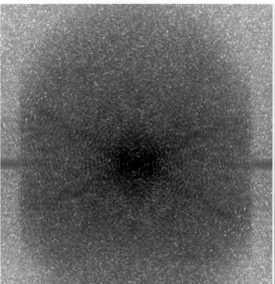
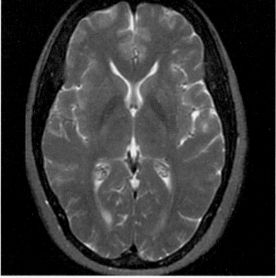

FIGURE 1–9. K-space *(left)* is a map of digital data that, when subjected to Fourier transform analysis, generates an image of physical space *(right)*. The image at right is a 256 × 192 fast spin echo image with TR/TE$_{ef}$ of 2317/90.

driver to a preamplifier, which prepares the signals for conversion to digital data.

Initially, the received signal consists of numerous analog (nondigital) radio waves that make up a composite waveform. This complex composite waveform contains many different frequencies, phases, and amplitudes. These data do not directly indicate the spatial location of the protons from which they originated. The MR signals undergo analog-to-digital conversion (ADC), producing digital data that consist of a set of numbers representing points along the waves. These data are filtered, stored in memory, and processed by the MR acquisition computer. The digital data are not mapped directly as points in a final image; rather, they are represented in a matrix referred to as *k-space*. Each point in k-space contains data from all portions of an MR image.

The k-space data are subjected to Fourier transform analysis, which produces pixel data with different gray-scale values. Fourier transform analysis consists of calculating the amplitude and phase of each individual frequency that is part of a complex wave that occurs over a specific time interval (Fig. 1-8).

Fourier analysis of k-space yields pixel data that allow construction of a two- or three-dimensional image. Each pixel is assigned a number that represents the MR signal amplitude (intensity) from that spatial location. These pixels form images that are sent to the host computer for display, printing, or further manipulation or analysis. Because signal intensity depends on the receiver gain and other factors, absolute signal intensity numbers, by themselves, are meaningless. The signal intensity of pixels in an image, relative to each other, are however, quite useful.

Details of MR image creation and how MR parameters can be adjusted to alter the appearance and information content of MR images are addressed throughout the remaining chapters of this book.

The center of k-space contains data that are used to derive most of the amplitude values for pixels throughout the image and, therefore, determines most contrast. The periphery of k-space has little effect on image contrast, but it contains data that determine fine detail. Figure 1-9 demonstrates an image and its corresponding k-space map. K-space is discussed and illustrated in greater detail in Chapter 6.

ESSENTIAL POINTS TO REMEMBER

1. In the presence of a magnetic field, protons spin at a frequency that is directly proportional to the strength of that magnetic field.
2. The net magnetization of protons at equilibrium is called *longitudinal magnetization*.
3. When excited by a radio pulse of comparable frequency the magnetization axis of spinning protons is rotated toward the transverse plane. The strength and duration of this excitation radio pulse determine how many degrees this axis is rotated.
4. A radio pulse that rotates the magnetization of spinning protons by 90° is referred to as *a 90° pulse*. A 90° pulse converts all *longitudinal magnetization* into *transverse magnetization*.
5. Equilibrium (longitudinal) magnetization cannot be measured. Magnetization must be rotated into the transverse axis if it is to be measured.
6. The source of MR signals is determined by applying magnetic field gradients, which cause the resonant frequency of protons to vary along the axis of the magnetic field.
7. The amplitude, frequency, and phase of MR signals are measured and used to create a map of k-space. The map of k-space undergoes Fourier transform analysis to create an MR image.

2 Proton Environments and Relaxation

If all other factors are equal, a higher density of mobile protons results in a stronger magnetic resonance (MR) signal, and therefore higher signal intensity, on MR images. This is also true for radiography and scintigraphy, wherein the major determinant of tissue contrast is density. However, there are other mechanisms for MR tissue contrast that often are more important than density and that do not have counterparts in other imaging modalities. These factors relate to the local environment of protons. That is, the signal arising from a given proton varies according to its position within a molecule and its relationship to other molecules.

First, we will consider water, the principal source of most signals used for MR imaging. The signal intensity from water protons varies greatly, depending on their physical relationship to other molecules and to certain magnetically active materials. Additionally, there are fundamental differences in the signals arising from water protons and those from protons within lipids and other macromolecules.

WATER STRUCTURE

The structure of water in biological tissues is surprisingly complex. For the purposes of understanding tissue contrast on MR images, a simplified two-compartment model is sufficient. These two water compartments are commonly referred to as *free water* and *bound water.*

Free water consists of simple water molecules in solution that are not in immediate proximity to macromolecules such as proteins, phospholipids, or DNA. Free water moves rapidly and is highly disorganized. Bound water, on the other hand, is close enough to macromolecules for its motion to be restricted, principally

through hydrogen bonding. Bound and free water are illustrated in Figure 2-1.

Following rotation toward the transverse plane by an excitation radio pulse, the net axis of proton magnetization returns toward equilibrium. This return to equilibrium is referred to as *relaxation.* Because of free water's rapid motion and lack of structure, the transfer of energy is inefficient. Following excitation by a radio pulse, the return to equilibrium of free water's net proton magnetization is slow. In other words, free water *relaxes slowly.* Protons in bound water, however, recover more rapidly after exposure to a radio pulse. The different magnetic and electric behaviors of bound and free water have profound effects on the appearance of MR images.

The relative amounts of free and bound water within tissues vary greatly throughout the body. Soft tissues with abundant intracellular organelles, such as brain, pancreas, and liver, have a large intracellular surface area and therefore contain a large proportion of bound water and have short relaxation times. In contrast, there is a large proportion of free water in urine and cerebrospinal fluid (CSF), as well as within cysts, follicles, and glands. Water in these locations thus looks different from water in solid tissues (Fig. 2-2).

T1 RELAXATION (RECOVERY)

Equilibrium is disrupted when a radio pulse rotates net magnetization away from its initial longitudinal plane. This disturbance of equilibrium, whereby transverse magnetization is produced, is termed *excitation.* Longitudinal magnetization is eliminated, or *saturated.* The saturation of longitudinal magnetization is complete for a 90° pulse.

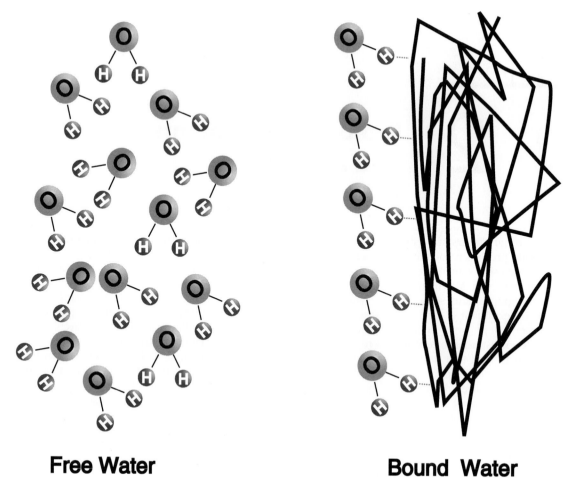

Free Water   ## Bound Water

FIGURE 2-1. Biological water can be considered as being in one of two compartments: free water *(left)*, or bound water *(right)*, which is closely associated with macromolecules.

Following exposure to a radio pulse, net magnetization returns to equilibrium. This return, which does not require any additional radio pulses or other events, is termed *relaxation.* In general, relaxation processes are slower for free water than for bound water, as described above. The process by which longitudinal magnetization recovers is referred to as *longitudinal relaxation,* or *T1 relaxation.* The time required for protons in a tissue to return to their equilibrium longitudinal orientation is expressed as a constant called a *relaxation time,* which at a given magnetic field strength is a property of that tissue and of the efficiency with which it can transfer energy to surrounding structures. The transfer of energy involved in T1 relaxation is referred to as *spin-lattice* interaction. T1 relaxation involves recovery of magnetization to the longitudinal plane (Fig. 2-3).

The rate at which longitudinal magnetization

recovers after saturation by an excitation radio pulse, the *T1 relaxation rate,* is determined by the properties of the material itself as well as by the magnetic field strength. The T1 relaxation rate is sometimes abbreviated as R1, or as the reciprocal of the T1 relaxation time, 1/T1. The *T1 relaxation time* is defined as the time required for longitudinal magnetization to recover to 63% of its original equilibrium level after complete saturation by a 90° pulse. After an interval twice that of the T1 relaxation time, longitudinal magnetization has recovered to 91% of its equilibrium value, and after three relaxation times, to 97% (Fig. 2-4). The levels of 63%, 91%, and 97% are based on the characteristics of logarithmic recovery curves; a level of 100% defines an asymptote, which, theoretically, is never reached.

The upper limit for biological T1 relaxation times is that of pure free water, approximately 3 seconds. In pure water and other nonviscous

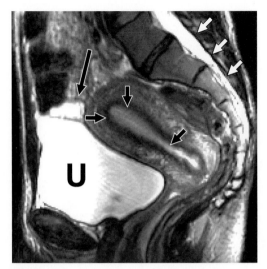

FIGURE 2–2. Sagittal T2-weighted image of the pelvis depicts free water in urine (U), endometrial glands *(short black arrows)*, bowel lumen *(long black arrow)*, and cerebrospinal fluid *(white arrows)* as having high signal intensity, owing to the long T2 relaxation time of free water. Solid tissues such as uterine myometrium and skeletal muscle have shorter relaxation times and, therefore, lower signal intensity on this image.

liquids, molecules move rapidly and thus transfer energy inefficiently, leading to long relaxation times. The T1 relaxation times of CSF and urine, which contain several electrolytes but few large molecules, are between 2 and 3 seconds.

Relaxation of protons in molecules other than water depends in part on the size of the molecules. Small molecules such as water move rapidly, which decreases the efficiency of relaxation, leading to long relaxation times. The motion of fatty acids within adipose tissue is restricted, increasing the efficiency of T1 relaxation and causing adipose tissue to have the shortest T1 relaxation times of all biological tissues. The T1 relaxation time of adipose tissue is approximately 100 to 150 msec, depending on magnetic field strength.

Protons in large macromolecules such as protein do not produce MR signal on currently used pulse sequences, because their transverse magnetization decays so rapidly that no signals are detected by must current clinical MR techniques. However, macromolecules restrict the motion of nearby water and thus shorten its T1 relaxation time. Fluids with high protein content, such as mucus and synovial fluid, have shorter T1 than do less viscous fluids.

Most benign cellular soft tissues have a large intracellular surface area, which results in a large proportion of bound water. Benign cellular tissues thus tend to have much shorter T1 relaxation times than do simple fluids such as urine and CSF (Fig. 2–5).

Most malignant neoplasms have larger and less organized cells than do benign tissues and thus contain more intracellular free water. Additionally, malignant neoplasms tend to have more extracellular fluid, principally in their in-

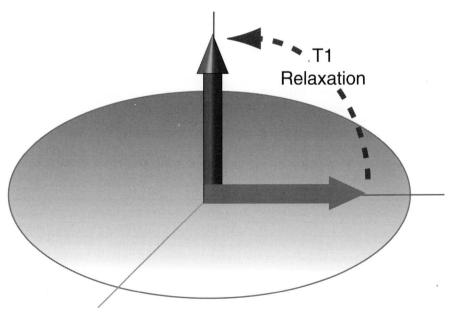

FIGURE 2–3. T1 relaxation (recovery) converts transverse magnetization back to longitudinal magnetization, its equilibrium state.

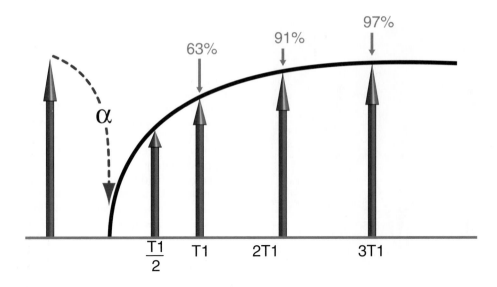

FIGURE 2–4. T1 relaxation following a 90° excitation pulse (α), shows the logarithmic recovery of longitudinal magnetization at T1/2, T1, 2T1, and 3T1.

terstitia. For both of these reasons, most neoplasms have more free water than most benign tissues and, thus, longer T1 relaxation times.

MAGNETIC FIELD STRENGTH

The T1 relaxation times of some materials are longer in stronger magnetic fields. This is not true for pure free water, which has a uniform T1 relaxation time regardless of magnetic field strength. In bound water, the reduction of the T1 of water protons by proximity to macromolecules diminishes as field strength increases; that is, a given amount of interaction between tissue macromolecules and water has a smaller effect at high magnetic field strength than at low field strength. The T1 relaxation

time of bound water within soft tissues, therefore, is longer at higher field strength. Thus, there is less difference between the T1 relaxation times of free and bound water and inherently less T1 contrast between many tissues as field strength increases.

The effects of magnetic field strength on T1 relaxation time are less pronounced for adipose tissue than for tissues rich in bound water. Therefore, as T1 relaxation times of most non-fatty soft tissues increase with field strength, the T1 contrast between these tissues and adipose tissue increases as well. Examples of T1 at 0.5 T and at 1.5 T, and the ratio of the T1s at the two different field strengths, are shown in Table 2-1. Table 2-2 describes contrast between different tissues at these two different field strengths.

In summary, as magnetic field strength increases, T1 relaxation times increase substan-

TABLE 2-1. REPRESENTATIVE T1 RELAXATION TIMES AT 0.5 T AND 1.5 T

	T1 at 0.5 T (msec)	T1 at 1.5 T (msec)	T1 Ratio: 1.5 T/0.5 T
Cerebrospinal fluid (free water)	> 4000	> 4000	1.0
Skeletal muscle (bound/free water)	600	870	1.4
Gray matter (bound/free water)	656	920	1.4
Liver (bound/free water)	323	490	1.5
Adipose tissue	215	260	1.2

Cerebrospinal fluid (free water) has long T1, which does not change with field strength. Skeletal muscle, gray matter, and liver, rich in bound water, have significantly longer T1 at 1.5 T. Adipose tissue also has longer T1 at 1.5 T, but the magnitude of the change is less than that for bound water. (Data from the SMRI and MResource Guide, 1994 Edition, Wood ML, Bronskill MJ, Mulkern RV, Santyr GE: Physical MR desktop data. JMRI 1993; 3(S):19–26.)

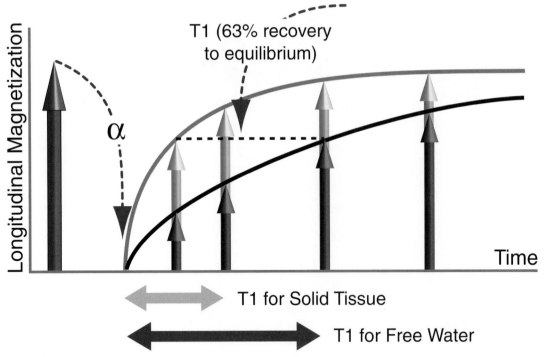

FIGURE 2–5. T1 relaxation for solid tissue *(gray)* and free water *(black)*. In this example, recovery to 63% of equilibrium longitudinal magnetization requires four times as much time for free water as for solid tissue. Therefore, T1 relaxation is four times as long for free water as for solid tissue.

tially for bound water, increase slightly for adipose tissue, and remain constant for free water. Therefore, at higher magnetic field strength, T1 contrast between free and bound water decreases and contrast between bound water and adipose tissue increases.

Magnetic field strength is also a major determinant of MR signal strength. For this reason, MR images obtained with comparable parameters are usually noisier at low field strength (Fig. 2–6).

T2 RELAXATION (DECAY)

Transverse magnetization, created by the rotation of longitudinal magnetization into the transverse plane, decays at a rate equal to or faster than the rate of T1 recovery. The decay of transverse magnetization is defined as *T2 relaxation,* and the rate of this T2 decay is defined by a tissue's T2 relaxation time. If T2 relaxation were simply a reconversion of transverse magnetization back into longitudinal magnetization, T1 and T2 relaxation times would always be equal and there would be no need to consider two separate relaxation processes. Indeed, T1 and T2 relaxation times are equal for pure water and are similar for many other fluids and for adipose tissue. In these tissues, there is little organized structure and motion is relatively random.

The absolute upper limit for the T2 relaxation time of any material is its T1 relaxation

TABLE 2–2. T1 CONTRAST AT 0.5 T AND 1.5 T

Tissues Imaged	T1 Contrast Ratio 0.5 T	T1 Contrast Ratio 1.5 T
Gray matter vs. cerebrospinal fluid	6.1	4.6
Skeletal muscle vs. adipose tissue	2.8	3.4
Skeletal muscle vs. liver	1.9	1.8

Data are based on the values from Table 2–1. Contrast between gray matter and CSF (bound versus free water) is greater at 0.5 T, whereas contrast between skeletal muscle and adipose tissue (bound water versus adipose tissue) is greater at 1.5 T. There is little change in contrast between skeletal muscle and liver, both of which contain abundant bound water.

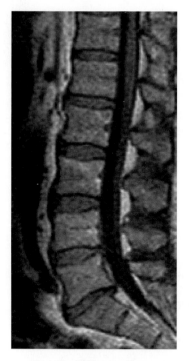 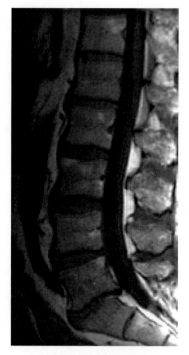

FIGURE 2–6. Comparison of T1-weighted spin echo images of the lumbar spine of one subject obtained with similar parameters at 0.2 T *(left)* and at 1.5 T *(right)*. The image obtained at 0.2 T is noisier but has greater contrast between cerebrospinal fluid and spinal cord or intervertebral discs. Contrast between cellular and fatty marrow in the vertebral bodies is greater at 1.5 T. (Courtesy of Lawrence Tannenbaum, M.D. and Edison Imaging, Edison, NJ.)

0.2 Tesla   1.5 Tesla

time. This is because it is not possible for any transverse magnetization to persist after all longitudinal magnetization has recovered to its equilibrium value. For most soft tissues in the body, however, T2 relaxation is faster than T1 relaxation, so T2 relaxation times are shorter than T1 relaxation times. The additional transverse relaxation occurs as a result of exchange of energy between protons, referred to as *spin-spin interaction.*

The rapid and random motion of free water molecules renders exchange of energy between protons inefficient. Therefore, transverse magnetization decays slowly in free water. For free water, the T2 relaxation time is long (i.e., comparable to its T1 relaxation time). Conversely, T2 relaxation is especially efficient in bound water, which has a more organized structure. Tissues composed of well-differentiated cells with large intracellular surface area contain abundant bound water. The motion of water in these tissues is nonrandom, and T2 relaxation times are much shorter than T1 relaxation times (Fig. 2-7).

T2 relaxation times are less affected by magnetic field strength than are T1 relaxation times. Additional decay of transverse magnetization secondary to local magnetic effects, however, depends much on magnetic field strength. The decay of transverse relaxation resulting from the combination of T2 relaxation and magnetic field heterogeneity, referred to as *T2* relaxation,* is discussed in the next section.

LOCAL MAGNETIC EFFECTS

The T1 and T2 relaxation of water protons is enhanced by proximity to paramagnetic materials, which contain atoms with unpaired electrons. Relaxation times are reduced for water protons in the vicinity of paramagnetic substances. Examples of T1 and T2 relaxation enhancement by paramagnetic materials include the effect of MRI contrast materials and signal alterations of tissues secondary to contained iron.

A magnetic field is altered by tissues and other materials within it. The ability of a material within a magnetic field to produce additional magnetism is referred to as *susceptibility.* This term causes some confusion because the material that produces the additional magnetic field is considered to have susceptibility, whereas it is the water protons that are susceptible to this added magnetic field.

The susceptibility of a vacuum is defined as

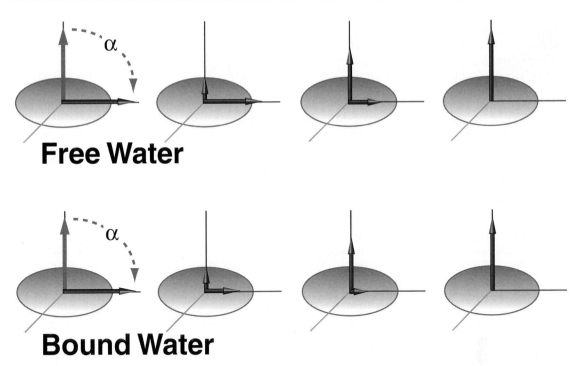

Free Water

Bound Water

FIGURE 2–7. T1 and T2 relaxation for free and bound water. For free water *(top)*, T2 is nearly equal to T1. Thus, transverse magnetization decays at a rate comparable to the rate at which longitudinal magnetization recovers. For bound water *(bottom)*, T2 is shorter than T1. Thus, transverse magnetization decays faster than longitudinal magnetization recovers.

zero. Most soft tissues have no susceptibility relative to water. Air and nonmetallic solids such as bone have negative susceptibility (i.e., they tend to induce weaker magnetic fields than does water). Materials with abundant unpaired electrons, including iron and paramag-netic elements, strengthen magnetic fields in their vicinity. Positive and negative susceptibility are illustrated in Figure 2–8.

Particles that have substantial positive susceptibility and therefore produce a strong supple-mentary magnetic field when exposed to

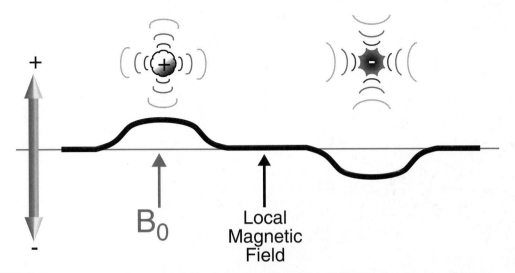

FIGURE 2–8. Effects on local magnetic field relative to main magnetic field (B_0) of positive (+, *left*) and negative (−, *right*) susceptibility. A superparamagnetic focus such as a particle of iron has positive susceptibility, increasing the local magnetic field in its vicinity. An air bubble or focus of calcium has negative susceptibility, decreasing the local magnetic field in its vicinity.

magnetic forces are referred to as *superpara-magnetic.* Superparamagnetic materials are said to have positive susceptibility because they increase the magnetic field in comparison to the magnetic field in water.

Magnetic fields are most heterogeneous near interfaces between substances with different susceptibilities. The most severe perturbation of the magnetic field seen in common clinical MRI arises from ferromagnetic objects within or adjacent to the patient, such as metallic prostheses, bullets, and bracelets (Fig. 2–9).

Somewhat less deleterious, but significant for some imaging applications, are the abundant and unavoidable interfaces between the patient and the surrounding air. The negative susceptibility of air relative to water is generally not as pronounced as is the positive susceptibility of metal, so the artifact near air tends to be less intense.

Some artifacts from air-tissue interfaces can be reduced by placing water or materials with similar susceptibility (e.g., fluorocarbons) adjacent to the patient, displacing the air away from the patient's skin. Other air-tissue interfaces, such as those within cranial sinuses, airways, lung, and bowel, cannot be eliminated. Bone also has negative susceptibility, and bone-tissue interfaces are present throughout the body.

Water protons are exposed to increasing magnetic fields as they come closer to superparamagnetic foci. Each superparamagnetic focus in a magnetic field thus produces local magnetic distortions, facilitating some forms of relaxation. The susceptibility effect, and thus the sensitivity to superparamagnetic substances, increases with the second power of the magnetic field strength (Fig. 2–10).

The effects of paramagnetic and superparamagnetic materials on MR images are completely unlike those of any material on images produced by any other modality. For instance, dense materials such as iodine and calcium prevent photons from reaching a radiographic detector or film and thus have direct effects on the final radiographic image. Similarly, radioactive materials emit photons that are detected directly and displayed on scintigraphic images. In contrast, paramagnetic and superparamagnetic materials are not detected directly; all current clinical MR images are derived from signals produced by protons. A compound containing paramagnetic materials is not depicted on an MR image unless that compound also contains protons.

The reduction of tissue relaxation times by magnetic materials depends on the concentration of these magnetic materials and on their

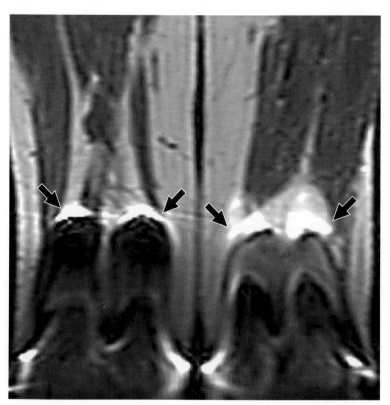

FIGURE 2–9. Coronal T1-weighted spin echo image of the lower thighs of a patient with bilateral metallic knee prostheses. Arrows indicate distortion due to susceptibility differences between stainless steel and body tissue.

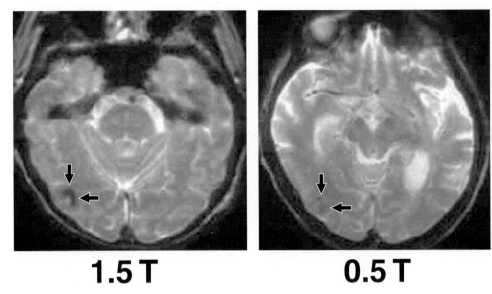

1.5 T   0.5 T

FIGURE 2–10. T2-weighted spin echo images of the brain show a small hemorrhagic infarction *(arrows)* with low signal intensity that is due to the susceptibility effects of the iron within hemosiderin. The lesion is better visualized at 1.5 T than at 0.5 T owing to the greater susceptibility at higher magnetic field strength. Both images are at the level of the hemorrhage, but other anatomy is different because of different patient positioning. (Courtesy of W. G. Bradley.)

microscopic interactions with water protons. For example, a paramagnetic substance may have little effect on a tissue if it is shielded from close contact with tissue water. Similarly, a superparamagnetic material has greater effect on a tissue if it is distributed heterogeneously, producing more pronounced variation of local magnetic fields. Thus, the concentration and microscopic distribution of magnetic materials are both important determinants of the resulting signal intensity on MR images (Fig. 2–11).

CHEMICAL SHIFTS

Chemical shifts are the differences in resonant frequency of protons based on their mo-lecular environment. Note that chemical shift, which defines the resonant frequency of protons, is *completely independent of relaxation time,* which defines the time it takes protons to recover after excitation by a radio pulse. For example, free and bound water have the same resonant frequency, and therefore the same chemical shift, whereas their relaxation times are quite different.

There is a single resonant frequency for protons in water at a given magnetic field strength, whereas protons in other molecules, such as silicone, lactate, and the various fatty acids, resonate at slightly different frequencies. In other words, the protons in these various molecules have slightly different chemical shifts. In fact, protons at different sites in a given complex molecule (e.g., methylene [CH_2] and methyl [CH_3] protons within triglycerides) may

FIGURE 2–11. Hepatic cavernous hemangioma *(arrows)*, on T1-weighted images before and 10 minutes after intravenous injection of iron oxide particulate contrast material. The paramagnetic effects of the contrast agent vary, depending on its distribution. After 10 minutes, many particles have been taken up heterogeneously by reticuloendothelial cells, decreasing hepatic signal intensity because of heterogeneous magnetic susceptibility. The intravascular distribution within the hemangioma is more homogeneous, decreasing susceptibility-induced signal loss. Additionally, the intravascular particles are in closer approximation to water, increasing the paramagnetic enhancement of T1 recovery and, in turn, increasing signal intensity of the hemangioma.

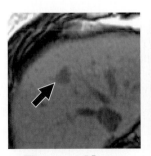
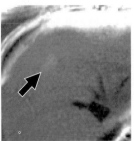

Baseline   10 min post

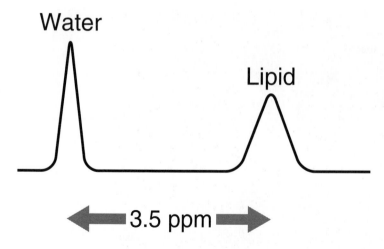

FIGURE 2-12. The difference in resonant frequency between water *(left)* and lipid *(right)* is approximately 3.5 ppm. There are several different lipid resonances, so the composite peak for lipids is broader than the simple peak for water.

have different chemical shifts. Protons in some components of adipose tissue, such as unsaturated olefinic acids (−CH=CH−) actually have resonant frequencies closer to that of water than to the resonant frequencies of most other lipid protons.

The most important chemical shift in most MRI applications is the shift between water protons and CH_2 protons within long-chain fatty acids (e.g., triglyceride) in adipose tissue. The chemical shift between protons in different magnetic environments is proportional to the main magnetic field wherein they lie. Therefore, the magnitude of chemical shifts is expressed in parts per million (ppm). For example, the chemical shift between water and methylene protons is expressed as approximately 3.5 ppm (Fig. 2-12).

The actual value of this chemical shift is directly proportional to the main magnetic field, so the chemical shift between water and lipid is larger at higher magnetic field strengths. For example, at 1.5 T, protons precess at 63.86 MHz; the chemical shift between water and CH_2 protons is 224 Hz. At 0.5 T, protons precess at approximately 21 MHz, and the chemical shift between water and CH_2 protons is 73.5 Hz. Chemically nonselective excitation pulses have a bandwidth large enough so that water and lipid are both excited. Chemical shift techniques that involve selective excitation or saturation of either water or CH_2 protons utilize radio pulses with a bandwidth narrow enough so that only one of these groups of protons is affected.

Theoretically, chemical shift MRI techniques are possible at any field strength, although they are technically difficult at lower field strengths, owing to the smaller differences between the resonant frequencies of lipid and water protons.

ESSENTIAL POINTS TO REMEMBER

1. Water in biologic tissues can be considered as being divided into free and bound compartments.
2. Bound water is associated with macromolecules; free water is not.
3. After exposure to an excitation radio pulse, transverse magnetization returns toward the longitudinal plane. This is referred to as *longitudinal relaxation* or *T1 relaxation*.
4. The T1 relaxation time is defined as the time required for recovery of approximately two thirds (63%) of longitudinal magnetization. The rate of T1 recovery is the inverse of a tissue's T1 relaxation time (i.e., 1/T1).
5. Transverse magnetization decays at a rate defined by a tissue's T2 relaxation time.
6. Bound water tends to have shorter T1 and T2 relaxation times than does free water.
7. The upper limit of T1 and T2 relaxation times is approximately 3 seconds for distilled water. T2 relaxation time can never be greater than T1 relaxation time. For structured tissues, T2 relaxation time is less than T1 relaxation time.
8. T2 relaxation times are less affected by magnetic field strength than are T1 relaxation times.
9. Paramagnetic materials contain unpaired electrons, which reduce the relaxation times of nearby water protons.

10. Aggregates of paramagnetic materials are superparamagnetic. Superparamagnetic materials have increased susceptibility, which means that they induce greater magnetic field strength in their vicinity. Heterogeneous distribution of superparamagnetic particles within a tissue decreases the homogeneity of the magnetic field, which can reduce the intensity of MR signals.

11. Paramagnetic and superparamagnetic materials are not demonstrated directly in MR images. Rather, their presence changes the T1 and T2 relaxation times of water protons and thus changes their signal intensity on MR images.

12. The resonant frequency of protons varies, depending on their position within a molecule. The difference between two such resonant frequencies is called *chemical shift*.

13. Protons in water, silicone, and lipid have different chemical shifts.

14. Chemical shift differences are independent of differences in relaxation times.

15. Chemical shifts are greater at higher magnetic field strengths.

3 Longitudinal Magnetization and T1 Contrast

In this section, we will concentrate on longitudinal magnetization and T1 recovery, postponing further consideration of transverse magnetization and T2 decay until Chapter 4. As a brief review, remember that, at equilibrium, net magnetization orients longitudinally, along the axis of the main magnetic field. Equilibrium is disturbed when an excitation radio pulse reduces net longitudinal magnetization. T1 relaxation occurs when longitudinal magnetization recovers (i.e., returns to equilibrium). Tissues that contain abundant intracellular surface area or paramagnetic materials relax more efficiently and therefore have shorter T1 relaxation times than do tissues that contain abundant free water.

The T1 relaxation time is a property of a tissue at a given magnetic field strength. MRI pulse sequence parameters can be manipulated so that differences between the T1 relaxation times of tissues can be either important or insignificant determinants of tissue contrast. The two major parameters in most pulse sequences that can be varied to control the T1 weighting of an image are the repetition time (TR) and the flip angle. (In inversion recovery pulse sequences, an additional parameter, the inversion time (TI), also has great effect on how T1 differences between tissues look. Discussion of TI, however, is postponed until Chapter 12.)

REPETITION TIME

For most pulse sequences, it is necessary to excite each slice repeatedly to acquire all the data needed to produce the images. Following each excitation pulse, longitudinal magnetization is reduced—or, in fact, eliminated if the pulse imparts 90° of rotation. The time between repetitions of the excitation pulse is defined as the *repetition time* (TR).

After each excitation, longitudinal magnetization begins to recover. If the TR is similar to or shorter than the T1 relaxation time of a tissue, recovery of longitudinal magnetization is only partial. Therefore, immediately before the second excitation pulse, the amount of longitudinal magnetization is less than it was at equilibrium before the first excitation pulse. Recovery of longitudinal magnetization following this pulse is also incomplete, resulting in even less longitudinal magnetization at the time of the third excitation pulse. After several pulses, the amount of magnetization that recovers before the next excitation pulse reaches a constant level, referred to as a *steady state.*

Before the steady state is achieved, each subsequent excitation radio pulse creates less transverse magnetization than the previous excitation pulse. If data acquisition for imaging began immediately, this varying magnetization would create artifacts. To prevent this, the echoes produced by the first several excitations are not measured. The excitation radio pulses that occur before the achievement of a steady state are sometimes referred to as *"dummy" pulses,* because no data are collected from them. Once the steady state is reached, following several dummy pulses, data acquisition begins (Fig. 3-1).

With short TR, longitudinal magnetization recovers more completely for tissues with short T1 than for tissues with long T1. At the time of the next excitation pulse, longitudinal magnetization is greater for tissues with short T1 than for those with long T1. The amount of transverse magnetization created is therefore greater for tissues with short T1.

Although only transverse magnetization is measured, the amount of transverse magnetization created by an excitation radio pulse in a

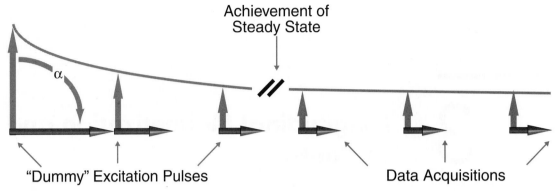

FIGURE 3–1. Achievement of a steady state following a series of "dummy" excitation pulses, which are identical to later excitation pulses except that no data are acquired. After several dummy pulses, the amount of longitudinal magnetization present at each excitation pulse reaches a steady state. Data are acquired only after a steady state is achieved.

T1-weighted pulse sequence is directly related to the amount of longitudinal magnetization that has recovered since the previous excitation pulse. In other words, the amount of recovered longitudinal magnetization is determined by first converting it to transverse magnetization and then measuring it.

With a pulse sequence of sufficiently short TR (typically one comparable to or less than the T1 of the tissues to be distinguished) contrast on the resulting images is affected by T1 differences between tissues. With such a pulse sequence, the amplitude of an echo, and the resulting signal intensity on an image, are low for tissues with long T1 and high for tissues

with short T1 (Fig. 3–2). Because images such as these are effective for depicting T1 differences between tissues, they are said to be *T1-weighted* (Figs. 3–3 and 3–4).

FLIP ANGLE

The degree of rotation of magnetization caused by an excitation radio pulse is a product of the strength and duration of that pulse. The amount of rotation that results from a radio pulse is referred to as the *flip angle*. With a flip angle of 90°, longitudinal magnetization is

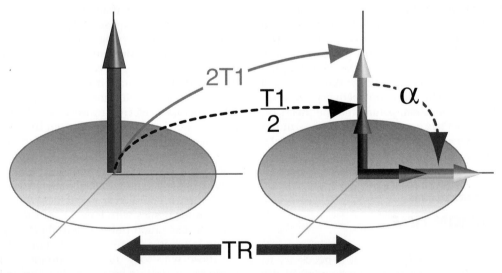

FIGURE 3–2. Effect of T1 differences on amount of transverse magnetization created. T1 for black is four times as long as it is for gray. The repetition time (TR) is half the T1 for black and twice that for gray. Different amounts of transverse magnetization are created by the next 90° excitation pulse (α) for each of the two tissues, directly reflecting the different amounts of longitudinal magnetization that had recovered. Thus, the differences in T1 between the two tissues produced different amounts of transverse magnetization and different intensities on the eventual image (T1 contrast).

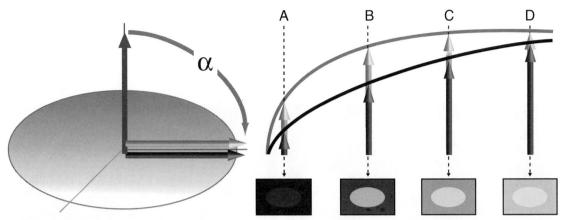

FIGURE 3–3. T1 relaxation curves of two tissues show contrast based on four different repetition time (TR) values *(A–D)*. The T1 relaxation time indicated by the black line is four times as long as that indicated by the gray line. If the TR is too short *(A)*, contrast may be subtle, owing to low signal intensity of both tissues. With more moderate TR *(B)*, contrast may be depicted optimally. As TR increases, magnetization of the tissue with long T1 continues to recover and contrast may become increasingly subtle *(C)* and *(D)*.

converted completely to transverse magnetization. Thus, the saturation of longitudinal magnetization and the creation of transverse magnetization are both maximal with a 90° excitation pulse.

The excitation flip angle can be decreased by reducing either the strength or the duration of the excitation radio pulse. The effect of flip angle reduction on the strength of the resulting MR signal depends on a balance between the amount of transverse magnetization created and the amount of longitudinal magnetization saturated by the excitation radio pulse.

The relationship between excitation flip angle and signal intensity can be appreciated by considering the competing effects of saturation of longitudinal magnetization and creation of transverse magnetization. A flip angle of 90° creates the most transverse magnetization, but it also saturates longitudinal magnetization most completely. Flip angles smaller than 90° create less transverse magnetization. This, *by itself,* results in *lower* signal intensity on the eventual MR images (Fig. 3–5).

If TR is less than T1, recovery of longitudinal magnetization between pulses is incomplete when a 90° flip angle is used. Use of a lower flip angle causes less saturation of longitudinal magnetization, so that longitudinal magnetization can recover closer to its equilibrium value during TR. The less complete saturation resulting from a reduced flip angle, *by itself,* results in *higher* signal intensity on the eventual MR images. The amount of signal intensity depends on the *combination* of these competing effects: creation of transverse magnetization

and saturation of longitudinal magnetization, both of which are maximal with 90° flip angles.

For a tissue with a given T1, at a given TR there is an optimal excitation flip angle that generates the greatest signal intensity. If the flip angle is too large, most longitudinal magnetization is saturated and recovery time is insufficient. There is thus little longitudinal magnetization present at the time of each excitation pulse, and little transverse magnetization is created. Conversely, if the flip angle is too small, even though there may be abundant longitudinal magnetization at the time of each excitation pulse, little of it is converted into transverse magnetization. Thus, there is an optimal flip angle that is small enough so that saturation of longitudinal magnetization is not too complete but large enough so that sufficient transverse magnetization is created (Fig. 3–6). This optimal flip angle for the highest resulting signal intensity, depending on the T1 of a tissue and the TR used, is referred to as the *Ernst angle*. This angle can be calculated (by the mathematically literate) based on the TR of the pulse sequence and the T1 of the tissue. Tissues with long T1 recover slowly after excitation, so Ernst angles are smaller than for tissues with short T1.

In most imaging situations, we are not necessarily interested in maximizing signal intensity of a specific tissue but rather in maximizing contrast between two or more tissues. To maximize contrast, it is important for the tissue with long T1 to have low signal intensity. Therefore, the optimal flip angle for depicting this contrast must be higher than its Ernst angle. T1

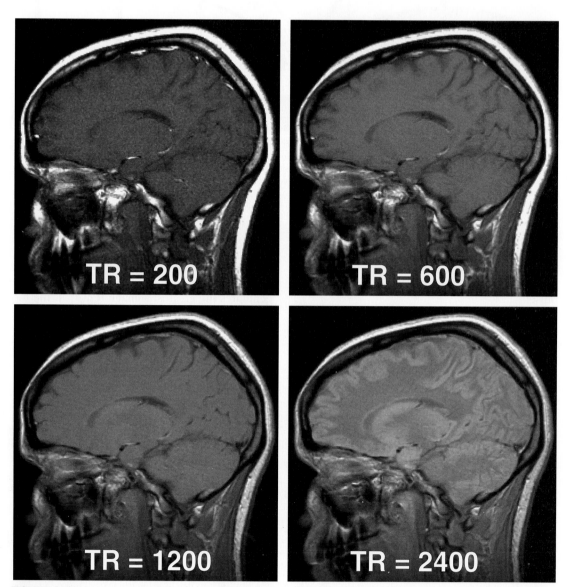

FIGURE 3–4. Effect of varying repetition time (TR) on tissue contrast. Sagittal fast spin echo images of the brain with TE of 15 msec and variable TR. With TR of 200 and 600 msec, there is substantial T1 contrast between gray and white matter and cerebrospinal fluid, but overall signal intensity is higher with TR of 600 msec. As TR increases to 1200 and 2400 msec, T1 contrast diminishes.

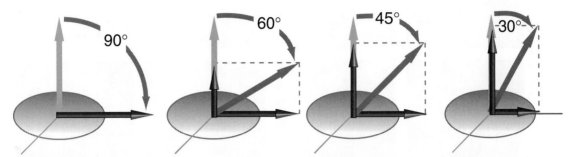

FIGURE 3–5. Diagram of 90°, 60°, 45°, and 30° excitation pulses, rotating different amounts of longitudinal magnetization into the transverse plane. With a reduced excitation flip angle, such as 30°, less transverse magnetization is created and more longitudinal magnetization remains.

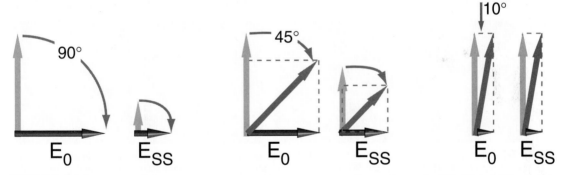

FIGURE 3–6. Comparison of the amount of transverse magnetization created at steady state by 90°, 45°, and 10° at a given short repetition time (TR) for a tissue with a given T1. Although the amount of transverse magnetization created by the initial excitation pulse (E_0) is greatest for the 90° excitation pulse, most magnetization remains saturated at the time of each excitation pulse during the steady state (E_{SS}). With 45° excitation pulses, T1 relaxation is more complete at the same TR, since less longitudinal magnetization is saturated with each excitation pulse. Thus, more transverse magnetization is created during the steady state by 45° pulses than by 90° pulses. With 10° pulses, although there is nearly complete T1 recovery between excitation pulses, little transverse magnetization is created by each excitation pulse. For the tissue and TR in this example, the optimal excitation angle (Ernst angle) is closer to 45° than to 90° or 10°.

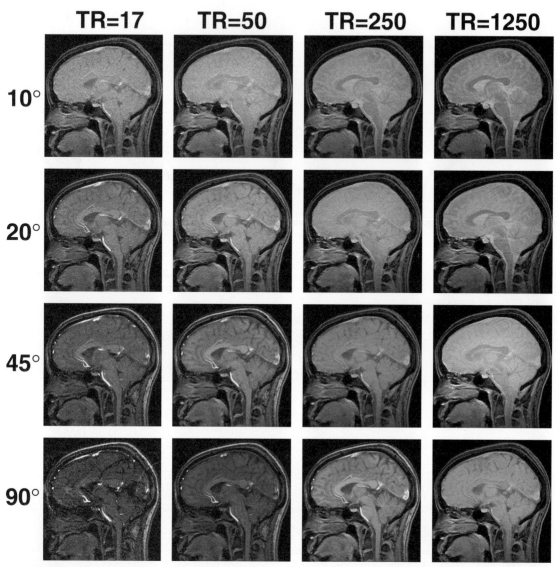

FIGURE 3–7. Effect of varying repetition time (TR) and flip angle on tissue contrast. Sagittal spoiled gradient echo images of the brain using variable TR and flip angle. With short TR and high flip angle *(bottom left)*, overall signal intensity is low. With long TR and low flip angle *(top right)*, signal intensity is higher but there is little T1 contrast. The best balance between adequate signal intensity and T1 contrast is achieved with TR–flip angle combinations of 17/20°, 50/45°, or 250/90°.

contrast at the chosen TR is optimal at or higher than the Ernst angle for the tissue with shorter T1. TR and flip angle should be considered together, because in many cases changes in one should be accompanied by changes in the other. Smaller flip angles should be chosen when using short TRs, especially for tissues with long T1 relaxation time (Fig. 3–7).

ESSENTIAL POINTS TO REMEMBER

1. T1 relaxation time is a property of a tissue at a given magnetic field strength.

2. The T1 relaxation time of a tissue is independent of pulse sequence, but T1 differences between tissues (T1 contrast) can be depicted by appropriate choice of the MRI pulse sequence.

3. Most pulse sequences involve exciting tissue repeatedly within a section. The time between excitation radio pulses is the TR.

4. Before data acquisition, several dummy excitation radio pulses are transmitted to allow the longitudinal magnetization present before each excitation radio pulse to reach steady state.

5. If the TR is similar to or less than the T1

of a tissue, relaxation during the TR is incomplete. This tissue therefore has less signal intensity on the resulting image than does a tissue with shorter T1.

6. Images that depict differences between tissues based on different T1 relaxation times are *T1-weighted images.*

7. For any two tissues, there is an optimal TR that produces the best contrast between them. If TR is too short, the MR signal strength is too low. If TR is too long, longitudinal magnetization recovers too completely for both tissues.

8. If the flip angle of the excitation radio pulse is less than 90°, conversion of longitudinal magnetization into transverse magnetization is incomplete. Less transverse magnetization is created, but less time is required for longitudinal magnetization to recover during the TR.

9. To obtain a desired degree of saturation in a tissue, decreases in TR should be accompanied by decreases in excitation flip angle. Smaller flip angles are generally used with short TR pulse sequences.

10. For a tissue with a given T1, at a given TR there is a specific flip angle, the Ernst angle, that results in maximal signal strength.

CHAPTER

4 Transverse Magnetization and T2 Contrast

In clinical MRI, transverse magnetization cannot be measured immediately, because it decays rapidly owing to magnetic field gradients applied to locate the source of MR signals. The rapid decay of transverse magnetization immediately after it is created is referred to as the *free induction decay* (FID). To measure coherent transverse magnetization, it is necessary to form an echo of the original signal by bringing the transverse magnetization back into phase (see Chapter 5). There is always a finite delay between the creation of transverse magnetization and the measurement of the resulting echo. During this delay, transverse magnetization decays at a rate defined by its T2 relaxation time. The time between the initial creation of transverse magnetization and its measurement is defined as the *echo time* (TE) (Fig. 4-1).

ECHO TIME

The decay of transverse magnetization during the TE reduces the signal intensity on the resulting image. This reduced signal intensity is especially significant for tissues with short T2 relaxation times. Images with a TE such that signal intensity is determined largely by T2 differences between tissues are referred to as *T2-weighted images*. Images with TEs much shorter than the T2s of the tissues of interest have little T2 weighting, so image contrast is determined principally by other factors. Images with TEs comparable to or slightly longer than the T2 relaxation times of the tissues of interest are considered to have significant T2 weighting. Images with TEs much longer than the T2s of the tissues of interest may exhibit such substantial decay of transverse magnetization that the ratio of signal intensity to noise (SNR) in the image may limit their clinical usefulness.

For optimal T2 contrast between two tissues, it is desirable for most of the signal intensity of the tissue with shorter T2 to have decayed. Conversely, it is essential for ample signal intensity to remain from the tissue with longer T2. Thus, to depict T2 contrast between two tissues, an optimal TE balances sufficient decay of transverse magnetization from one tissue against sufficient remaining transverse magnetization from the other (Figs. 4-2 and 4-3).

NON–T2 CAUSES OF TRANSVERSE MAGNETIZATION DECAY

Each tissue has a characteristic T2 relaxation time that is independent of magnetic field strength. This T2 relaxation time can be considered an upper limit of the time before which two thirds of the transverse magnetization has decayed. The actual rate of decay of transverse magnetization manifested on MR images, however, is augmented by additional factors, including magnetic field strength and chemical shift heterogeneity.

When the transverse magnetization is first created by excitation of longitudinal magnetization, the spins in the transverse plane are coherent (i.e., they resonate in phase with each other). Anything that causes spins to resonate at different frequencies causes dephasing, which causes the transverse magnetization to decay. Purposefully applied imaging gradients, one such cause of dephasing, can be compensated for by applying a rephasing lobe of the gradient (see Chapter 5). Two causes of dephasing that are not corrected by the rephasing lobe of the imaging gradients are heterogeneity of the local magnetic field and heterogeneity of the chemical shifts of the tissue itself.

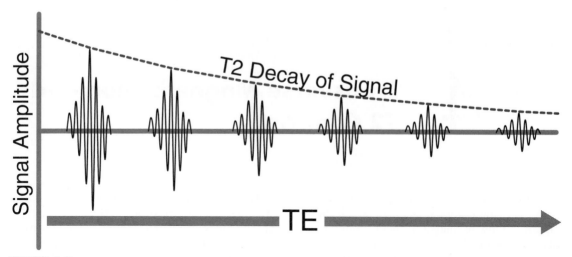

FIGURE 4-1. Logarithmic decay of MR signal due to T2 relaxation. The signal strength is weaker as the echo time (TE) increases.

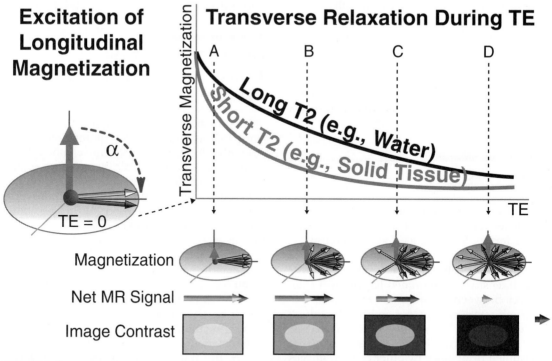

FIGURE 4-2. T2 relaxation curves of two tissues show contrast based on four different TEs. The T2 decay of solid tissue *(gray curve)* is faster than that of free water *(black curve)*. If the TE is too short *(A)*, SNR is high but contrast may be poor owing to insufficient decay of transverse magnetization from either tissue. With more moderate TE *(B)*, contrast may be optimal. As TE increases further, transverse magnetization of the tissue with long TE continues to decay, and contrast may become increasingly subtle *(C and D)*. The vertical gray arrows indicate longitudinal magnetization, which recovers more slowly than transverse magnetization decays.

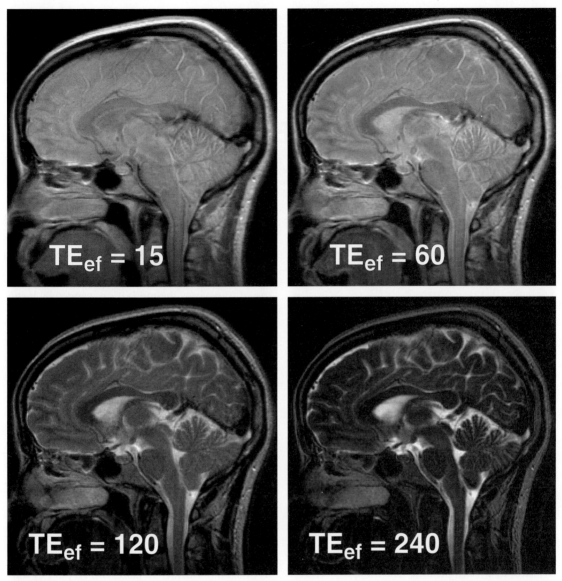

FIGURE 4–3. Effect of varying TE on tissue contrast. Sagittal fast spin echo images of the brain with increasing effective TE (TE_{ef}) show minimal T2 contrast at 15 msec. T2 contrast increases up to 120 msec. With an effective TE of 240 msec, there is good T2 contrast between brain and CSF, but signal intensity of "non–CSF" tissues is too low for adequate contrast.

Heterogeneous Magnetic Field and Susceptibility

When the magnetic field that affects a tissue is not homogeneous, the magnetic forces vary from proton to proton. Protons exposed to stronger magnetic fields resonate faster than protons exposed to weaker magnetic fields, causing dephasing and accelerated decay of transverse magnetization during TE (Fig. 4-4). Figure 4-5 illustrates the exacerbation of susceptibility effects with increasing TE. The combined decay of transverse magnetization from

T2 relaxation and heterogeneous magnetic field is referred to as *T2* relaxation.*

Every effort is made to construct homogeneous magnets for use in MRI units. Weak supplemental gradients, referred to as *shim gradients,* are adjusted to correct for minor heterogeneities in the main magnetic field. Even if shimming is perfect, however, the magnetic field is disturbed once a patient lies within it. This is largely because of differences in magnetic susceptibility between tissues within the patient relative to each other and relative to air or other substances. With some MRI systems,

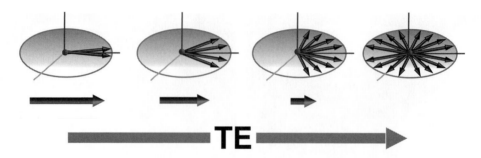

FIGURE 4-4. Progressive loss of coherent transverse magnetization results from magnetic field heterogeneity during the interval between creation of transverse magnetization by the excitation pulse and measurement of the echo at the echo time (TE). The horizontal arrows above the TE indicate the decreasing net transverse magnetization.

patient-induced magnetic field heterogeneity is minimized by applying additional shimming while the patient lies within the magnetic field and before imaging begins.

Heterogeneous Chemical Shift

Even in a perfectly homogeneous magnetic field, not all protons resonate at the same frequency. The motion of a proton within a magnetic field is affected by its local molecular environment, a property referred to as *chemical shift*. Protons within water and different components of lipids (e.g., methyl [CH_3], methylene [(CH_2], and carboxyl [$COOH$]) and similar molecules experience different magnetic environments and therefore resonate at different frequencies. Thus, often there is some dephasing of transverse magnetization in tissues that contain protons with two or more different chemical shifts, such as adipose tissue.

MR signal from adipose tissue is dominated by saturated CH_2 protons within triglyceride, although unsaturated fatty acids and water in blood vessels and connective tissue also contain protons. If this chemical shift within adipose tissue is not corrected for, it produces dephasing of transverse magnetization, especially if the chemical shifts between water and saturated CH_2 protons are maximally out of phase with respect to each other.

Since water protons resonate faster than the protons in these saturated fatty acids, they gain phase relative to fatty acid protons. When first created, the transverse magnetizations of water and CH_2 protons are in phase with respect to each other, but the phase gain of water relative to CH_2 protons increases with time until the phases are maximally opposed with respect to each other (i.e., 180°). At this time, destructive interference between these two different populations with opposite phases reduces the net transverse magnetization and results in low signal intensity (Fig. 4-6).

As TE increases beyond the time of 180° opposed phase, the phase of water proton magnetization continues to gain with respect to that

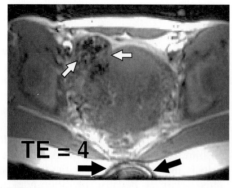
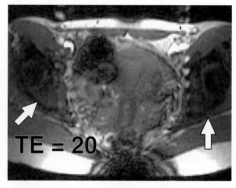

FIGURE 4-5. Effect of increasing TE on susceptibility effects. Spoiled gradient echo images were obtained at 1.5 T. With TE of 4 msec *(left)*, air and stool are visible in the sigmoid colon *(small white arrows)*. Artifact due to metal is noted posteriorly *(black arrows)*. Increasing TE to 20 msec *(right)* intensifies these susceptibility artifacts and susceptibility-induced signal intensity loss from bone trabeculae in the acetabula *(large white arrows)*.

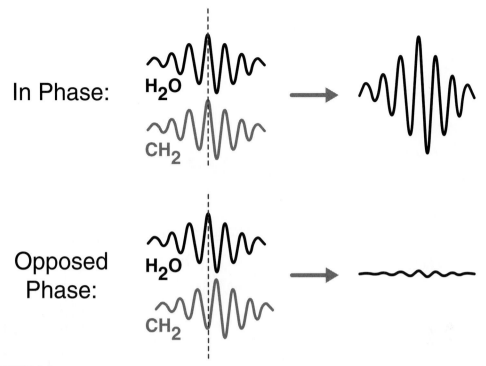

FIGURE 4–6. Summation of two in-phase waves *(top)*, and cancellation of two opposed-phase waves *(bottom)*.

of CH_2 protons, so that the phase difference between them reaches 360°, which is equivalent to 0°, and is, again, in phase (Fig. 4–7).

As TE increases, transverse magnetization can vary owing to the combined effects of cyclic dephasing from chemical shift heterogeneity and the logarithmic decay from a heterogeneous magnetic field (T2* decay). Figure 4–8 graphically depicts these combined effects. In this figure, T2* decay is represented as a logarithmic curve drawn along the peaks of a graph depicting cyclic variations of signal intensity as TE increases. This latter curve represents signal loss due to the combined effects of T2* and chemical shift heterogeneity. An example of this oscillation of signal intensity with increasing TE is shown in Figure 4–9.

REFOCUSING RADIO PULSES AND THE SPIN ECHO

There are some applications in which decay of transverse magnetization from heterogeneous susceptibility and/or heterogeneous chemical shift is acceptable or even desirable. In other applications, such loss of coherent transverse magnetization produces unaccept- able image degradation. In such situations, additional radio pulses can be applied to refocus transverse magnetization that has begun to decay because of factors other than T2 relaxation. These additional radio pulses are called *refocusing pulses.* Refocusing pulses are applied at or near the center of the chosen TE (i.e., halfway between the excitation and the time of the peak of the resulting echo). The refocusing pulse is maximally effective when it imparts a rotation of 180°.

Consider a tissue that contains tiny foci of iron like those that may be present in hemosiderin following hemorrhage. These foci of iron have positive susceptibility and in their immediate proximity induce a supplemental magnetic field, which increases to total local field strength beyond that of the main magnetic field. The protons nearest to the iron foci resonate faster than other protons. Thus, shortly after creation of transverse magnetization by the excitation radio pulse, protons near the focus of iron gain phase relative to other protons. At a time halfway between the excitation pulse and the echo peak, a 180° refocusing pulse can be applied, which rotates all spins within the transverse plane, reversing the phases of these protons relative to each other. The protons near the focus of iron still resonate

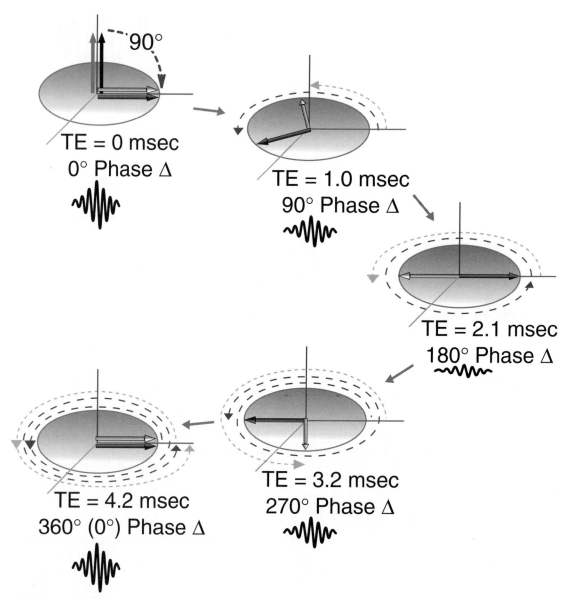

FIGURE 4–7. Phase differences between water and lipid with changing TE. In this example, the TEs are appropriate for a field strength of 1.5 T. At a TE of 2.1 msec, water *(black arrow)* and lipid *(gray arrow)* magnetizations are 180° out of phase with respect to each other, leading to maximal phase cancellation. At TEs of 0 and 4.2 msec, water and lipid magnetizations are in phase with respect to each other, leading to maximal summation of signal.

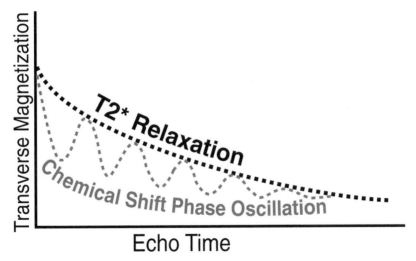

FIGURE 4–8. Decay of transverse magnetization due to T2* relaxation, corresponding to the peaks of the decay of transverse magnetization of a tissue with heterogeneous chemical shift. The light gray curve represents the combined effects of T2* decay and superimposed oscillations due to chemical shift heterogeneity.

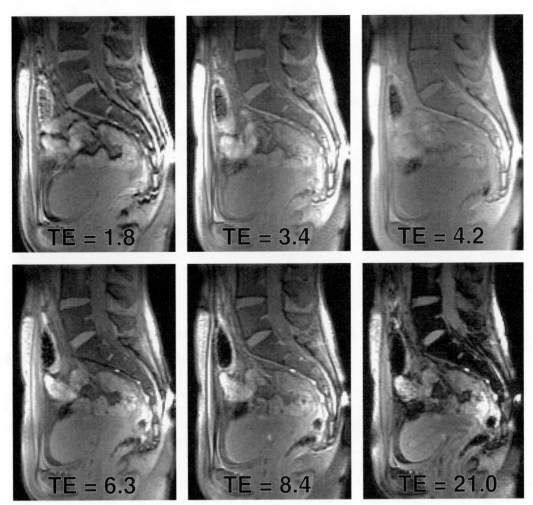

FIGURE 4–9. Sagittal gradient echo images of the pelvis and lower lumber spine with increasing TE show a combination of T2* and chemical shift effects. At TE of 1.8 msec, the phases of lipid and water proton magnetizations are opposed; at 4.2 msec they are in phase. Thus, the signal intensity of bone marrow increases through this range of TEs. At 8.4 and 21 msec, lipid and water proton magnetizations are also in phase, but the heterogeneous magnetic susceptibility of trabecular bone causes a short T2*, and therefore low signal intensity, with increasing TE.

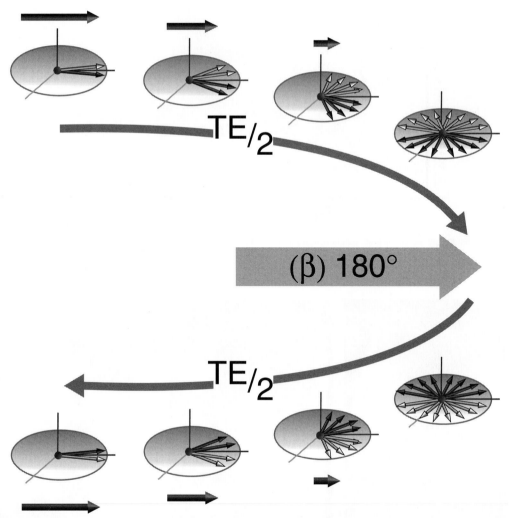

FIGURE 4–10. Effect of a 180° refocusing pulse (β), which reverses the phase accumulation of spins at the midpoint of the TE. Spins that resonate at relatively high frequency *(light arrows)* gain phase relative to other spins *(dark arrows)*. During the second half of the TE, after being rotated 180° in the transverse plane by the refocusing pulse the spins represented by light arrows are behind in phase but continue to resonate faster relative to the spins represented by dark arrows. At TE all spins are back in phase (0°).

faster than other protons, but their phase lags behind. As the TE approaches, the rapidly resonating protons near the iron focus regain this phase, "catching up" at the TE. This forms an echo referred to as a *spin echo* (Fig. 4–10).

Refocusing pulses also correct for dephasing in tissues containing protons with different chemical shifts such as adipose tissue. A 180° pulse, applied in the middle of the TE, reverses the relative phases of water and lipid protons, so that water protons fall behind in phase relative to lipid protons. During the second half of the TE, the phase of water protons approaches the phase of fatty acid protons, so that net magnetization reaches a crescendo at the spin echo.

ESSENTIAL POINTS TO REMEMBER

1. The interval between creation of transverse magnetization and its measurement is the TE. Transverse magnetization decays during this interval.
2. For depiction of T2 differences between tissues (T2 contrast), there is an optimal TE that is long enough to allow sufficient decay of transverse magnetization of short-T2 tissues but short enough to minimize decay of transverse magnetization of long-T2 tissues.
3. When protons in a tissue resonate at the same frequency, transverse magnetization

decays at a rate defined by the tissue's T2 relaxation time. When protons in a tissue resonate at a range of frequencies, transverse magnetization of the tissue decays faster than its T2 relaxation time would predict.

4. Protons at a given site resonate at different frequencies when the local magnetic field is heterogeneous, resulting in rapid decay of transverse magnetization.

5. Protons at a given site resonate at different frequencies when they have different chemical shifts, resulting in cycles of dephasing and rephasing of transverse magnetization.

6. Decay of transverse magnetization by T2 relaxation and magnetic field heterogeneity, considered together, is referred to as T2* relaxation.

7. A 180° refocusing pulse applied at mid–TE (TE/2) corrects for both magnetic field and chemical shift heterogeneity. Echoes sampled after a 180° refocusing pulse are called *spin echoes*.

5 Spatial Localization: Magnetic Field Gradients

Thus far we have been considering the MR properties of tissues without considering how tissues at different locations are resolved and depicted in their correct positions. To move beyond analysis of bulk tissue properties toward creation of useful diagnostic images, a reliable method of locating the source of MR signals is needed. This is not a simple process, since the MR signal itself, like other radio waves, does not possess any directional information. When we listen to a radio, we cannot determine from which direction the radio station is broadcasting. Thus, a variety of clever techniques in combination allow us to resolve the complex collection of radio signals in three dimensions, producing useful MR images.

The fundamental process used to determine the location of MR signal sources is the application of supplemental magnetic field gradients, referred to as *imaging gradients.* In a homogeneous magnetic field that is not subjected to imaging gradients, protons with identical chemical shift resonate at the same frequency, regardless of location. If we superimpose upon the main magnetic field a supplemental magnetic field we purposefully cause a predictable variation in the magnetic field along a predetermined axis. The resulting total magnetic field (the sum of the main and gradient magnetic fields) is strongest at one end, weakest at the other, and intermediate between those points along the axis of the gradient. Since the resonant frequency of a proton is directly proportional to the magnetic field to which it is exposed, the magnetic field gradient produces a predictable variation in resonant frequency along this axis. Thus, application of the magnetic field gradient causes protons at one end of the gradient to spin slower, and those at the other end to spin faster, relative to protons between these two extremes. The concept of using supplemental magnetic field gradients for

spatial localization of MR signals was introduced and illustrated in Chapter 1, Spatial Localization.

BASIC PULSE SEQUENCE ANNOTATION

Further discussion of imaging gradients, particularly their timing in relation to other events inherent in generating and measuring MR signals, is facilitated by use of a simple form of annotation that describes the timing and configuration of MR pulse sequence events. A pulse sequence is defined by a set of horizontally oriented lines. The horizontal axis indicates time, the scale of which is identical for all lines in a given example. Each line describes a sequence of radio pulses, image gradients, or MRI signals.

The top line, abbreviated as *RF* (radiofrequency), describes the radio pulses. Each radio pulse is indicated by a solid vertical bar whose height indicates the degree of rotation imparted to the affected magnetization. (Some alternative annotation systems indicate the radio pulse as a wave, similar to our annotation for the MR signal, illustrated later.) The purpose of the radio pulse is often indicated below the bar. Excitation pulses are referred to as α *pulses* and refocusing pulses as β *pulses.* The degree of rotation imparted by the radio pulses is sometimes indicated above the vertical bar. For example, in Figure 5–1, note that the 180° refocusing pulse (β) is twice as tall as the 90° excitation pulse (α).

Most of the remaining lines in a pulse sequence diagram describe the timing of the various imaging gradients. A flat line, in "neutral" position, indicates that the imaging gradient is turned off. When the imaging gradient is turned

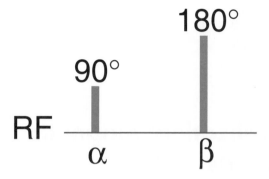

FIGURE 5-1. Radiofrequency (RF) pulse annotation, showing a 90° excitation (α) pulse followed by a 180° refocusing (β) pulse. This is the standard sequence of radio pulses used to produce a spin echo.

on, the level of the line changes to above neutral for positive polarity or below neutral for negative polarity (Fig. 5-2). The identity of the particular gradient illustrated (e.g., slice selection or frequency encoding) is indicated to the left of the diagram of the gradient.

Below the imaging gradient lines, or on the same line as the RF pulses, the MR echo is indicated as a brief wave. The wave has its maximum amplitude at the peak of the echo, which corresponds to the time of greatest phase coherence as determined by the timing of the refocusing lobe of the frequency-encoding gradient. The oscillations of the wave diminish toward the "tails" of the echo, both before and after the echo peak (Fig. 5-3).

SECTION SELECTION

If we transmit an excitation radio pulse into a tissue during the application of a magnetic field gradient, not all tissue is excited. The excitation radio pulse excites only tissues that resonate at the appropriate frequency, corresponding to a particular position along the axis of the imaging gradient. Thus, only a certain section is excited. An imaging gradient applied during

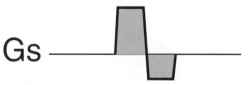

FIGURE 5-2. Basic annotation for an imaging gradient. This example shows two lobes of the section-select gradient (Gs) with, respectively, positive and negative polarity.

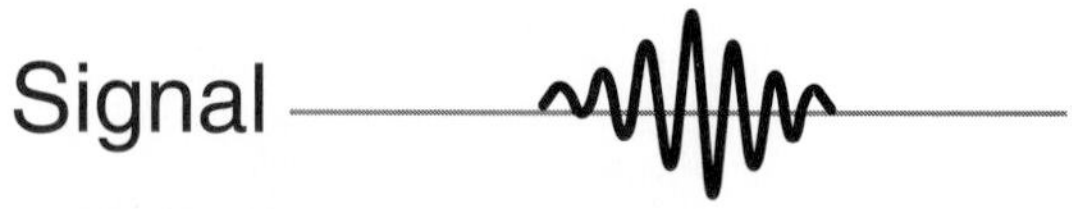

FIGURE 5-3. Basic annotation of an MRI echo.

exposure to an excitation or refocusing radio pulse is referred to as a *section-select gradient.* Appropriately oriented section-select gradients can be applied to selectively excite protons in an axial plane (Fig. 5-4), a coronal plane (Fig. 5-5), or a sagittal plane. Two or more section-select gradients can be applied simultaneously to selectively excite protons in an oblique section (Fig. 5-6). Figure 5-7 shows annotation for section-select gradients applied during the 90° and 180° radio pulses of a standard spin echo pulse sequence.

FREQUENCY ENCODING

In the absence of imaging gradients, all protons in an imaging plane resonate at identical frequencies, except for small variations that are due to magnetic field heterogeneity and differences in chemical shift. If an imaging gradient is applied along one axis of an image plane while the MR signal is being measured, additional variations in resonant frequency are created. During the application of such a gradient, the frequency of MR signals being measured (the readout) is higher at one end and lower at the other end along the axis of this gradient. This provides an opportunity to localize the source of MR signals in one dimension within a previously selected section. This process of encoding the spatial location of protons based on their positions relative to a gradient applied during their measurement is referred to as *frequency encoding,* and this gradient may be referred to as the *frequency-encoding gradient* or the *readout gradient.*

The process of in-plane frequency encoding described is based on principles similar to those of section selection. Both involve spatial localization based on resonant frequency. Sections are *selected* by applying an imaging gradient during radio *excitation.* Frequency is *encoded* by applying an imaging gradient during *measurement* of MR signals. While it is possible to use frequency encoding to locate the sources of MR signals in a third axis, this method has not provided satisfactory results. Instead, a method referred to as *phase encoding* is used

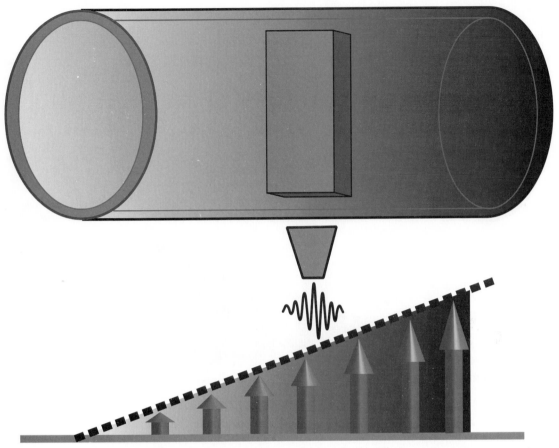

FIGURE 5–4. Section-select gradient. The magnetic field at one end of the magnet bore is weaker than at the other. A frequency of a transmitted radio pulse is chosen that matches the frequency of the desired image section, resulting in an axial section.

for this third axis. This is described later. First, however, we consider some issues and artifacts related to frequency encoding.

The information required for localizing the source of MR signals along the frequency-encoding axis is contained in each echo. The MR signal is an analog wave, which is digitized to a series of numbers from which the wave can be inferred. The conversion of the analog wave to digital data is called *analog-to-digital conversion* (ADC). The duration of echo sampling and the rate of ADC determine the number of differ-

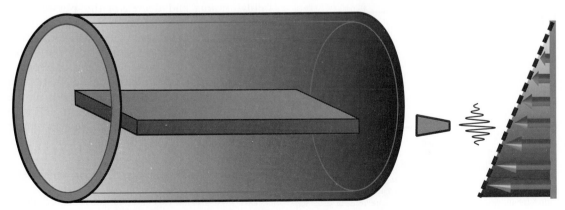

FIGURE 5–5. Section-select gradient used to generate a coronal image section.

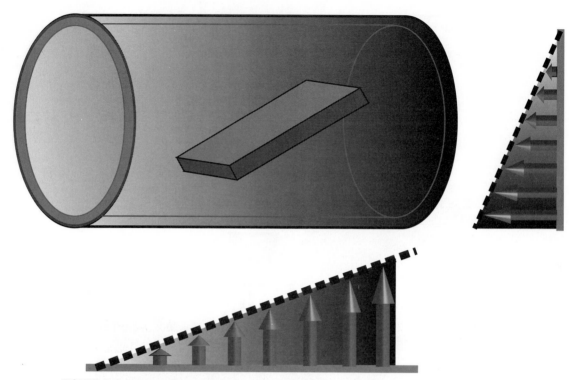

FIGURE 5–6. Simultaneous application of two section-select gradients generates an oblique section.

ent locations that can be resolved along this axis. If the image field of view (FOV) is not changed, increasing the number of frequency-encoding samples increases the imaging matrix,

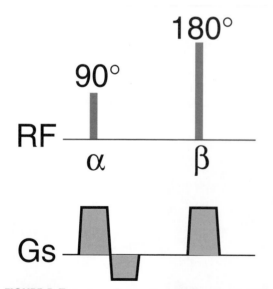

FIGURE 5–7. Section-select gradients (Gs) applied for 90° excitation and 180° refocusing radio pulses. The polarity (direction of strong versus weak) of each gradient is indicated by its position above or below the neutral line. RF, radiofrequency.

and therefore the FOV. An image of a given size is divided into a larger number of smaller picture elements (pixels), increasing spatial resolution. To increase the number of locations mapped along the frequency-encoding gradient (i.e., increase spatial resolution along the frequency-encoding axis), it is necessary to sample either longer or faster (Fig. 5–8).

Spatial resolution can also be increased by keeping constant the number of locations along the frequency-encoding gradient while increasing the strength of that gradient. The use of a stronger frequency-encoding gradient increases the differences in frequency between two particular points and decreases the physical distance between two particular resonant frequencies. With a stronger frequency-encoding gradient, small distances can be resolved better because they correspond to greater differences in frequency. Therefore, the spatial resolution improves as gradient strength increases. If the number of samples remains constant, increasing gradient strength results in smaller image FOV (Figs. 5–9 and 5–10).

Chemical Shift Misregistration Artifact

The sources of MR signals are mapped along the axis of the frequency-encoding gradient

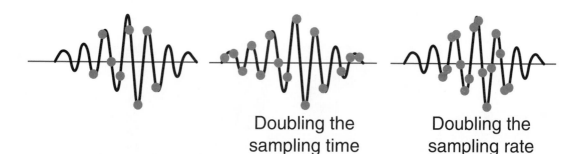

Doubling the
sampling time

Doubling the
sampling rate

FIGURE 5–8. Data acquisition in the frequency-encoding axis can be increased by doubling the sampling time or the sampling rate. Each sample of the wave is indicated by a gray dot.

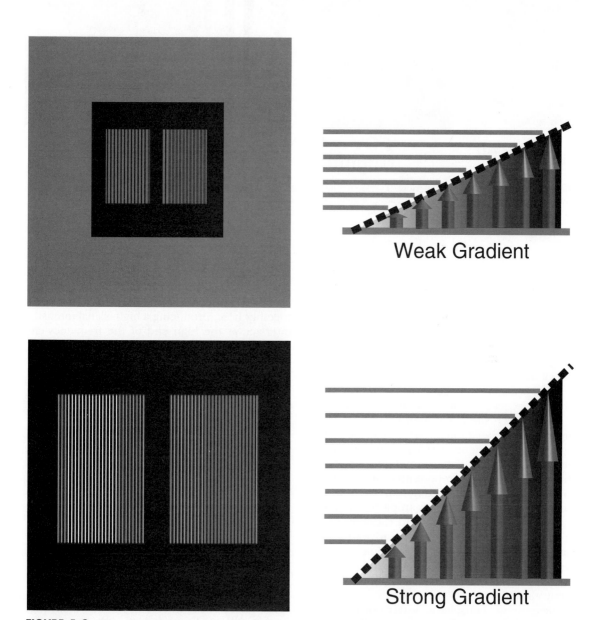

Weak Gradient

Strong Gradient

FIGURE 5–9. Effect of gradient strength on spatial resolution. In this example, the black squares with vertical lines represent the areas of interest and the larger gray square *(top)* represents surrounding space of no interest. The use of a stronger frequency-encoding gradient *(bottom)* results in greater frequency differences between two points. This results in smaller pixel size and finer spatial resolution. If the same number of pixels along the frequency-encoding axis is depicted, the image will have a smaller field of view (FOV), since each pixel is smaller, so smaller structures will be resolved. A square image is maintained by also increasing the strength of the phase encoding gradient (see Phase Encoding).

43

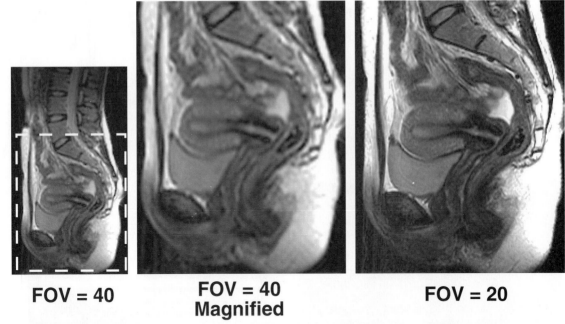

FOV = 40   FOV = 40   FOV = 20
                            Magnified

FIGURE 5-10. Effect of field of view (FOV) on spatial resolution. Sagittal T2-weighted images of the pelvis acquired without changing the number of frequency-encoding views (unchanged matrix). The image at left was acquired using a FOV of 40 cm^2 and magnified by 200% *(middle)*, so that anatomic structures correspond to those acquired using a 20 cm^2 FOV *(right)*. With a smaller FOV *(right)* spatial resolution is improved.

based on their frequencies during readout. The assumption inherent in this method is that any difference in frequency between spins is due to a difference in location along the frequency-encoding gradient. Any additional cause of differences in resonant frequency produces frequency-encoding errors. One salient example of such a frequency-encoding error is signal misregistration secondary to chemical shift differences, producing chemical shift misregistration artifact.

At any given site along the frequency-encoding axis, all water protons precess at the same frequency. Methylene (CH$_2$) protons in lipids precess at a lower frequency, however; thus, these lipid signals are represented on the eventual MR image at a site different from water signals from the same region. In particular, lipid signals are misregistered toward the lower end of the frequency-encoding axis relative to water signals arising from the same location. Thus, a typical MR image actually consists of superimposed water and lipid images that are not perfectly aligned.

For example, consider a "water object" such as a kidney surrounded by lipid (adipose tissue). The water image of the kidney shifts relative to the fat image from adipose tissue toward the high end of the frequency-encoding axis. At the high end of the axis, water signals from

kidney are misregistered so that they are mapped at the same location as perinephric fat signals. The signals of water and fat are added together here, producing a high–signal intensity interface at the high end of the frequency-encoding axis. At the low end of the frequency-encoding axis, signals from renal water are shifted away from adjacent fat, leaving a void (i.e., no signals). This is shown graphically in Figure 5-11, and an example of chemical shift artifact at the edges of a kidney is shown in Figure 5-12. As an example, using a 32-kHz sampling bandwidth and 256 frequency-encoding pixels (125 Hz per pixel) at 1.5 T, the chemical shift between water and CH$_2$ of 224 Hz is equivalent to approximately 2 pixels.

Chemical shift misregistration can also produce image aberrations when water and fat are not immediately adjacent to each other, as when they are separated by a thin low–signal intensity structure. Examples of this include cortical bone such as vertebral end-plates separating vertebral fat from water in intervertebral discs. Water in the intervertebral disc is misregistered toward the high end of the frequency-encoding axis relative to fat on the other side of the vertebral end-plate, decreasing its apparent thickness on the MR image. The water in the disc is misregistered *away* from the opposite

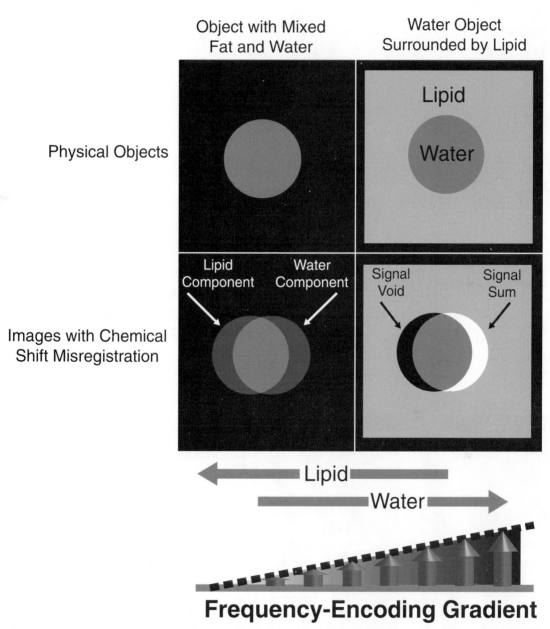

FIGURE 5–11. Chemical shift misregistration artifact. The left column shows smearing of a round object that contains a mixture of lipid and water. The right column shows the typical artifact that results at the edges of "water objects" such as kidneys that are surrounded by adipose tissue. Relative to surrounding lipid, the round water-containing object is mapped toward the right, producing a crescent-shaped set of high–signal intensity pixels to the right, which represents signals from both lipid and water. The crescentic signal void to the left reflects absence of signal mapped to this region.

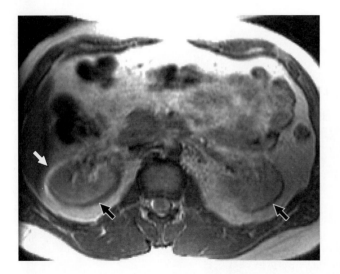

FIGURE 5-12. Chemical shift misregistration artifact. Water in the kidneys is misregistered along the frequency axis toward the right relative to adipose tissue. This causes black signal voids at the kidneys' left margins *(black arrows)* and white summation lines at their right margins *(white arrow).*

end-plate, *increasing* its apparent thickness on the MR image (Fig. 5-13). Similarly, fat in the medullary cavity of a long bone is misregistered along the frequency axis relative to surrounding muscle (Fig. 5-14) or articular cartilage (Fig. 5-15), producing errors in the apparent thickness of cortical bone in these sites.

Silicone (Si) is an elongated molecule consisting of a siloxane (−Si−O−Si−O−) backbone, with 2 or 3 methyl (CH_3) molecules attached to

each Si atom. The chemical shift between silicone and water protons is even larger than the shift between fat and water (Fig. 5-16).

GRADIENT DEPHASING AND REPHASING

To select the appropriate section, the section-select gradient determines that only a slice of

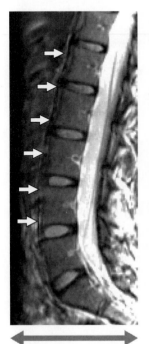
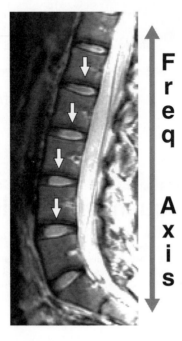

Freq. Axis

FIGURE 5-13. Chemical shift misregistration artifact affecting vertebral bodies. With the frequency axis anteroposterior *(left),* the anterior and posterior vertebral cortices *(arrows)* appear indistinct owing to misregistration of fat within vertebral marrow relative to water. With the frequency axis superoinferior *(right),* misregistration of water in intervertebral discs relative to vertebral fat has produced indistinct images of the vertebral end-plates *(arrows).*

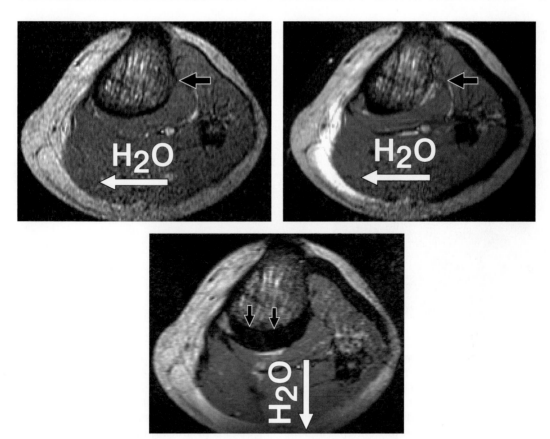

FIGURE 5-14. Erroneous depiction of cortical bone thickness results from chemical shift misregistration between muscle and fatty marrow on axial gradient echo 100/40/45° images. Water in muscle is shifted toward the right relative to lipid *(white arrows)*. With a sampling bandwidth of 32 kHz *(top left)*, the shift is about 1 pixel, resulting in thinning and indistinctness of the left side of the cortex *(black arrow)*. With a sampling bandwidth of 4 kHz *(top right)*, chemical shift misregistration is several pixels. When the axis of frequency encoding is switched to anteroposterior *(bottom)*, muscle is misregistered several pixels posteriorly relative to fatty marrow, producing a large signal void and exaggerating the thickness of posterior cortex *(small black arrows)*.

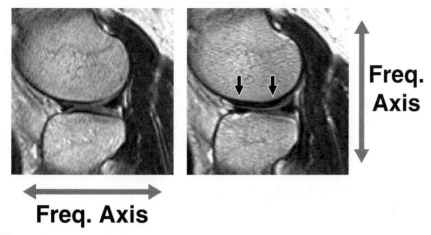

FIGURE 5-15. Example of chemical shift misregistration artifact in a sagittal image of the knee. In the image on the right, with a superoinferior frequency-encoding axis, lipid signals of bone marrow are misregistered superiorly relative to water signal of hyaline cartilage *(arrows)*, exaggerating the thickness of femoral articular cortex and decreasing the apparent thickness of tibial articular cortex.

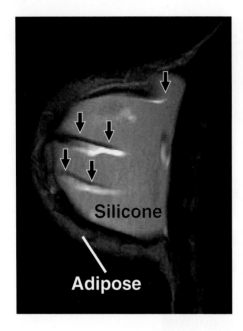

FIGURE 5-16. Chemical shift misregistration between water and silicone in a breast implant. Water within folds of the silicone capsule *(arrows)* is misregistered inferiorly relative to the silicone.

tissue with a certain range of frequencies along this axis is excited. Next, for spatial localization along one axis of this slice, a frequency-encoding gradient is applied while the MR signals are being measured. During the application of each of these imaging gradients, protons spin at non-uniform frequencies; therefore, these gradients rapidly destroy phase coherence of spins. This gradient dephasing causes a potential problem, because it is essential that the MR signals have maximum phase coherence to generate enough signal for producing images.

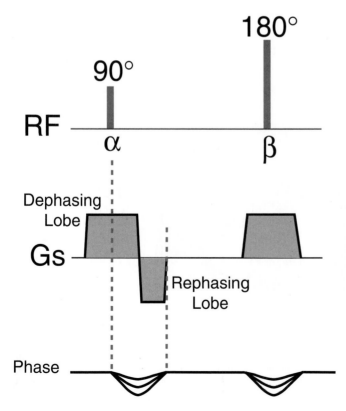

FIGURE 5-17. Phase of transverse magnetization during application of the dephasing and rephasing lobes of a section-select gradient (Gs). Once transverse magnetization is created by the 90° pulse, the continued presence of the dephasing lobe of the gradient causes phase dispersion. This is reversed by application of the rephasing lobe. All spins are in phase when the effects of the dephasing and rephasing lobes are balanced. RF, radiofrequency.

The problem of gradient-dephasing secondary to the section-select gradient and frequency-encoding gradient is solved by applying additional gradients in both of these axes, with reversed polarity. The section-select gradient is applied initially while the image section is excited. Once this transverse magnetization is created, protons in the section are dephased until the section-select gradient is turned off. The section-select gradient is then reapplied in the reverse direction to bring the spins in the excited section back into phase. The initial application of the section-select gradient is called the *dephasing lobe* of the section-select gradient, because it dephases the resonating spins. The repeated but reversed application of the section-select gradient is referred to as the *rephasing lobe*.

The dephasing and rephasing lobes of the section-select gradient, and the accompanying phase changes of the transverse magnetization, are shown in Figure 5-17. The product of the amplitude and duration of the rephasing lobe is equal to the comparable product *after the application of the excitation pulse*. In Figure 5-17, the amplitudes of the dephasing and rephasing lobes are identical, while the duration of the rephasing lobe is half that of the dephasing lobe (corresponding to the time after the excitation pulse). Alternatively, the rephasing lobe could have the same duration and half the amplitude. A rephasing lobe is not needed after the 180° refocusing pulse; the portion of the gradient lobe after the 180° pulse corrects the phase changes caused before the 180° pulse.

For in-plane frequency encoding, the challenge is to measure MR signals with a wide range of frequencies while the phases of these signals are coherent. This is accomplished by applying a dephasing lobe of the frequency-encoding gradient before the rephasing lobe, which in turn occurs during measurement of the MR signals.

While the dephasing lobe of an imaging gradient is being applied, spins at one end of the gradient are faster and thus gain phase relative to spins at the other end. When the dephasing lobe of the frequency-encoding gradient is turned off, the frequencies of the spins within the image section become identical once more (except for differences due to magnetic field heterogeneity and chemical shift differences), so they remain out of phase with each other, neither gaining nor losing phase. Then, near the echo time (TE), the rephasing lobe of the frequency-encoding gradient is applied. Spins that have gained phase now resonate slower

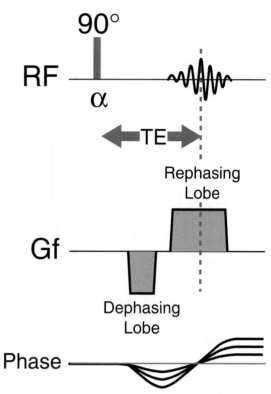

FIGURE 5-18. Effects on phase coherence of the dephasing and rephasing lobes of a frequency-encoding gradient (Gf), and the signal that results at the echo time. RF, radiofrequency.

and thus lose phase relative to spins at the opposite edge. As with the section-select gradient, the dephasing and rephasing lobes of the frequency-encoding gradient have opposite polarities but comparable products of strength and duration. The rephasing lobe thus compensates for the dephasing lobe, and spins come back into phase, producing an echo that peaks at the TE, allowing measurement. The timing of the dephasing and rephasing lobes with respect to the echo is shown in Figures 5-18 and 5-19.

GRADIENT ECHOES AND SPIN ECHOES

As described above, an echo is created by applying two frequency-encoding gradient lobes with opposite polarities. Because this echo is created by reapplication of a magnetic gradient, it is referred to as a *gradient echo*. If a refocusing radio pulse (usually 180°) is applied during the interval between these two fre-

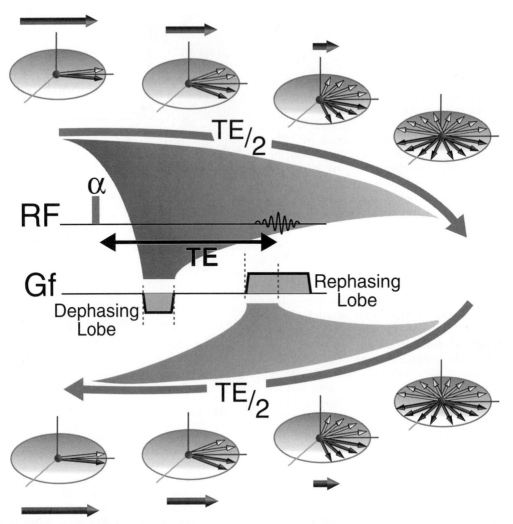

FIGURE 5–19. Gradient echo technique shows phase dispersion and refocusing caused by, respectively, the dephasing and rephasing lobes of the frequency-encoding gradient (Gf). The dephasing lobe causes some protons *(dark arrows)* to resonate faster than others *(light arrows)*. The rephasing lobe, with opposite polarity, causes the spins that have lost phase to resonate faster, so that their phase "catches up," forming a gradient echo at the echo time (TE). RF, radiofrequency.

quency-encoding gradient lobes, the echo obtained is called a *spin echo.*

Application of a 180° refocusing pulse compensates for frequency variations that are due to magnetic field and chemical shift heterogeneity. Variations due to magnetic field heterogeneity include those imposed by main magnetic field imperfections and heterogeneous susceptibility (a combination called T2* effects). In contrast, the reapplication of an imaging gradient compensates only for itself. If there is no 180° refocusing pulse, a gradient echo is formed by reapplying the frequency-encoding gradient with *reversed* polarity, compensating for its dephasing lobe. If a 180° refocusing pulse is applied, the phase differences between spins are reversed. In this situation, an echo is created

by applying a rephasing lobe that has the *same* polarity as the dephasing lobe (Fig. 5–20).

An echo generated by a 180° refocusing pulse, which rephases signal that had decayed owing to heterogeneous susceptibility and chemical shift, is defined as a *spin echo.* Whether or not a 180° refocusing pulse is applied, an MR echo is created by applying dephasing and rephasing lobes of the frequency-encoding gradient; this echo can therefore be considered a *gradient echo.* In common usage, however, this echo is not always called a gradient echo. In most applications where a 180° refocusing pulse is applied, the echo is referred to as a spin echo. When a 180° refocusing pulse is not applied, the echo is referred to as a gradient echo.

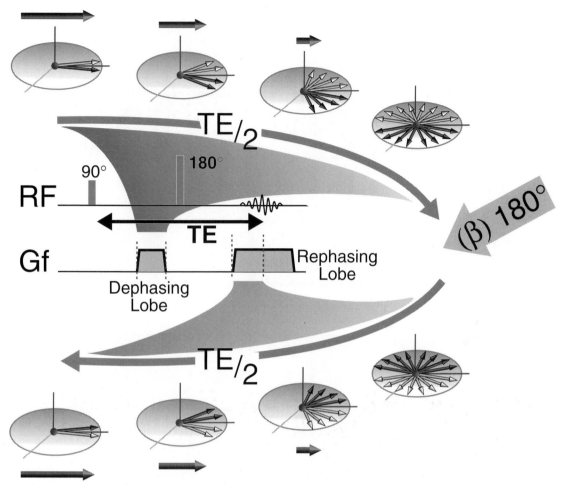

FIGURE 5–20. Spin echo technique, showing refocusing of transverse magnetization by a 180° radio pulse, which occurs at the middle of the echo time (TE) (compare Fig. 5-19). The 180° pulse corrects for differences in resonant frequency that are due to heterogeneous chemical shift or heterogeneous magnetic field. During the first half of the TE, some protons *(dark arrows)* resonate faster than others *(light arrows)*. The 180° pulse reverses the phases of the fast and slow spins. During the second half of the TE, the frequency-encoding gradient (Gf) is reapplied using the same polarity. The phase of the fast spins "catches up" to the phase of the slow spins, forming a spin echo at the TE. RF, radiofrequency.

PHASE ENCODING

Thus far, we have discussed spatial localization using frequency differences, which depend on position along the axis of a magnetic field gradient. This includes selective excitation to choose an image section, and frequency encoding, which is used to encode one axis within an image. The second in-plane axis of the image is localized by a different technique, *phase encoding,* which involves mapping the location of the sources of MR signals based, not on their frequency at readout, but on their phase.

The phase-encoding gradient is established by applying a single brief magnetic field pulse perpendicular to the axes of section-selection and frequency encoding. This brief gradient pulse causes resonant frequencies to vary momentarily along this axis. Once the phase-encoding gradient pulse has ended, resonant frequencies return to uniformity. The signal acquired during echo readout contains phase differences caused by the phase-encoding gradient.

The phase-encoding gradient must be applied repeatedly, at different strengths, to locate different sources of MR signals along the phase-encoding axis. This is quite different from the process of frequency encoding, which allows the mapping of all points along the frequency-encoding axis based on information contained within each echo. Although each echo contains data from throughout the entire two-dimen-

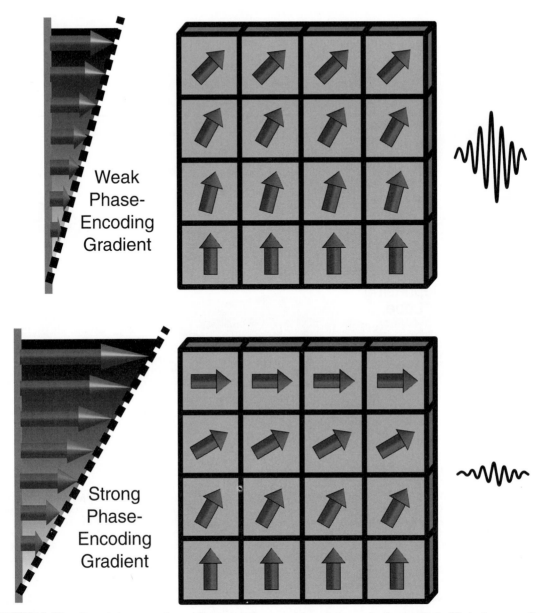

FIGURE 5–21. Effect of phase-encoding gradient strength on spatial resolution and echo amplitude. Weak phase-encoding gradients cause mild dephasing across the phase-encoding axis and thus give rise to strong echoes. Strong phase-encoding gradients accentuate differences between nearby points and thus help to resolve fine detail; however, the increased phase differences across the image secondary to the stronger phase-encoding gradients cause dephasing of these echoes. Thus, the echoes obtained using stronger phase-encoding gradients have lower amplitude.

sional image section, data from multiple echoes are needed to solve a complex equation by two-dimensional Fourier transform (2D-FT). Strong phase-encoding gradients accentuate differences between two structures that are near each other; thus, they are useful for resolving fine detail. However, the greater differences in phase that result cause these echoes to have lower-amplitude MR signal than do echoes pro-

duced with weaker phase-encoding gradients (Fig. 5–21). The number of different phase-encoding gradient strengths determines directly the number of different locations mapped along the phase-encoding axis. This is discussed in greater detail in Chapter 6.

The section-select gradient and frequency-encoding gradient include dephasing and rephasing lobes to ensure that the phases of MR sig-

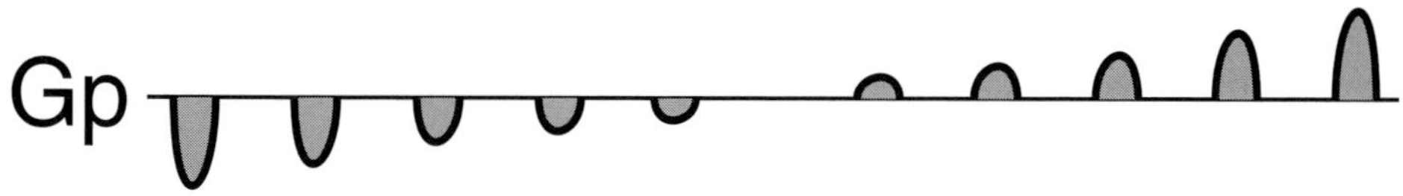

Gp

FIGURE 5–22. Annotation for multiple phase-encoding gradient (Gp) pulses, each occurring after a different excitation. In this example, eleven Gp pulses are applied, beginning with the strongest negative pulses and ending with the strongest positive pulses; the middle pulse has an amplitude of 0.

nals are coherent while they are sampled. Since the phase-encoding gradient pulse is quite brief and generally rather weak, the disturbance in phase is small enough so that the signals are sufficiently coherent. There is no rephasing lobe before measurement of the MR signal, since a rephasing lobe would eliminate phase differences and thus prevent phase encoding.

Typically, the brief phase-encoding pulse is indicated by a short curved line rather than by the rectangular shape used to approximate the timing and amplitude of the other, more sustained, imaging gradients. The variable amplitude of the phase-encoding gradient throughout multiple repetitions can be indicated by repeating it with a different height further along the time scale (Fig. 5-22). Alternatively, phase-encoding gradient pulses of varying amplitudes within successive repetitions are indicated in Figure 5-23.

PULSE SEQUENCE BASICS

Combinations of the characteristics and timing of the radio pulses and magnetic field gradients are referred to as *pulse sequences.* Classification and analysis of pulse sequences are greatly facilitated by the use of a standard set of pulse sequence annotations. Throughout the remainder of this book, we utilize the standard pulse sequence annotation, introduced in the section—Basic Pulse Sequence Annotation.

The first line in the pulse sequence diagram indicates the transmitted radiofrequency (RF) pulses and, usually, the RF echo, which is the MR signal. Sometimes, the RF echo is indicated

separately on the bottom line. The next three lines indicate the timing, amplitude, and polarity of the section-select (Gs), frequency-encoding (Gf), and phase-encoding (Gp) gradients. The frequency-encoding gradient is referred to by some authors as *Gr,* for *readout gradient.* Some authors use an alternative "xyz" notation, referring to the section-select gradient as Gz, frequency-encoding gradient as Gx, and phase-encoding gradient as Gy. Although this notation is popular, we do not favor it because these axes may be confused with the physical axes of the magnet bore. (If, for example, one mentions the *z axis,* does this indicate the long axis of the magnet bore or the axis of section selection? Only for axial imaging are these axes identical.)

The scale for amplitude of the three imaging gradients varies. For example, the frequency-encoding gradient is typically much stronger than the phase-encoding gradient, and the amplitude of the section-select gradient varies with section thickness. While the time scale for application of the three gradients on their respective lines is identical, the duration of the phase-encoding gradient is generally exaggerated relative to the duration of other gradients. This is because the phase-encoding gradient pulse is so brief. Precise indication of the relative amplitude of the imaging gradients would also complicate annotation. Generally, pulse sequence diagrams are used to indicate the *timing* of the dephasing and rephasing lobes of imaging gradients, relative to each other and to radio pulses and echoes. Figure 5-24 is a diagram that describes the timing of radio pulses and imaging gradients relative to the production of a signal for a standard spin echo pulse sequence.

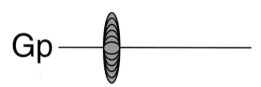

FIGURE 5–23. Condensed annotation for multiple phase-encoding gradient (Gp) pulses.

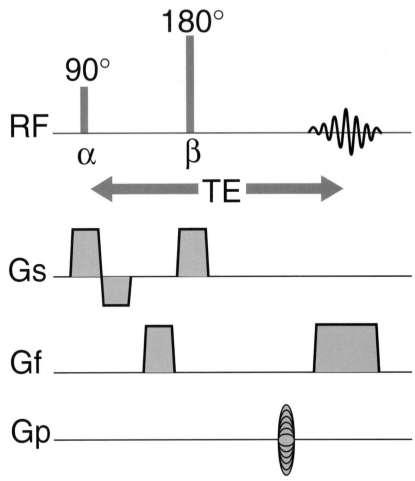

FIGURE 5–24. Pulse sequence annotation for a conventional spin echo pulse sequence. The first line (RF) describes the sequence of radio pulses (90° and 180°) followed by the radio echo that occurs at a time (TE) after the α (90°) pulse. The next two lines (Gs and Gf) describe the timing of, respectively, the section-select and frequency-encoding gradients. Deflection above the baseline indicates positive polarity; deflection below the baseline indicates negative polarity. The final line (Gp) indicates multiple pulses, with varying strengths, of the phase-encoding gradient.

ESSENTIAL POINTS TO REMEMBER

1. Position along an axis can be determined by applying a magnetic field gradient along this axis, so that the resonant frequency of protons will depend on their position along this axis.

2. Image sections are selected by applying a section-select gradient during application of radio pulses, so that the frequency of the radio pulse corresponds to the frequency of protons within the desired image section, but not to protons outside this section.

3. The position of protons along one axis in an MR image can be determined by

obtaining the MR data during application of a frequency-encoding gradient.

4. Since CH_2 protons resonate at a frequency different from that of water protons, signals from these lipid protons are misregistered relative to signals from water protons in the MR image along the frequency-encoding gradient. This is called *chemical shift misregistration artifact.*

5. The timing and polarity of magnetic field gradients can be annotated using a line, with deflections above and below baseline indicating the application of a magnetic field gradient with, respectively, positive and negative polarity.

6. Application of a magnetic field gradient dephases the MR signal. Reapplication of a comparable gradient with reversed po-

larity rephases the MR signal, restoring phase coherence.

7. To produce a coherent echo during frequency encoding, it is necessary first to apply a dephasing lobe of the frequency-encoding gradient. The rephasing lobe of the frequency-encoding gradient forms an echo that provides the signal that is measured to create the MR image.

8. A 180° refocusing pulse applied between the dephasing and rephasing lobes of the frequency-encoding gradient can correct for heterogeneous chemical shift and magnetic field.

9. If a 180° refocusing pulse is applied, the two lobes of the frequency-encoding gradient must have the same polarity to form an echo. This echo is called a *spin echo*.

10. The other axis of an image is encoded by applying a brief phase-encoding pulse to change the phase of signals along this axis. The phase-encoding gradient must be repeated for the generation of each echo, each time with a slightly different amplitude.

6   K-Space: A Graphic Guide

K-space is a formalism created to provide a graphic explanation for some of the important points about Fourier transform image reconstruction without resorting to complex mathematics. It is sometimes perceived as intimidating, since it is even less familiar to many than *outer* space. This book is written for those who wish to understand MRI without being confronted with equations. Avoidance of k-space, however, actually makes this more difficult.

Computed tomography (CT) and MRI share some similarities. In both, data from multiple views are used to calculate pixel data of the final images, and each "view" contains data that contribute to the entire image. With CT, the different views are obtained using different angles of the x-ray path, whereas with MRI the different views represent nondirectional signals generated using different values of the phase-encoding gradient. Perhaps the most nonintuitive concept of Fourier transform reconstruction is that some views are used principally to calculate image intensity and contrast, and others mainly determine fine detail.

BASICS OF K-SPACE

K-space is represented as a grid of points, each one representing a complex number. While this two-dimensional grid of k-space resembles a two-dimensional image of physical space, it must be remembered that k-space does not correspond directly to physical space.

Each MR echo is obtained while the rephasing lobe of the frequency-encoding gradient is turned on. The echo begins prior to complete rephasing, at which time the overall signal amplitude is weak. As rephasing becomes complete, the signal amplitude builds to a peak, after which the amplitude decreases.

The analog signal from the echo is converted to digital data, yielding a specific number of data points. These are used to fill a line of data in k-space corresponding to the frequency-encoding axis. Remember, this line along the frequency-encoding axis of k-space does not correspond directly to the frequency-encoding axis of the final MR image. The left and right extremes of the frequency-encoding axis in k-space correspond to the fine detail in this axis, not the left and right portions of the MR image.

The center of k-space represents data that determine most of the overall signal intensity and tissue contrast of the image, but with poor spatial resolution. The periphery of k-space represents data that determine the fine detail of the image. To emphasize this point, our representation of k-space uses larger points for the center of k-space, and finer points for the periphery of k-space (Fig. 6–1). Figure 6–2 shows a map of k-space and its corresponding MR image.

Different echoes are obtained using different strengths of the phase-encoding gradient. To resolve points close to each other, strong phase-encoding gradients are necessary. Thus, echoes obtained after strong phase-encoding gradients principally provide information about fine detail of the image. The data from these echoes are represented at the superior and inferior extremes of k-space. Stronger phase-encoding gradients dephase the MR signal somewhat, reducing its overall intensity. Thus, most information about signal intensity and gross contrast is obtained using weaker phase-encoding gradients. These data are represented by the horizontal lines near the center of k-space.

Note that k-space is not divided neatly into gross-contrast portions and fine-detail portions. The relative contributions to contrast and detail

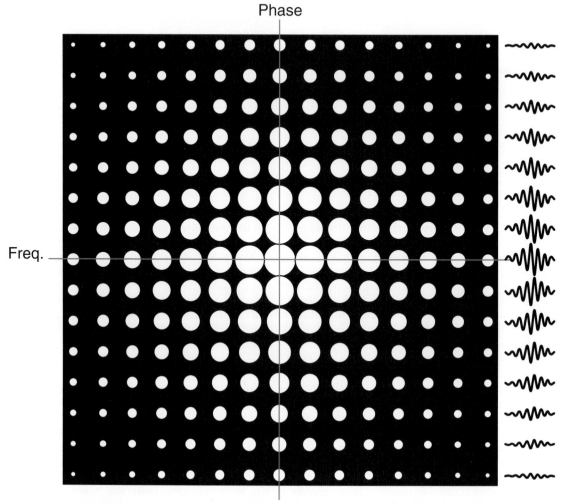

FIGURE 6–1. The k-space for a square field of view image with a 15 × 15 matrix. The horizontal axis indicates frequency encoding and the vertical axis, phase encoding. The large dots at the center of the matrix represent data at the center of k-space. The small dots at the periphery of the matrix determine the fine detail of the image. Echoes that correspond to the center of k-space have greater amplitude.

change gradually between the center and periphery of k-space, intermediate portions of k-space providing significant contributions to both.

K-SPACE REPRESENTATION OF IMAGE RESOLUTION AND FIELD OF VIEW

Diagrams of k-space are helpful for describing the effects of pulse sequence changes on image resolution and field of view (FOV). The depiction of resolution and FOV in k-space is, however, the opposite of their depiction as pixel data in physical MR images. Two points that are close together can best be resolved by the use of strong imaging gradients; the phase difference between two points increases with stronger phase-encoding gradient. Echoes acquired with strong phase-encoding gradients are represented at the edges of k-space. Thus, increasing the spatial resolution of an image involves obtaining echoes farther from the center of k-space. In other words, increased spatial resolution is represented as increased *size* of k-space. In the physical MR image, however, increasing the spatial resolution of an image means obtaining more pixel data per square centimeter of tissue.

The resolution (distance between points) in k-space is not affected by a change in spatial

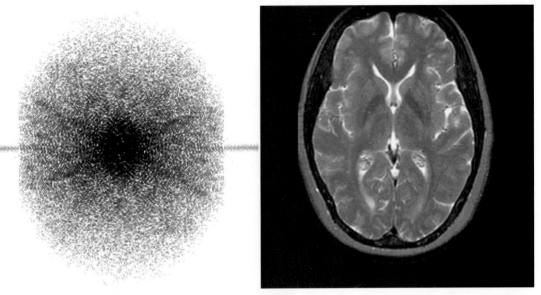

FIGURE 6–2. At left is a k-space map of digital data acquired from an axial T2-weighted fast spin echo pulse sequence with a 256 × 192 matrix, interpolated to a 256 × 256 map of k-space. At right is the image that results from Fourier transform analysis.

resolution of the physical image. As an example, the effect of a 50% reduction of image matrix of Figures 6-1 and 6-2, without changing the FOV, is shown in Figures 6-3 and 6-4. An even greater reduction in image matrix is demonstrated in Figure 6-5. Decreased image matrix is represented as k-space of decreased size.

Note that Figures 6-4 and 6-5 show increas-

ing blurring as more of the data from the periphery of k-space are eliminated. Figures 6-6 and 6-7 show the k-space maps and corresponding images reconstructed solely from the periphery of k-space. These images represent the edge information that was absent in Figures 6-4 and 6-5, without the image contrast from the center of k-space that was present in these images.

FIGURE 6–3. The k-space for an image with field of view identical to that of Figure 6-1, but with lower spatial resolution (i.e., 7 × 7 matrix). The points at the periphery of k-space, which account for the fine detail in Figure 6-2, have not been acquired in this example.

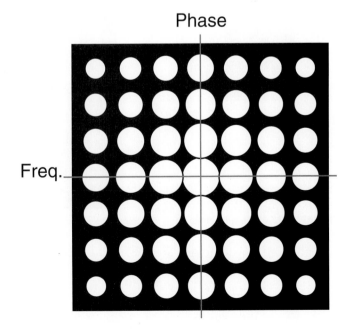

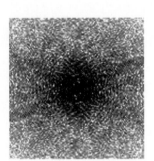

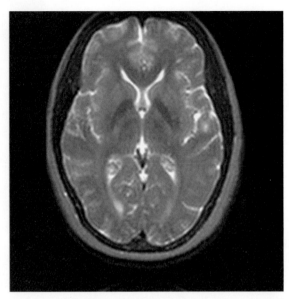

FIGURE 6–4. At left, the central 128 × 128 points of k-space from Figure 6-2 were used to construct the 128 × 128 image at right.

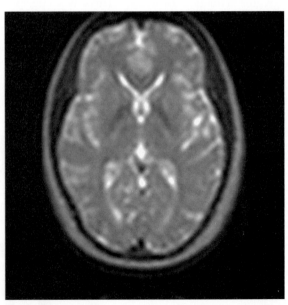

FIGURE 6–5. At left, the central 64 × 64 points of k-space from Figure 6-2 were used to construct the 64 × 64 image at right.

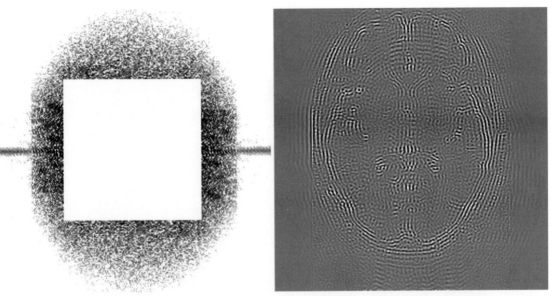

FIGURE 6–6. At left, the central 128 × 128 points of k-space from Figure 6-2 were eliminated. The remainder of k-space was used to construct the image at right, which consists entirely of fine detail—and no image contrast.

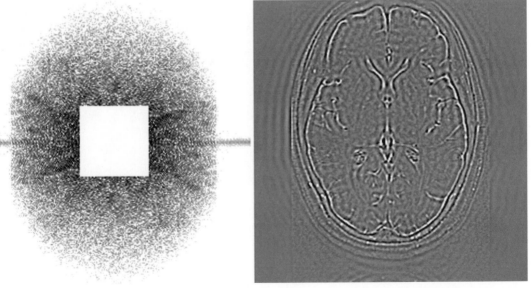

FIGURE 6–7. At left, the central 64 × 64 points of k-space from Figure 6-2 were eliminated. The remainder of k-space was used to construct the image at right, which consists principally of fine detail—and minimal image contrast.

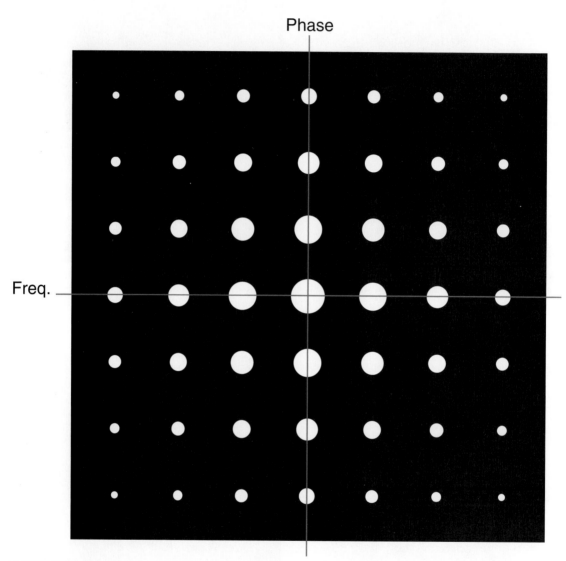

FIGURE 6–8. The k-space for a square field of view (FOV) image with identical resolution but with dimensions half that of Figure 6-1. The k-space is sampled as far toward the periphery as in Figure 6-1, so spatial resolution is not changed. There is more space between points of k-space, however, so the FOV is reduced.

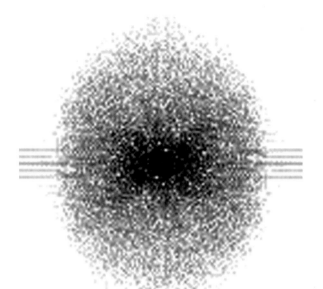
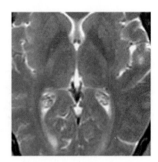

FIGURE 6–9. The k-space map *(left)* is filled less densely than the map in Figure 6-2, generating an image *(right)* with field of view half that of the image in Figure 6-2 but with identical spatial resolution.

Increasing image FOV involves obtaining additional pixels at the periphery of the physical image. If spatial resolution is not changed, these pixels have the same size; thus, no additional lines are obtained farther from the center of k-space. Increased physical FOV is represented in k-space by decreasing the distance between the points of k-space. To increase the FOV of the physical image, k-space is filled more densely. For decreased FOV, k-space is filled less densely. A 50% reduction in FOV relative to Figures 6-1 and 6-2, without changing pixel size, is shown in Figures 6-8 and 6-9.

In summary, the representations of image resolution and FOV are inversely related for physical image space as opposed to k-space. A larger map of k-space indicates higher spatial resolution, whereas a map of k-space with points spaced more closely indicates a larger FOV.

ESSENTIAL POINTS TO REMEMBER

1. K-space is a graphic matrix of digitized MRI data that represents the image prior to Fourier transform analysis. The Fourier transform of k-space is the image.
2. All points in k-space contain data from all locations within an MR image.
3. Points in the center of k-space provide most of the MR image signal intensity and, so, determine gross tissue contrast throughout the image.
4. Points at the periphery of k-space provide fine edge detail throughout the image, but these points have little effect on image contrast.

CHAPTER

7

Creating MR Images

Most of our previous discussion has addressed the sequence of events involved in the generation of one echo in a typical MR pulse sequence. These events are repeated several times, keeping all factors constant except for the value of the phase-encoding gradient. The time between repetitions is the repetition time (TR), defined earlier, during our discussion of T1 relaxation. Within certain constraints, the MR user can choose the TR. The various techniques for acquiring MR images differ in how section selection and phase encoding are changed for successive excitations.

SINGLE-SECTION ACQUISITIONS

For single-section techniques, the acquisition time of an image is directly proportional to the TR. When a single image is created using one repetition for each value of the phase-encoding gradient, the acquisition time is simply the number of phase-encoding values multiplied by the TR. Therefore, single-section acquisitions usually have short TRs, typically 50 msec or less. If a short TR is acceptable or desirable, single-section acquisitions may be appropriate. The TR, phase-encoding pulses, and echo amplitudes for single-section acquisition are illustrated in Figure 7–1. Acquisition of one section does not begin until acquisition of the previous section is complete.

For some applications, short image acquisition time is considered paramount. In such situations, TR is chosen as the minimum interval achievable within the constraints of the pulse sequence and MRI hardware. In these situations, the TR is defined by the echo time (TE) and the time required for application of the radio pulses and imaging gradients, plus any delays between these that may be necessary.

For rapid techniques such as these, minimizing TR, and thus acquisition time, requires the use of the shortest possible TE.

TWO-DIMENSIONAL MULTISECTION ACQUISITIONS

For many applications, longer TR is desirable or essential, for example, to increase the signal intensity of tissues that have long T1 relaxation times. For images with long TR, single-section acquisition techniques are unacceptably inefficient, since the time between measurement of the echo and the next excitation radio pulse (the difference between the TE and the TR) is dead time. Rather than waste the time during the interval between the TE and the next excitation pulse, a different section can be excited by reapplying an excitation pulse of slightly different frequency so that it corresponds to the frequency of a different location along the section-select gradient. This results in excitation of a second section, which is followed by measurement of the echo from this second section at its TE. If time permits, additional sections can be thus excited in an "interleaved" manner during each TR, followed each time by measurement of the resulting echo. Typically, the sections are not excited exactly in sequential order (i.e., 1, 2, 3 . . .) but in such a way as to maximize the time elapsing between excitation of adjacent sections to reduce the effects of cross-talk (see Cross-Talk). Figure 7–2 illustrates an example of four different sections being excited during each TR.

As an example, let us assume that, for Figure 7–2, TR is 40 msec and TE 5 msec. Section #1 is first excited by a radio pulse, during application of the section-select gradient, and an echo is sampled whose peak is 5 msec after the

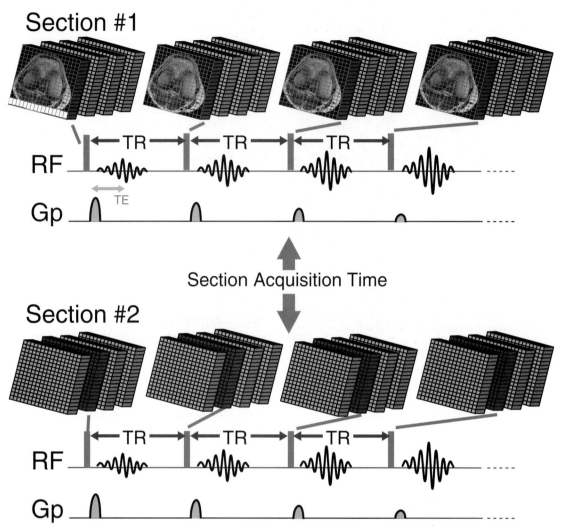

FIGURE 7–1. Sequence of radiofrequency (RF) and phase-encoding gradient (Gp) events involved in imaging a stack of sections using single-section acquisition. A given section is excited repeatedly, varying the strength of the phase-encoding gradient. As the phase-encoding gradient strength decreases, the magnitude of the echo increases. After enough echoes have been obtained to complete acquisition of a given section, the process is repeated for a different section.

excitation radio pulse. Next, the section-select gradient is reapplied along with an excitation pulse with a slightly different frequency that matches the frequency of section #3. In practice, an excitation pulse cannot occur immediately after the echo peak, because time is required to finish sampling the echo and to apply additional (spoiling and crushing) gradients to reduce artifacts. In this example, let us assume a delay of 5 msec between each echo peak and the next excitation pulse. Thus, section #3 is excited 10 msec after section #1. Next in order, the frequency of the excitation pulse is changed so that sections #2 and #4 are excited, generating their respective echoes 5 msec after each excitation pulse. Finally, at the TR, 40 msec

after the initial excitation pulse, the value of the phase-encoding gradient is changed and section #1 receives its second excitation pulse. Figure 7–3 illustrates a comparison of images acquired using single-section and multisection gradient echo techniques.

Cross-Talk

One potential consequence of multisection acquisitions is inadvertent excitation of tissue outside the intended image section owing to imperfection of the slice profile of the excitation radio pulse. This can reduce longitudinal magnetization and thus decrease signal inten-

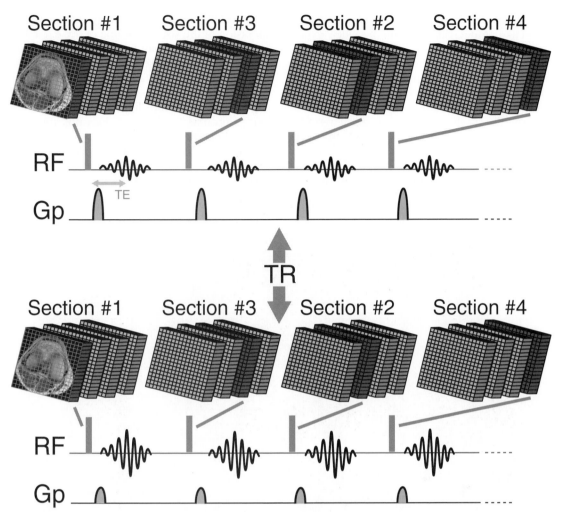

FIGURE 7–2. Sequence of radiofrequency (RF) and phase-encoding gradient (Gp) events involved in imaging a stack of sections using multisection acquisition. Each section is excited using a given phase-encoding gradient strength. After each section has been excited once, all sections are excited a second time, using a different phase-encoding gradient strength.

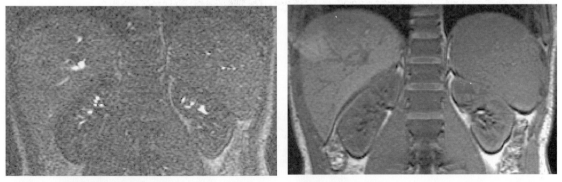

Single Section; TR = 7 msec   Multisection; TR = 100 msec

FIGURE 7–3. Coronal gradient echo images of the abdomen acquired using single-section *(left)* and multisection *(right)* techniques, with 90° excitation flip angles. With multisection technique, longer repetition time (TR) is possible without longer acquisition time for the stack of images. The use of longer TR results in improved signal-to-noise ratio.

sity in the resulting image. In other words, cross-talk can decrease the time between exposures of a section to excitation radio pulses, thus reducing the "effective TR," since the time between excitations of protons at the section surfaces is shorter than the specified TR (Fig. 7–4).

Cross-talk results in reduced signal-to-noise ratio (SNR), particularly for tissues with long T1 relaxation times, since these recover more slowly from cross-excitation. Cross-talk is especially likely when the gaps between image sections of a multisection acquisition are too small relative to the precision of the excitation radio pulses or where sections are contiguous.

Cross-talk can be reduced by improving the precision of the section profile of the excitation radio pulses. This may require increased radio energy and/or increased time and is not usually an operator-selected variable. More commonly, cross-talk is reduced or avoided by choosing gaps between sections large enough so that the excitation that "spills over" does not affect the nearest section (Fig. 7–5).

If contiguous sections are needed, cross-talk can be avoided by first acquiring half of the image sections with 100% gaps (e.g., 5-mm thick with 5-mm gaps) and then acquiring the other half of the image sections during a separate acquisition, filling in the gaps to achieve a

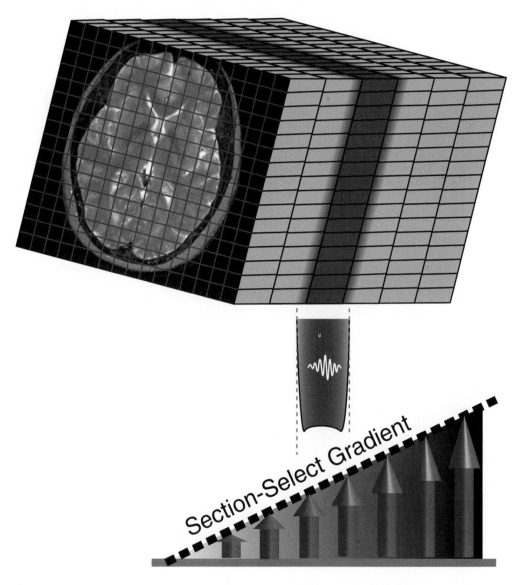

FIGURE 7–4. Cross-talk. Because the range of frequencies of a radio pulse is not perfectly precise, its section profile is less than perfect. Thus, adjacent tissue outside the intended image section is partially excited.

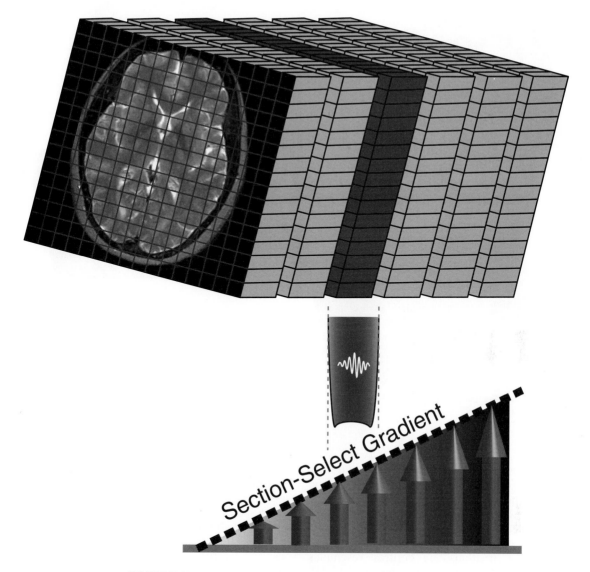

FIGURE 7-5. Cross-talk is avoided by using gaps between image sections.

contiguous set of image sections (Fig. 7-6). This is sometimes referred to as *concatenation.*

Magnetization Transfer

Magnetization transfer (MT) results from excitation of macromolecular protons that do not contribute directly to signal intensity in MR images. Macromolecular protons have a much broader range of resonant frequencies than free water protons. Macromolecular protons can therefore be excited by radio pulses that are several thousand kilohertz greater or smaller than the resonant frequency of water protons. These macromolecular protons then transfer saturated magnetization to the surrounding water protons, which, in turn, reduce the observable MR signal. This transfer of saturated magnetization causes signal loss, which is greatest in tissues containing abundant macromolecules.

MT affects tissue contrast in multisection acquisitions, since radio pulses targeted to different image sections partially saturate the magnetization of all macromolecular protons within the volume of interest. Figure 7-7 illustrates the saturation of water, methylene (CH_2), and macromolecular protons by a radio pulse. The longitudinal magnetization of macromolecular protons can also be saturated deliberately by applying appropriate saturation pulses before each excitation pulse (see Chapter 12).

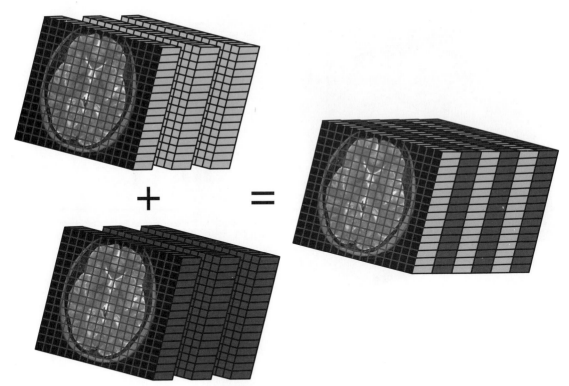

FIGURE 7–6. Contiguous sections free of cross-talk can be obtained by interleaving two separate sets of sections, each with 100% gaps.

Solid tissues lose substantial signal intensity because of MT, whereas fluid and adipose tissue do not. This loss of signal intensity is generally greater for tissues that have long T1 relaxation times, since their longitudinal magnetization recovers more slowly after saturation. In many but not all situations, MT contrast resembles T2 contrast. The effects of cross-talk and MT contrast in fast spin echo technique are illustrated in Figure 7–8.

Considerations of Time

One might think that the TR of a simple multisection pulse sequence could be as short as the TE multiplied by the number of sections; that is, as soon as an echo is sampled at the TE, the next section could be excited. Thus, with a TE of 5 msec, a TR of 60 msec should be long enough to obtain 12 image sections. In practice, however, the actual number of sections obtained is often half this or even less. There are several additional factors that contribute to reducing the time within a TR available for exciting sections and generating echoes.

An MR echo is not instantaneous; rather, it occurs over a period of a few milliseconds, during which the frequency-encoding gradient is on. TE refers to the time of the echo peak; echo sampling begins before the TE and continues after the TE. Once the echo is sampled, there is still transverse magnetization, which, if excited by the next radio pulse, can lead to unwanted signals that degrade the image. Thus, after echo sampling is completed, a series of crushing, spoiling, or rewinding gradients is applied to either eliminate this magnetization or otherwise prevent it from producing image degradation.

The overall efficiencies of two-dimensional Fourier transform (2D-FT) single-section and of multisection techniques are comparable; that is, for a given TE, spatial resolution, number of signal averages, and number of image sections, single-section and multisection acquisitions require about the same amount of time. For example, a single-section technique might allow acquisition of one image section per second, whereas a comparable multisection technique might require 20 seconds for acquisition of a stack of 20 image sections. Both techniques require 20 seconds to complete acquisition for the entire volume of interest.

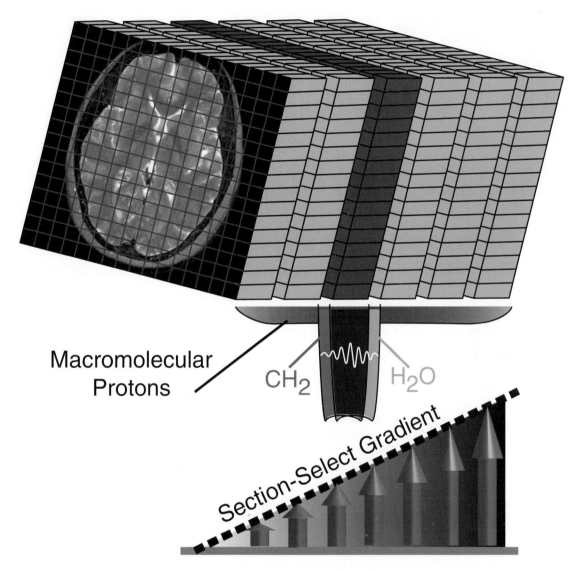

FIGURE 7–7. Range of frequencies within an image section for H_2O *(light gray)*, CH_2 *(dark gray)*, and macromolecular *(shaded)* protons. H_2O and CH_2 protons have similar ranges of frequencies, corresponding to the range of frequencies of the excitation pulse. The range of frequencies is much greater for macromolecular protons, so they are excited by every excitation and refocusing pulse, including those targeted to other sections. This excited magnetization is then transferred to nearby H_2O protons.

With the single-section technique, 10 images have been completely acquired after 10 seconds. With the multisection technique, however, 20 images have been partially acquired after 10 seconds and no acquisition has been completed. If severe motion occurs in the middle of a 20-image acquisition, one image is degraded with single-section technique whereas with multisection technique all images are affected. This is one reason why single-section techniques tend to be less sensitive than multi-section techniques to motion artifact. Motion sensitivity is explored further in Chapter 10.

TWO- AND THREE-DIMENSIONAL FOURIER TECHNIQUES

Fourier analysis involves using data from the frequency, phase, and amplitude of waves to compute a detailed spatial map, or picture.

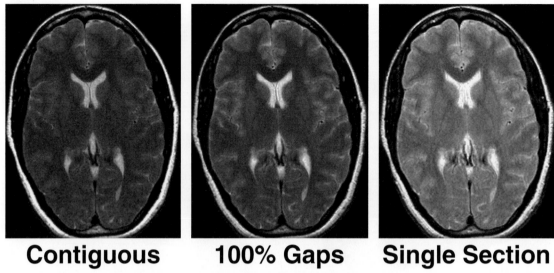

Contiguous   100% Gaps   Single Section

FIGURE 7–8. T2-weighted fast spin echo image of the brain obtained using contiguous multisection *(left)*, interleaved acquisitions with 100% gaps *(middle)* and single-section techniques *(right)*. Cross-talk is eliminated by using 100% gaps, resulting in increased signal intensity and improved contrast between gray and white matter. With single-section technique *(right)*, cross-talk and magnetization transfer are both eliminated, further increasing signal intensity of both gray and white matter.

Thus far we have restricted our discussions to 2D-FT imaging, which involves using frequency-selective excitation of one or more discrete image sections and encoding a two-dimensional image via phase encoding in one axis and frequency encoding in the other (Fig. 7–9).

Alternatively, it is possible to construct a three-dimensional picture using a single frequency-encoding gradient for one in-plane axis and phase encoding for the two other axes. This process, whereby multiple signals are acquired using different values of phase-encoding gradients along two different axes, is termed

three-dimensional Fourier transform (3D-FT) imaging. The pulse sequence annotation for 3D-FT is illustrated in Figure 7–10, and the events are shown graphically in Figure 7–11.

A three-dimensional data set resulting from 3D-FT techniques is usually defined by an in-plane field of view (FOV) (e.g., 20 cm²) and matrix (e.g., 256 × 192), and by the thickness of image sections (often called *partitions*). This is similar to the description of 2D-FT images, except that 2D-FT sections may be separated by gaps whereas 3D-FT partitions are contiguous. The process by which image sections or

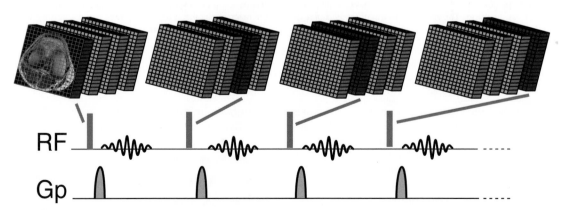

FIGURE 7–9. Two-dimensional Fourier transform (2D-FT) multisection acquisition of a stack of sections. A given section is not excited again until each section in the stack has been excited. TR is therefore equal to the product of the time between excitations of different sections and the number of sections.

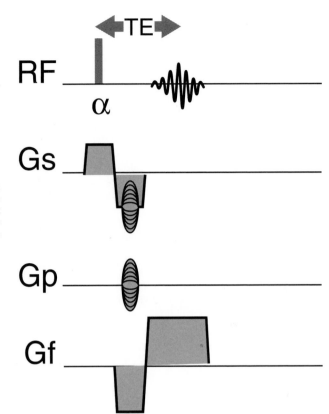

FIGURE 7-10. Pulse sequence for 3-dimensional Fourier transform (3D-FT) volume acquisition. The volume is selected by the section-select gradient (Gs), the rephasing lobe of which has variable strength. Thus there is phase encoding in both the phase-encoding and section-select axes.

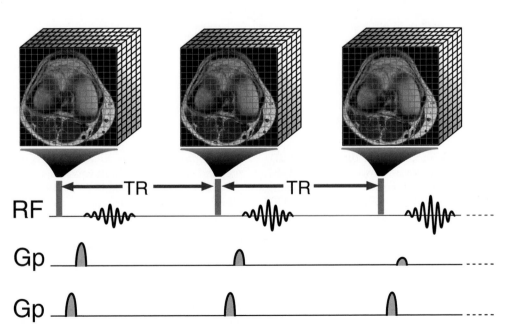

FIGURE 7-11. 3D-FT volume acquisition. The entire volume is excited by each excitation pulse. TR is the time between successive excitations and is therefore usually much shorter than the TR for 2D-FT multisection acquisitions. Phase encoding is performed in two different axes.

Phase

Freq.

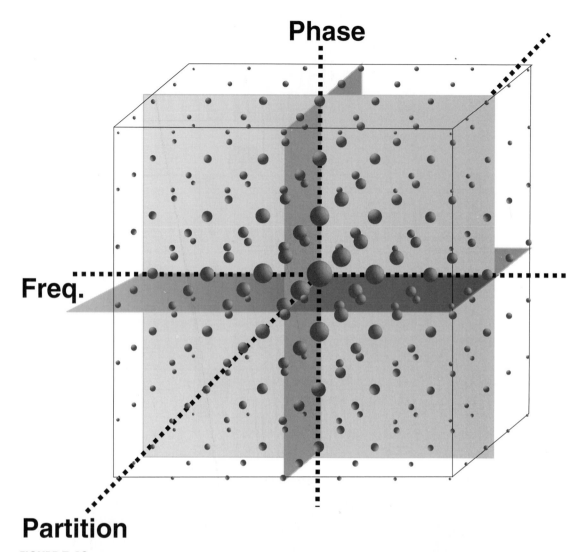

Partition

FIGURE 7–12. Three-dimensional map of k-space. Each point in k-space is represented by a sphere. Each echo provides a line of data along the frequency-encoding axis.

partitions are defined is quite different for 2D-FT and 3D-FT techniques, however. With 2D-FT techniques, image sections are *excited* by using a section-select gradient, whereas with 3D-FT techniques volume partitions are *encoded* by using a phase-encoding gradient, similar to the method by which one axis of an image is phase encoded. A three-dimensional representation of k-space for 3D-FT techniques is shown in Figure 7–12.

With 2D-FT imaging, the excitation pulse is targeted to a single image section by the section-select gradient, and each resulting echo contains signals from throughout that single section. With 3D-FT imaging, however, each excitation pulse excites the entire volume, and *each resulting echo contains signals from*

throughout the entire volume. Thus, each image, and each pixel within each image, is based on a much greater number of MR signals for 3D-FT techniques than for 2D-FT techniques. For this reason, 3D-FT techniques generate images with much higher signal-to-noise ratio (SNR) than do 2D-FT single-section images of comparable voxel size and other imaging parameters (Fig. 7–13). On some occasions, however, the longer TR of 2D-FT *multisection* techniques allows SNR comparable to that of 3D-FT techniques. In general, the increased imaging time of 3D-FT relative to 2D-FT techniques is equal to the number of partitions. A general comparison between 2D-FT single-section, 2D-FT multisection, and 3D-FT techniques is presented in Table 7–1.

TABLE 7–1. GENERAL FEATURES OF 2D-FT SINGLE-SECTION, 2D-FT MULTISECTION, AND 3D-FT TECHNIQUES

Characteristic	Single-Section 2D-FT	Multisection 2D-FT	3D-FT
TR	Short	Intermediate to long	Short
SNR	Low	Intermediate to high	High
Cross-talk	None	Possible	None
MT	Usually none	Some to substantial	None
Motion sensitivity	Low	Substantial	Substantial

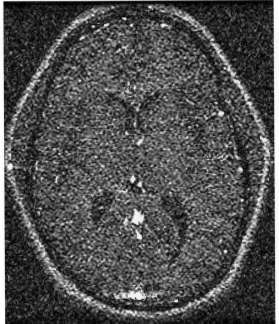
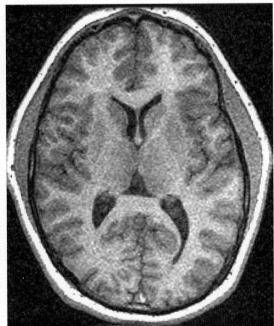

2D Spoiled GRE   3D Spoiled GRE

FIGURE 7–13. A comparison of 2D *(left)* and 3D *(right)* spoiled gradient echo 25/5/45° images. For both techniques, 1.5-mm thick slices were imaged. Signal-to-noise ratio is much better with the 3D technique.

ESSENTIAL POINTS TO REMEMBER

1. For single-section acquisitions, a section is excited repeatedly, changing the phase-encode value until echoes of all values have been obtained. During this period, no additional sections are excited.
2. Single-section acquisitions are most appropriate when short or minimal TR is acceptable or desirable.
3. Two-dimensional multisection acquisitions involve exciting several different sections using a particular value of the phase-encoding gradient, not usually reexciting the first section until after all other sections have been excited.
4. Two-dimensional multisection acquisitions are most appropriate when longer TR is considered desirable or necessary, as to increase SNR of tissues that have long T1 relaxation times.
5. Partial saturation of protons in an image section during excitation of an adjacent image section—cross-talk—reduces the effective TR for the pulse sequence.
6. Protons in macromolecules are partially saturated by radio pulses targeted to different image sections. This saturated magnetization is transferred to nearby water molecules, reducing signal intensity of tissues with abundant macromolecules without affecting the signal intensity of free fluid or lipid. This phenomenon is *magnetization transfer.*
7. Anatomic coverage and imaging efficiency can be similar for both single-section and multisection acquisitions, as long as the rates at which echoes are acquired are comparable.
8. Single-section acquisitions are usually less sensitive to motion. A brief episode of motion that occurs during a multisection acquisition may degrade every section of that acquisition.
9. 2D-FT techniques involve selecting sections by applying a magnetic field gradient during excitation radio pulses.
10. 3D-FT techniques involve encoding partitions by applying a second series of phase-encoding magnetic field gradient pulses along the section-select axis.

CHAPTER

8 Signal-to-Noise Ratio, Spatial Resolution, and Acquisition Time

MRI pulse sequences can be chosen with great flexibility, to optimize contrast between two or more tissues. Once this is done, most other choices relate to the competing concerns of signal-to-noise ratio (SNR), spatial resolution, and acquisition time.

SIGNAL-TO-NOISE RATIO

Thus far, we have considered the sources of MR signals and the manner by which these signals provide information to be encoded into MR images. These images can be degraded by noise. *Noise* consists of random or systematic errors caused by (1) imperfections in the MR system, (2) the process by which images are acquired, or (3) factors arising from the patient, such as motion. In general, image clarity is optimized by increasing the amount of data (signal) and decreasing the amount of noise. This relationship between data and noise is expressed as the SNR. It is always desirable to increase the overall SNR of an image, but this is commonly prevented because of important tradeoffs between SNR, spatial resolution, and acquisition time.

SPATIAL RESOLUTION (PIXEL AND VOXEL SIZE)

Spatial resolution is generally determined directly by the size of the volume elements (voxels) that make up the image. A *voxel* is a three-dimensional unit of an image, consisting of a width in two axes; the third axis is the image section thickness (Fig. 8–1).

The actual in-plane spatial resolution is determined by the size of the picture elements (pixels) that make up the image. The size of each of these pixels is determined by dividing the area of the image by the number of pixels. For example, an image with a 200×200-mm field of view (FOV) has an area of $40,000$ mm^2. If the image matrix is 256×256 pixels, this results in a total of $65,536$ pixels, each with an area of 0.6 mm^2. If the section thickness is 5 mm, then the volume of each voxel is 3 mm^3. The ability to resolve small structures is determined by the in-plane resolution plus the section thickness; small objects can be obscured in thick image sections if their signal intensity is averaged with that of surrounding tissues.

For an image with a given FOV and section thickness, spatial resolution can be increased by dividing the image into a larger number of pixels (Figs. 8–2 and 8–3). Alternatively, for an image with a given number of pixels, higher spatial resolution can be obtained by choosing a smaller FOV (Figs. 8–4 and 8–5). Use of finer matrix or smaller FOV involves acquiring an image of smaller voxel size.

Spatial resolution is also affected by section thickness. Even with fine in-plane resolution, small structures can be obscured by partial volume averaging within the voxels of a thick image section (Fig. 8–6). The direct effects on spatial resolution of the pulse sequence parameters that determine voxel size are described in Table 8–1.

There are two reasons why voxel size cannot be decreased with impunity, frequently forcing operators to settle for an image with less spatial resolution than might be desired. Decreases in voxel size are generally associated with decreases in SNR and increases in acquisition time, as discussed later.

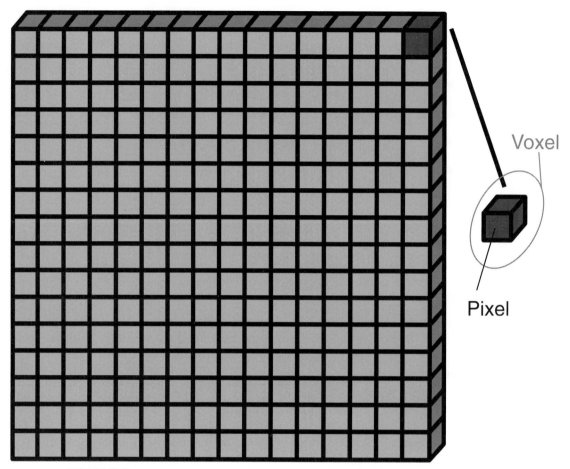

Voxel

Pixel

FIGURE 8–1. A voxel represents the volume of tissue that is depicted as a pixel in a 2D image.

Relationship to Signal-to-Noise Ratio

Voxels are volumes of tissue from which the pixels of an image are derived. The clarity of an image is best when the signal data for each voxel are much greater than the unwanted random or systematic fluctuations that combine to create image noise. As an image is divided into smaller voxels to increase spatial resolution, the amount of data used to determine the value of each voxel decreases. As the amount of data determining voxel signal values decreases, the

relative importance of noise increases. Thus, an image composed of small voxels has the desirable attribute of high spatial resolution but with the potentially deleterious attribute of low SNR.

The relationship between voxel size and SNR may seem counterintuitive. The total amount of data in an image is not reduced when it is divided into smaller voxels, and noise does not necessarily increase. Why, then, does SNR decrease when an image is divided into smaller voxels?

It may help to consider the following example. Consider a crowd of 100 persons, each 66 inches tall. If our measurement accuracy, limited by noise, is ± 1 inch, the range of actual measurements will be 65 to 67 inches. If errors are random, it is likely that the average height of this section of the crowd will be quite close to 66 inches. If the same crowd is divided into smaller groups of 10 persons each, the effect of this imprecision in measurement is likely to be greater. For example, in one group, the

TABLE 8–1. EFFECTS OF ACQUISITION MATRIX, SECTION THICKNESS, AND FIELD OF VIEW

Pulse Sequence Parameter Change	Effect on Spatial Resolution
Increased acquisition matrix	↑
Increased section thickness	↓
Increased FOV	↓

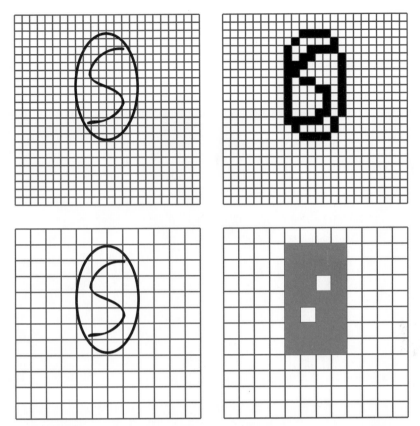

FIGURE 8–2. Effect of matrix size on spatial resolution. A finer matrix *(top row)*, results in smaller and more numerous pixels for a given field of view, improving spatial resolution. The images at the left show an object consisting of the letter "S" enclosed in an oval; the images at the right depict the pixels that are darkened if they contain part of the object. The intensity of the darkening is less with the lower-resolution image *(bottom right)*, because a smaller proportion of each voxel contains part of the object than in the higher-resolution image *(top right)*. In the lower-resolution image *(bottom right)*, all but two pixels in the region of the object contain part of the object and are thus darkened, so the structure of the object cannot be resolved.

height of four persons might be underestimated and the height of one might be overestimated, yielding a mean of 65.7 inches. In a different group, overestimation of four heights and underestimation of one would yield a mean of 66.3 inches, a difference between these two groups of more than 1/2 inch. As an extreme example, if each "group" contained only one person, groups could differ from each other by as much as 2 inches. The random variability between groups is, therefore considerably greater if the groups are small than if they are large, owing to the smaller amount of data from each small group.

Another example is illustrated in (Fig. 8–7). A 12 × 12 grid was constructed by randomly assigning values of 1 through 6. A value of 3 was added to the central 36 squares. The random variation is greater than the minimally darker shade of gray in the center, so it partially

obscures it. When 9 pixels are averaged together to form larger pixels, the random variations become less than the difference in shades of gray.

In conclusion, there is a direct relationship between voxel size and SNR. When all other factors are held constant, decreasing voxel size decreases SNR. In other words, for each application it is usually necessary to balance the desires for high spatial resolution and adequate SNR.

ACQUISITION TIME

If there is a single most important "currency" for tradeoffs between different pulse sequence considerations, it is acquisition time. Measures that increase spatial resolution and/or SNR usu-

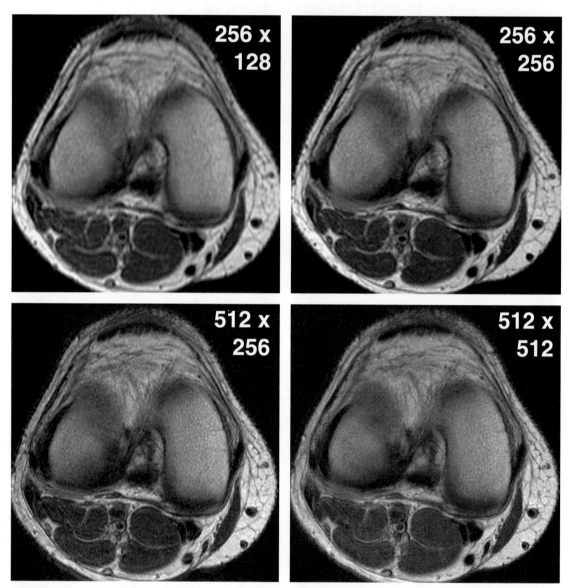

FIGURE 8–3. Axial T1-weighted images of the knee with increasing spatial resolution. As matrix is increased from 256 × 128 to 512 × 512, finer anatomic structures can be resolved; however, smaller pixel size also renders image noise more conspicuous.

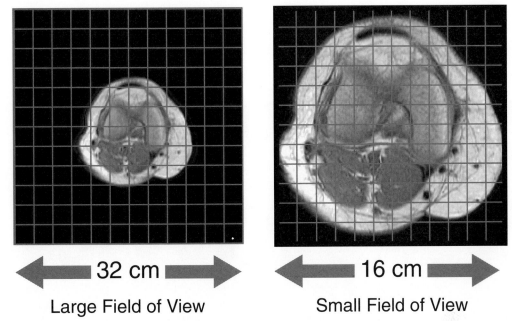

FIGURE 8–4. Effect of field of view on pixel size. The use of a smaller FOV (e.g., 16 cm²) results in smaller pixels and finer spatial resolution without changing the number of pixels. Although the number of pixels in the entire image is not changed, a larger number of pixels is used to depict the object of interest in the 16 cm² FOV image. Each pixel represents a smaller volume of tissue.

ally increase acquisition time. Acquisition time limits the ability of MRI to depict, or resist artifacts related to, physiologic motion and administration of contrast media. Finally, long acquisition time has significant adverse effects on patient tolerance and patient "throughput." The costs of long acquisition time include suboptimal resolution, SNR, and control of artifacts, and financial viability of an MRI center. Each radio pulse and each application of an imaging gradient, plus any necessary or unnecessary delays between them, take time. When efforts to increase spatial resolution and SNR prolong echo sampling or require sampling of more echoes, acquisition time increases.

Relationship to Spatial Resolution

A finite amount of time is needed to acquire each point in k-space, which is filled differently, and at different rates, for the phase-encoding and frequency-encoding axes, respectively. Each analog echo is sampled digitally (Fig. 8–8), usually during an interval of a few milliseconds. Each sample consists of a portion of the analog signal that is digitized and represented by a point along the frequency-encoding axis of k-space. A point in k-space does not correspond to a specific point in physical space; however,

the *number* of points along the frequency-encoding axis of k-space corresponds to the number of pixels along the frequency-encoding axis of the image.

This number can be increased, to increase the spatial resolution of the MR image, by spending more time sampling the echo (Fig. 8–9). Each echo can be sampled for a longer time during a similar gradient application (e.g., 8 msec rather than 4 msec per echo). The spatial resolution along the frequency-encoding axis can be increased by increasing the *number of samples* per echo. Although this does not increase the *number of echoes* that must be sampled, the sampling of each echo takes longer. This increases the echo time (TE), if the echo is sampled at the same rate (Fig. 8–10).

Acquisition time is determined by the repetition time (TR) and the total number of echoes sampled. Acquisition time is not affected by spatial resolution in the frequency-encoding axis *when TR remains constant*; however, increasing the spatial resolution in the frequency-encoding axis increases the duration of echo sampling, which increases the TE. Increased TE allows less time for exciting different image sections. Thus, when all other acquisition parameters are unchanged, increasing the spatial resolution in the frequency axis decreases the number of sections that can be imaged during

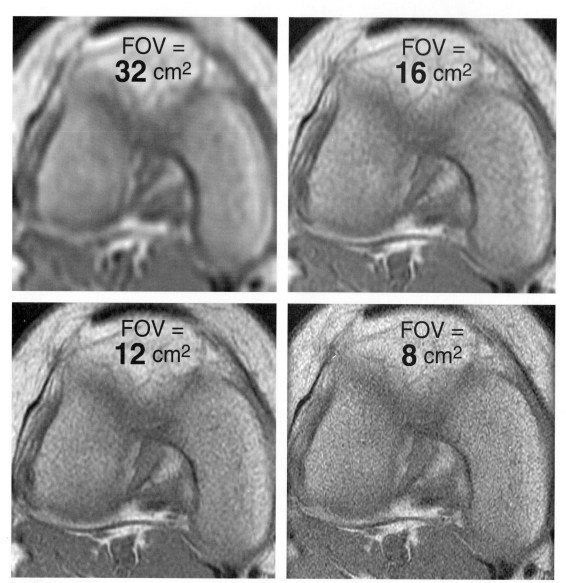

FIGURE 8-5. Effect of variation in field of view (FOV) on axial T1-weighted images of the knee. Images have been magnified so that anatomic structures are of comparable size. As FOV decreases from 32 to 8 cm², maintaining matrix at 256 × 160, smaller structures can be resolved; however, image noise increases because of the smaller pixel sizes.

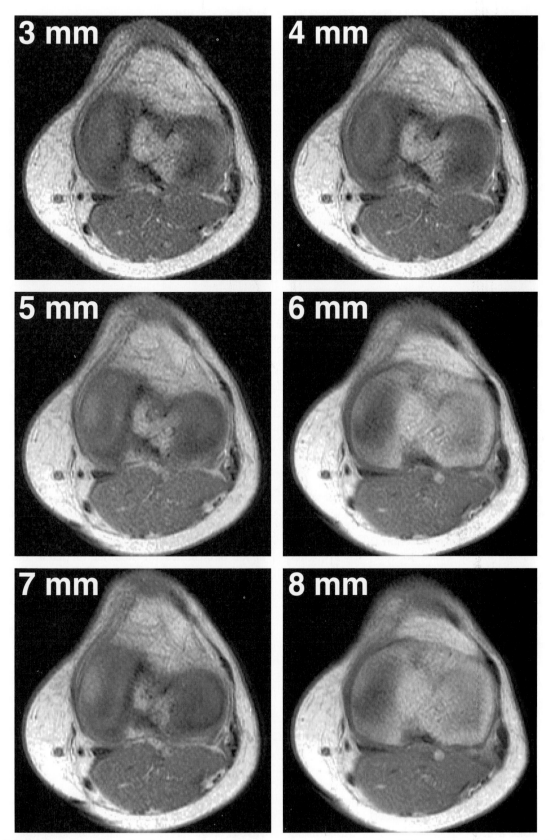

FIGURE 8–6. Effect of section thickness on axial MR images of the knee. As section thickness is increased from 3 to 8 mm, all other factors being constant, the larger voxels improve SNR. However, it becomes more difficult to perceive fine detail; spatial resolution is degraded owing to larger voxel size.

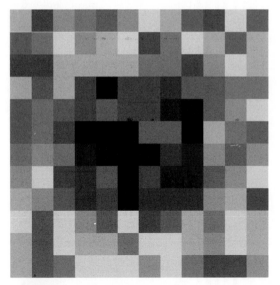 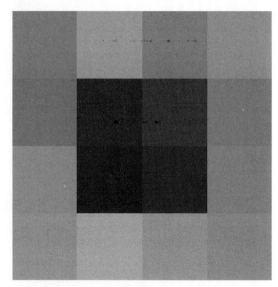

FIGURE 8–7. When nine adjacent pixels from the image at left are averaged mathematically to produce larger pixels at right, random variations in noise are de-emphasized, allowing the dark square at the center of the image to be depicted with greater clarity.

a given TR. This is illustrated in a comparison between Figures 8–11 and 8–12.

More images per TR can be obtained if TE is reduced. Methods of reducing TE include faster sampling of each echo and obtaining fewer samples per echo. Echoes can be sampled faster by using a greater sampling bandwidth, but this reduces SNR. The number of samples obtained per echo can be decreased, but this decreases resolution in the frequency-encoding axis.

The effect of image section thickness on acquisition time of a multisection pulse sequence is analogous to the effect of TE. Neither section thickness nor TE directly affects acquisition time when TR is constant; however, both variables affect coverage in the section select axis. If section thickness is reduced, more image sections are needed to cover the anatomy of interest, which requires either longer TR or additional pulse sequence acquisitions.

Relationship to k-Space

Each echo provides data for one horizontal line of k-space. Additional lines are obtained by repeating the acquisition using a different value for the phase-encoding gradient (Gp). The number of lines along the phase-encoding axis of k-space determines the number of pixels along the phase-encoding axis of the MR image. Each line of k-space, and each MR echo, requires an additional unit of time. Thus, reducing the spatial resolution along the phase-encoding axis generally reduces image acquisition time. An illustration of voxel matrix in such an image is

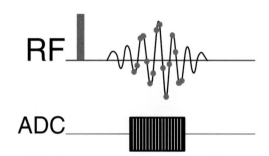 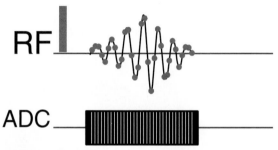

FIGURE 8–8. The echo is sampled for analog-to-digital conversion (ADC). In this example, 16 samples are indicated by white vertical lines, which would lead to a frequency-encoding resolution of 16. RF, radiofrequency.

FIGURE 8–9. The echo is sampled for analog-to-digital conversion (ADC) at the same rate as in Figure 8-8, but for twice as long, obtaining data for a frequency-encoding resolution of 32. RF, radiofrequency.

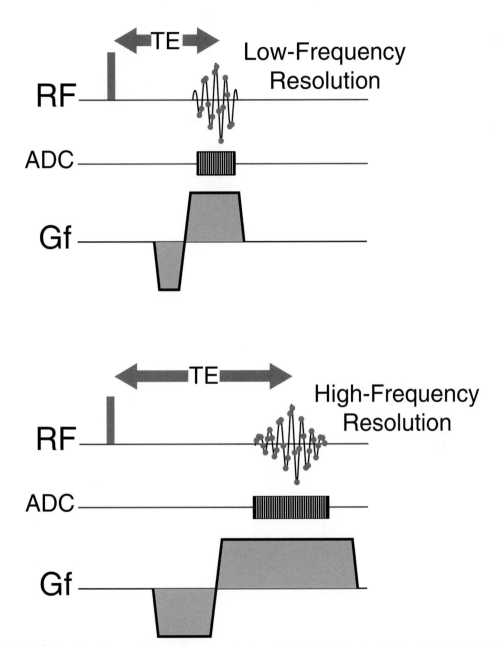

FIGURE 8-10. Doubling the number of samples per echo from 16 *(top)* to 32 *(bottom)* without changing the sampling rate doubles the frequency-encoding resolution and doubles the sampling time. The longer application of the frequency-encoding gradient (Gf) allows longer sampling of the echo, including more data from the tails. This increases the echo time (TE). ADC, analog-to-digital conversion; RF, radiofrequency.

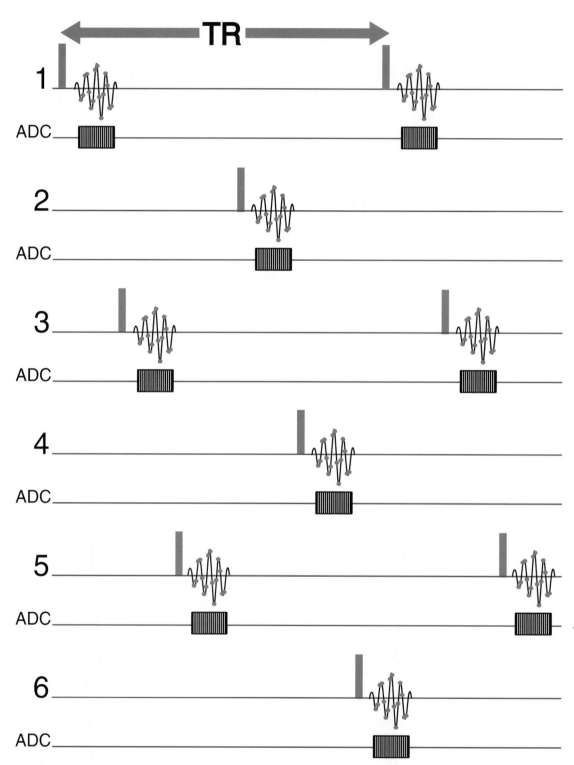

FIGURE 8–11. Multisection acquisition of six sections at 16 samples per echo. ADC, analog-to-digital conversion; TR, repetition time.

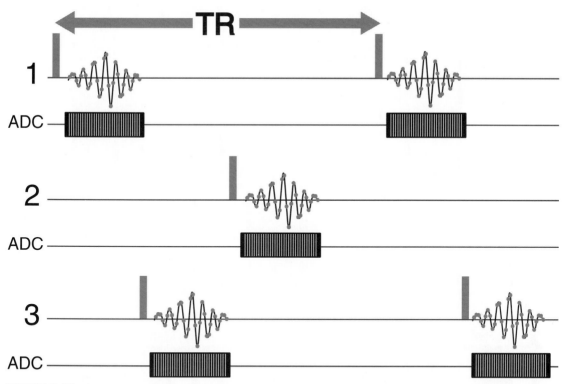

FIGURE 8–12. Multisection acquisition of three sections, obtaining 32 samples per echo. Compared with Figure 8–11 the duration of echo sampling has increased, which allows less time for obtaining additional sections during the TR.

presented in Figure 8–13, and the corresponding map of k-space is shown in Figure 8–14.

It is possible to reduce acquisition time without changing voxel dimensions by taking advantage of the symmetry of k-space. For example, slightly more than half of the phase-encoding lines of k-space can be sampled, and the remaining phase-encoding values can be interpolated, or zero filled. This method involves acquiring less than a single acquisition for Fourier transformation, so it is referred to as *partial Fourier technique* (Fig. 8–15).

Alternatively, slightly more than half of each echo may be sampled for analog-to-digital conversion (ADC). With this method, only part of k-space in the frequency-encoding axis is sampled directly, the remainder being interpolated. This method allows the use of shorter TE (Figs. 8–16 and 8–17).

Some MRI techniques (e.g., echo planar and fast spin echo) involve creating images from more than one echo per excitation. Each echo is used to fill a line of k-space. The number of echoes acquired per excitation radio pulse is referred to as the *echo train.* For example, a pulse sequence that involves acquisition of four echoes and four lines of k-space after each exci-

tation pulse is considered to have an echo train of 4. At a given TR and number of signals averaged, the total acquisition time is reduced by a factor of the echo train. For example, if TR and averaging are held constant, the use of an echo train of 4 would reduce acquisition time to one fourth that required for a single echo technique. Multiecho techniques are described in further detail in Chapter 13.

Relationship to Signal-to-Noise Ratio

The simplest method of increasing SNR is to obtain redundant additional data. The impact of random errors (noise) on a measurement (signal) can be reduced by averaging together two or more measurements. The signal intensity of a given pixel may be increased slightly by noise during one measurement and decreased slightly during another; averaging multiple signals reduces the impact of random noise on each pixel and on the image as a whole. For MRI, this involves acquiring two echoes, rather than only one, for each value of the phase-encoding gradient. This doubles the image acquisition time. The number of echoes sampled for each

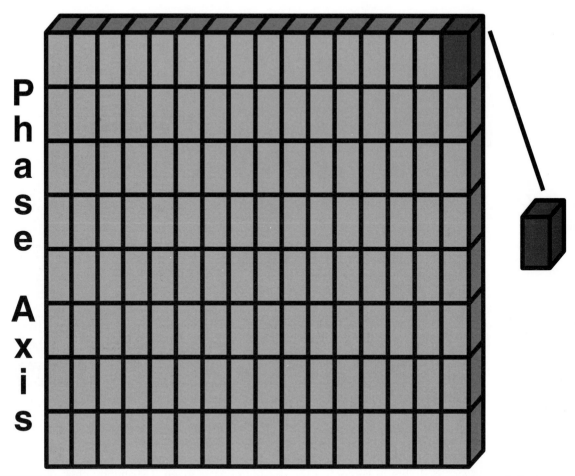

FIGURE 8–13. Representation of asymmetric pixel size, with reduced spatial resolution in the phase axis. If all other parameters are unchanged, acquisition time would be half that of the image section represented in Figure 8–1.

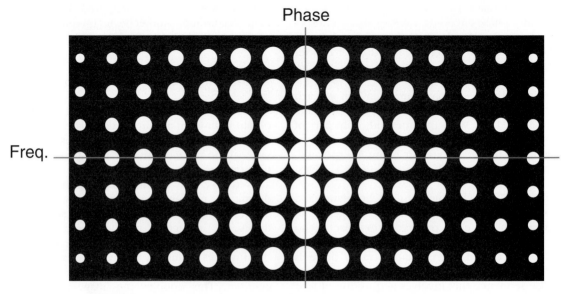

FIGURE 8–14. A k-space representation of the image section depicted in Figure 8–13.

Phase

Freq.

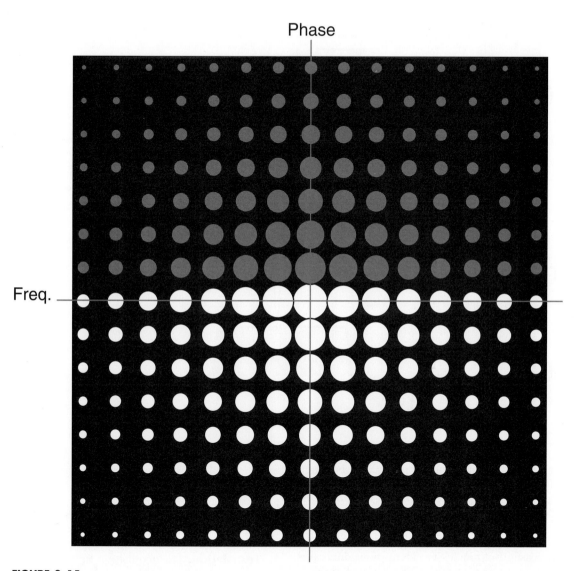

FIGURE 8–15. A k-space representation of a partial Fourier image. Nearly half of k-space is not sampled *(gray)* but is extrapolated on the basis of symmetry with the other half. Acquisition time is only slightly longer than that for Figure 8–14, although pixels are smaller and symmetric.

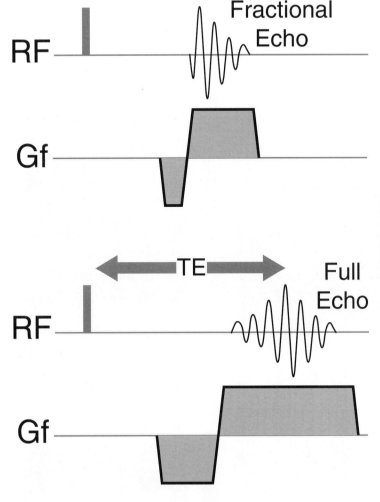

FIGURE 8–16. In fractional echo sampling *(top)* principally the latter portion of the echo is sampled. The peak of the echo can thus be sampled sooner than if the full echo is sampled *(bottom)*, resulting in shorter TE.

value of the phase-encoding gradient is generally referred to as the *number of signals averaged (NSA)* or the *number of excitations (NEX)*.

If two signals are obtained and added, the signal component of SNR is doubled. Noise also increases, but to a lesser extent; noise increases by the square root of the NSA because noise is random. Thus, doubling the NSA increases SNR by $\sqrt{2}$, approximately 1.4. Thus, SNR can be improved by a factor of about 1.4 by doubling image acquisition time.

Some Simple Equations

These few equations summarize some of the relationships between SNR, spatial resolution, and acquisition time explained in this chapter.

$$\text{Acquisition time} = \frac{\text{TR} \times \text{Np} \times \text{NSA}}{\text{ET}} \quad (1)$$

where TR is repetition time; Np, number of phase-encoding views; NSA, number of signals averaged; and ET, echo train.

Translation. The acquisition time of a pulse sequence is determined by the time between excitations (TR), multiplied by the number of excitations. The number of excitations, in turn, is determined by the number of phase-encoding views (Np) and the number of signals averaged for each phase-encoding value (NSA), divided by the number of echoes per excitation (ET).

$$\text{SNR} \; \alpha \; V \times \sqrt{N} \quad (2)$$

where V is voxel volume and $\sqrt{N}$, the square root of the total number of echoes.

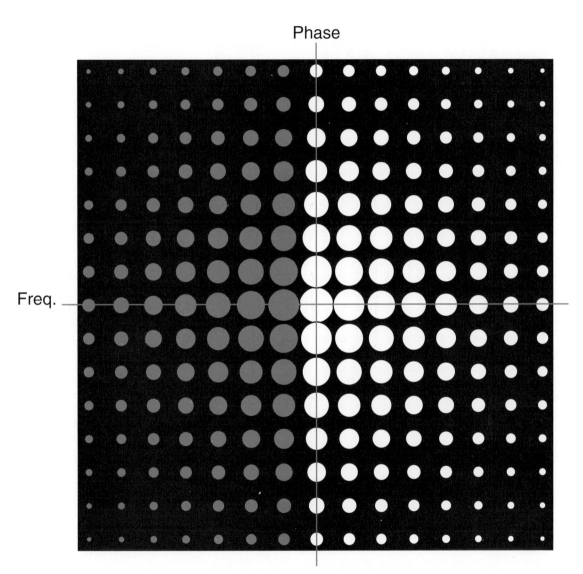

FIGURE 8-17. A k-space representation of fractional echo sampling. Nearly half of k-space *(gray)* is not filled directly, corresponding to the fraction of the echo that is not sampled. These k-space values are extrapolated based on symmetry with the other half. The resulting image section will have spatial resolution comparable to that of Figure 8–1, although SNR will be lower (less true data) and minimum TE will be lower (shorter echo sampling).

Translation. SNR is proportional to the product of volume of each voxel and the square root of the total number of echoes contributing to each image. The number of echoes equals, in turn, the product of the number of phase-encoding views (Np) and the number of averages for each phase-encoding view (NSA); that is, N = Np × NSA. For example, doubling NSA increases SNR by $\sqrt{2}$, or approximately 1.4.

A more complex example of the relationship between spatial resolution, SNR, and acquisition time involves increasing spatial resolution by doubling the matrix in the phase-encoding axis. This is accomplished by doubling the number of phase-encoding views obtained, which involves reducing each voxel by half as well as doubling the total number of echoes obtained. According to equation 2, doubling the number of echoes *increases* SNR by $\sqrt{2}$; however, doubling the number of phase-encoding views also involves reducing voxel volume (V) by half, which, also according to equation 2, reduces SNR by a factor of 2. These two effects, *combined, reduce* SNR by $\sqrt{2}$ ($2 \times \sqrt{2} = \sqrt{2}$), or 1.4. Thus, improving resolution in the phase-encoding axis by doubling the number of phase-encoding views reduces SNR by a factor of 1.4. Additionally, according to equation 1 above, doubling the number of echoes obtained doubles acquisition time. This example demonstrates that spatial resolution in MRI can be quite "expensive," in terms of both SNR and acquisition time.

The effect on acquisition time of various pulse sequence parameters is summarized in Table 8–2.

TABLE 8–2. EFFECT OF VARIOUS PULSE SEQUENCE PARAMETERS ON ACQUISITION TIME

Pulse Sequence Parameter Change	Effect on Acquisition Time
Increased section thickness	Decrease
Increased total field of view	No direct effect
Decreased (rectangular) *phase* field of view	Decrease
Increased TR	Increase
Increased TE	Increase
Increased frequency resolution	Increase
Increased phase resolution	Increase
Partial-Fourier technique	Decrease
Fractional echo sampling	Decrease
Increased signal averaging	Increase

ESSENTIAL POINTS TO REMEMBER

1. SNR, spatial resolution, and acquisition time are image attributes that compete with each other; efforts to improve one of these features usually worsen the other two.
2. Decreasing voxel size by decreasing FOV improves spatial resolution but decreases SNR.
3. Increasing the number of voxels by increasing matrix improves spatial resolution, decreases SNR, and increases acquisition time.
4. Obtaining multiple signal averages increases SNR and acquisition time.

9 Additional Determinants of Signal-to-Noise Ratio

In the previous chapter we discussed how signal-to-noise ratio (SNR) is affected by changes in spatial resolution and acquisition time. In this chapter, other determinants of SNR are addressed.

MAGNETIC FIELD STRENGTH

As magnetic field strength increases, a larger proportion of a tissue's protons align with the axis of the main magnetic field. This increases longitudinal magnetization, and therefore the signal intensity, of most tissues on MR images. Generally, SNR increases linearly with magnetic field strength (Fig. 9–1).

It is essential, at all field strengths, to be aware of the many tradeoffs in SNR so that protocol adjustments can be made most appropriately. Voxel size, number of signal excita-

tions, receiver bandwidth, and receiver coil can be changed to produce noisy high-field images or crisp low-field images. Users of low–magnetic field strength MRI instruments commonly increase SNR by reducing the receiver sampling bandwidth (see below). Conversely, users of high–magnetic field strength MRI instruments may increase the receiver sampling bandwidth, which reduces many artifacts and facilitates high-speed imaging.

The increased SNR available by imaging at high magnetic field provides options to increase spatial resolution and/or decrease examination time. Conversely, the low-field MR user must be more concerned with maintaining adequate SNR. Indeed, higher SNR is one of the greatest advantages of high magnetic field strength, which must be weighed against multiple disadvantages. These include generally higher purchase and maintenance costs, the requirement for increased radio pulse amplitudes, longer T1

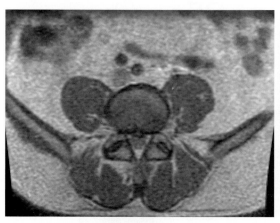 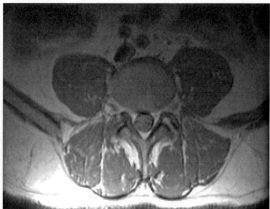

0.2 T   1.5 T

FIGURE 9–1. Axial intermediate-weighted images of the lumbar spine, showing lower SNR at 0.2T *(left)* than at 1.5T *(right).*

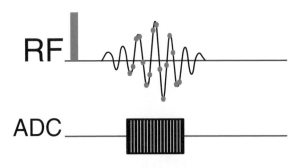

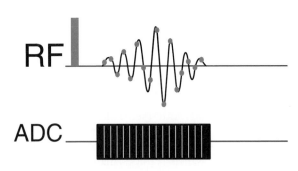

FIGURE 9–2. Relationship between the rate and duration of echo sampling. The same number of samples are obtained for analog-to-digital conversion (ADC) at top and bottom. The sampling rate at top is twice as rapid, so sampling takes half as long. RF, radiofrequency.

relaxation times and reduced T1 contrast for some tissues, and increased sensitivity to artifacts from chemical shift, magnetic field heterogeneity, and motion. The costs of high-field MRI can, however, be offset by greater patient throughput and perhaps by more comprehensive examinations, whereas the potential for artifacts at high field strength can be decreased by appropriate choice of imaging parameters and by artifact-reducing software.

The controversy over which field strength is best for clinical imaging has not been resolved, but this is beyond the scope of this text. Most importantly, users of MR—at any and all field strengths—must become familiar with the basic principles of MRI and with the methods for optimizing the diagnostic content of MR images on their equipment.

SAMPLING BANDWIDTH OF THE RECEIVER

The MR signal is an analog set of radio waves with a combination of frequencies, phases, and amplitudes. The phases of these waves come together in a momentary crescendo at the peak of each echo. Each echo is sampled for a finite interval, during which it is converted to digital data by a process called *analog-to-digital con-*

version (ADC). The rate at which an echo is sampled is referred to as the *sampling bandwidth,* or sampling rate, of the receiver. As the sampling bandwidth (rate) decreases, the sampling time increases (Fig. 9–2) if the frequency-encoding resolution is not changed. In a simplified example, an MR image with a reso-

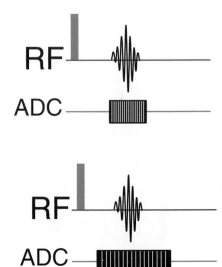

FIGURE 9–3. The sampling bandwidth (sampling rate) at bottom is half that at top, doubling the sampling time. Much of this sampling occurs during the tails of the echo, where signal is negligible.

lution of 256 in the frequency-encoding axis requires 256 samples of each echo. If the entire echo is sampled at a rate of 32 kHz (32,000 cycles per second), 8 msec is needed to digitize the 256 samples. If the sampling bandwidth is reduced to 16 kHz, 16 msec is needed.

Reduced sampling bandwidth results in less sampling of high-frequency noise, which is excluded from the sampling range of the receiver when bandwidth is decreased. The decreased noise sampled potentially improves SNR proportionally to the square root of the change in sampling time.

The SNR of tissues with short T2 relaxation time may not be increased by the use of low-bandwidth technique. If the T2 relaxation time is comparable to or shorter than the sampling time, it may not be possible to detect additional signal by sampling longer, as signal may decay markedly during sampling (Fig. 9-3). For this reason, images of tissues with short T2 relaxation times such as muscle may show blurring and decreased SNR when they are acquired using long sampling times (reduced sampling bandwidth).

To maintain a constant field of view (FOV) and pixel size in an image, changes in sampling bandwidth must be complemented by proportional changes in frequency-encoding gradient (Gf) strength (Fig. 9-4). For example, if sam-

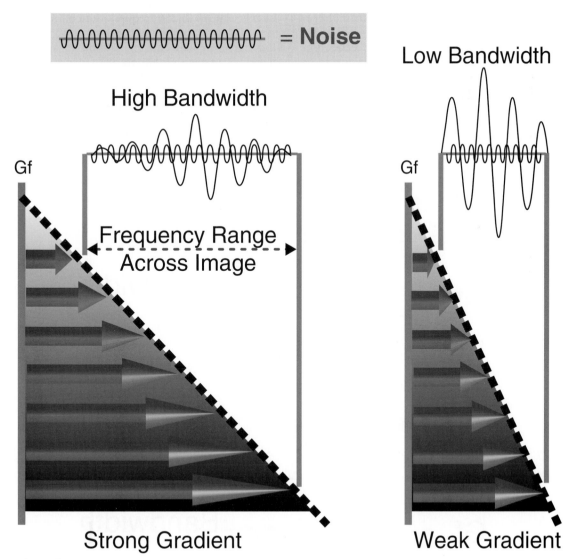

FIGURE 9–4. For a given field of view, the frequency range across the frequency-encoding axis of an image is greater with a high sampling bandwidth than with a low one. Thus, the frequency-encoding gradient (Gf) is weaker for low–bandwidth techniques. Less noise is sampled with the low–bandwidth technique, so SNR is higher.

pling bandwidth is reduced by half, gradient strength must also be reduced by half and gradient duration (sampling time) doubled.

If gradient strength remains unchanged while sampling bandwidth is reduced, FOV and pixel size are reduced by a proportional amount. Thus, reduced bandwidth can be used to reduce pixel size (increase spatial resolution) without increasing the frequency-encoding gradient strength. Pixel dimensions in the frequency-encoding axis can be reduced either by decreasing the FOV or increasing the number of pixels in this axis. Both of these changes require either increased frequency-encoding gradient strength or reduced sampling bandwidth.

For many applications, the major disadvantage of reduced sampling bandwidth is the increased time needed for sampling each echo. This causes significant increases in echo time (TE; Fig. 9-5), which can introduce unwanted T2 or T2* contrast into an otherwise T1-weighted image (T2* contrast discussed in Chapter 4). Additionally, greater image degradation from physiologic motion or decay of signal can occur during the longer TE. Increased sam-

pling time usually leads to increased acquisition time or a decreased number of image sections at a given TR (Fig. 9-6).

Increased chemical shift misregistration artifact is another disadvantage of reduced sampling bandwidth. Since weaker frequency-encoding gradients are used when sampling bandwidth is reduced, the difference in frequency from one pixel to the next is reduced. The frequency difference between water and methylene (CH_2) protons, however, is constant at a given field strength. The chemical shift differences between them thus cause a shift of more pixels when sampling bandwidth is reduced (Fig. 9-7).

As an example, the chemical shift between water and CH_2 protons at 1.5 T is approximately 240 Hz. If 256 frequency-encoding steps are used with a sampling bandwidth of 32 kHz, the chemical shift misregistration is approximately 2 pixels (32,000 Hz/256 pixels = 125 Hz/pixel; 2 pixels = 250 Hz). If the sampling bandwidth is reduced to 16 kHz, the chemical shift misregistration is doubled, to more than 4 pixels (500 Hz; Fig. 9-8).

At lower magnetic field strength, chemical

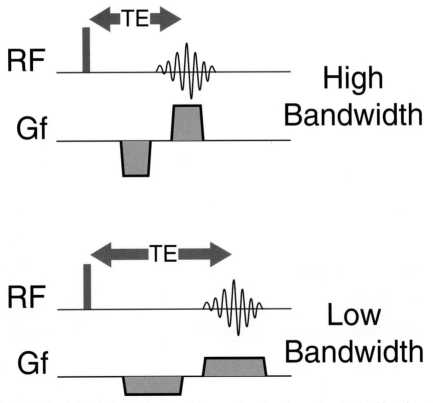

FIGURE 9–5. A high–bandwidth technique involves faster sampling than does a low–bandwidth technique, so TE can be shorter.

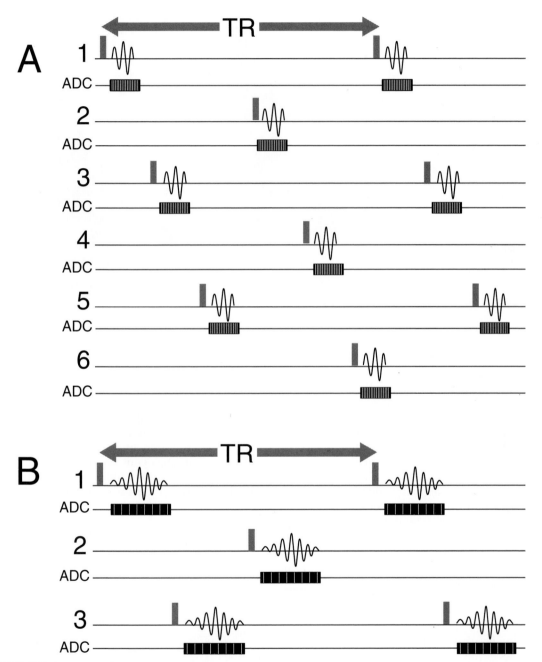

FIGURE 9–6. Lower sampling bandwidth *(B)* involves slower sampling, resulting in a longer time between excitations of different image sections. Therefore, with lower sampling bandwidth, fewer image sections can be obtained at a given TR.

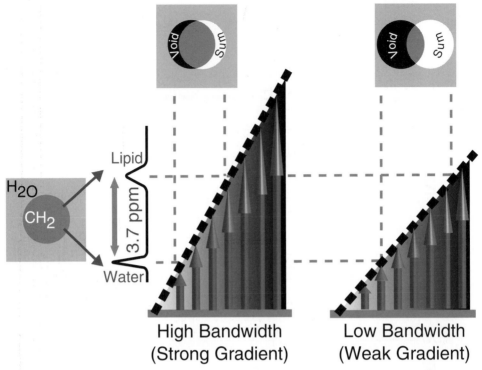

FIGURE 9–7. The frequency difference between lipid and water corresponds to a smaller distance along a strong frequency-encoded gradient (Gf) (high bandwidth, *left*) than it does along a weak frequency-encoded gradient (low bandwidth, *right*). Therefore, the misregistration on an image obtained with low bandwidth *(right)* corresponds to a greater portion of the image than it does with high bandwidth *(left)*.

shift misregistration artifact and motion artifact are less intense than at high field strength; however, reduced sampling bandwidth is used commonly at low field strength to compensate for low SNR. The increased SNR resulting is accompanied by exacerbated chemical shift misregistration and motion artifacts. Thus, one may think of modified sampling bandwidth as a form of "magnetic field strength compensation," rendering SNR and artifacts more similar between high- and low–magnetic field instruments (Table 9-1).

LOCAL RECEIVER COILS

In the previous chapter and in the initial two sections of this chapter, we discussed how SNR can be affected by changing voxel size, image acquisition time, and/or sampling bandwidth. Each of these changes involves making carefully considered tradeoffs between SNR and other attributes of MR image quality or acquisition time. None of these can be considered a "free lunch."

It is possible, however, to increase SNR without increasing voxel size or acquisition time. SNR can be improved directly by using a local radio receiver coil, which is better-configured for a specific region of interest. The local receiver coil is analogous to the antenna of a radio, except that, with MRI, we are interested only in MR signals that arise within centimeters

TABLE 9–1. EFFECTS OF VARIOUS PULSE SEQUENCE PARAMETERS ON SNR

Pulse Sequence Parameter Change	Effect on SNR
Increased section thickness	Increase
Increased total field-of-view	Increase
Reduced (rectangular) *phase* field-of-view	Decrease
Increased TR	Increase
Increased TE	Decrease
Increased frequency resolution	Decrease
Increased phase resolution	Decrease
Partial-Fourier technique	Decrease
Fractional echo sampling	Decrease
Increased signal averaging	Increase
Increased magnetic field strength	Increase
Increased sampling bandwidth	Decrease
Use of local receiver coil	Increase

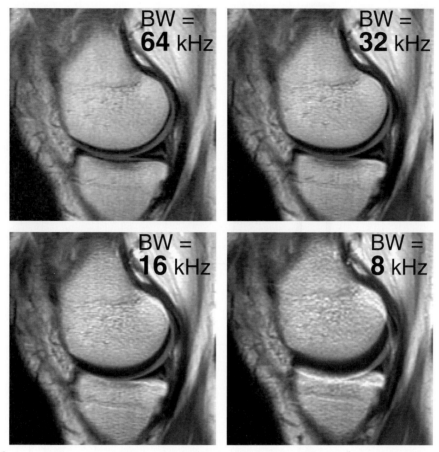

FIGURE 9–8. As sampling bandwidth (BW) is decreased from 64 to 8 kHz, SNR improves but the images are increasingly degraded by severe chemical shift misregistration artifact along the frequency-encoding (superoinferior) axis, obscuring intraarticular anatomy.

of the antenna. The local receiver coil is designed to detect radio waves and to transmit the induced electric current to the signal receiver, where the signal is processed and converted to digital data (Fig. 9-9).

Most early local coils were flat receiver coils that were placed on the surface of the body part of interest. For this reason, local coils are often referred to as *surface coils.* Many local coils have been designed, however, to image deep structures optimally. This can be accomplished by completely encircling the body part of interest or even inserting a local coil into a body cavity. Because of the wide range of specialized configurations that can be used, a more generic term such as *local coils* is more suitable.

There is a tendency to consider the use of local coils as a way of decreasing image FOV and improving spatial resolution. Although local coils are often used as a component of a strategy for obtaining high-resolution images, the use of the local coil does not by itself directly affect voxel size. Voxel size is chosen by the user.

One of the principal obstacles to improving the spatial resolution of MR images is limited SNR. By definition, improvement of spatial resolution involves reducing voxel size, which in turn decreases SNR. The major reason to use local coils is to improve SNR for the region of interest. This increased SNR, in turn, allows the MR operator to decrease FOV and/or increase image matrix without generating unacceptably noisy images.

The importance of changes in the local receiver coil can best be appreciated by first reviewing some basic principles of MR signals and local receiver coils.

MR signal is strongest from tissue closest to the MR receiver coil (Fig. 9-10). Thus, a local coil is designed to be placed as close as possible to the region of interest.

Larger local coils are sensitive to radio

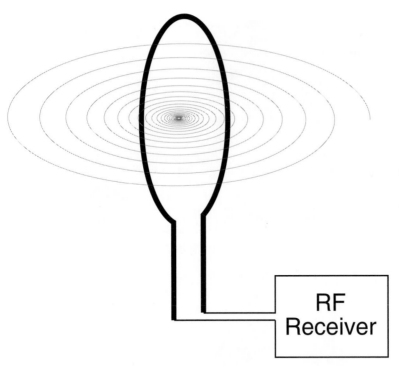

FIGURE 9–9. Simple loop radiofrequency (RF) coil for reception of MR signals. The received radio signal induces electric currents that are transmitted to the RF receiver.

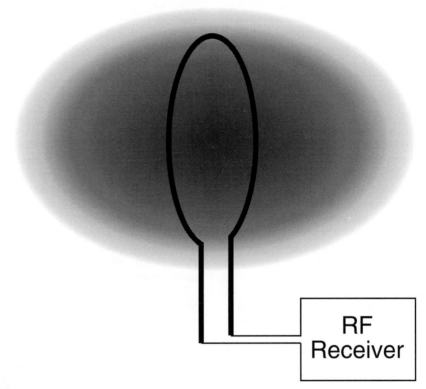

FIGURE 9–10. Sensitivity range of a simple loop coil. Lighter shades of gray distant from the coil indicate decreased sensitivity to MR signals.

signals arising from a greater distance. Thus, the diameter of a local coil must be increased to detect MR signals arising from deeper tissues.

System noise and motion-induced noise in an image are present in all MR signals that are detected by the local coil and transmitted to the receiver. Thus, detection of MR signals from a larger region of interest results in more noise (Fig. 9–11).

Optimal SNR thus involves matching the size and shape of the local coil as closely as possible to the anatomy of interest. If the coil is too small, signal is weak at the edges of the region of interest. If the coil is larger than the region of interest, noise is detected from tissue outside the region of interest. In other words, SNR is less than optimal if the local receiver coil is larger or smaller than the region of interest.

Transmit/Receive Coils

There are a few basic categories of local coils that can be used in appropriate situations. A single coil or coil array can be used both for transmitting the excitation and refocusing radio pulses and for receiving the radio signals from the resulting MR echoes. This involves switching the mode of the coil from transmitting to

receiving, a procedure similar to the switching that occurs in sonic transducers for B-mode and pulsed Doppler ultrasound. MR coils such as these are called *transmit/receive coils.*

Most currently used transmit/receive coils are circumferential (volume) coils used for body, head, or extremity imaging (Fig. 9–12). These coils are ideally suited for imaging entire objects or body parts that they can encircle completely. One particular advantage of circumferential transmit/receive coils is the pleasing uniformity of signal intensity across the resulting MR images. Flat (surface) transmit/receive coils have been unsatisfactory for most clinical applications because the resulting signal intensity profile has a banded appearance.

Receive-Only Coils

Most successful flat or curved surface coils are receive-only coils. When such coils are used, a separate coil is needed to generate the excitation and refocusing radio pulses. In most current MRI units, the built-in body coil is used to transmit radio pulses and the MR unit is set to receive signals from the local coil rather than from the built-in coil. Receive-only coils are ideal for superficial structures, but the signal intensity profile of images acquired when using these coils tends to be nonuniform unless im-

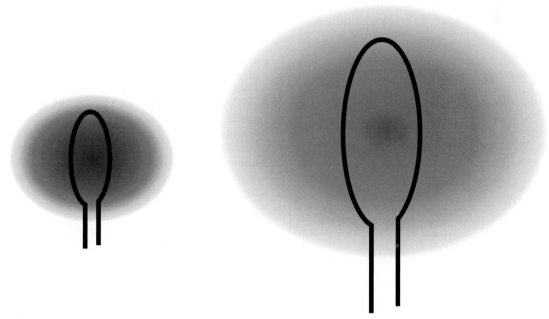

FIGURE 9–11. Sensitivity profiles of small and large loop RF coils. Sensitivity is greatest near the small coil, depicted as dark shades of gray. The larger coil is less sensitive, but its range extends over a greater volume.

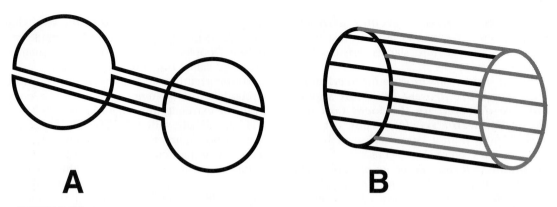

FIGURE 9–12. Two common geometries for transmit-receive volume coils: *(A)* saddle-shaped coil; *(B)* birdcage coil.

ages are acquired parallel to the axis of the coil. Uniformity perpendicular to the axis of the coil can be improved somewhat by using a curved, rather than flat, coil, but fall-off of signal intensity with greater distance from the coil is unavoidable.

Quadrature (Circularly Polarized) Coils

Quadrature coils are usually transmit/receive coils. This type of coil transmits radiofrequency to and detects radiofrequency from two orthogonal components of the precessing transverse magnetization. This generates a circularly polarized field within the antenna. The advantages of a quadrature coil include a 50% reduction in radiofrequency power deposition and increased SNR. The increased SNR varies, depending on the shape of the body part, but can be as much as 40%.

Intracavity Coils

Optimizing SNR for deep tissues has presented an enduring challenge to MR users and designers of MR equipment. One creative approach for imaging small structures deep within the body is to place a small receive-only surface coil in a body cavity on or near the surface of the structure of interest. Thus far, the most successful intracavitary coils have been intrarectal ones for imaging the prostate gland, cervix, or rectal mucosa (Fig. 9–13). Intracavitary coils have also been investigated for use in the vagina, the esophagus, and blood vessels.

Multicoil Arrays

The greatest challenge in coil design has been to maximize SNR for a large region of interest.

One approach is to optimize the size and design of a transmit/receive coil. This has been implemented most successfully for imaging the head and extremities. Because of the wide variety of body sizes and shapes, however, it has been far more difficult to image the pelvis, abdomen, and chest.

Another approach for increasing SNR for large structures has been to combine two coils, typically placed parallel to each other and on either side of the body part of interest. This coil configuration is sometimes referred to as a *Helmholtz coil.* The MR signals detected by both components of this composite coil are processed together by one receiver. In effect, the two individual coil components have been combined to produce a single larger local coil that is sensitive to deeper tissues, at the expense of increased noise for depiction of superficial structures. In other words, a compromise is made relative to the use of a single surface coil, involving improved SNR for deep structures and decreased SNR for superficial structures. Compared to a standard transmit/receive body coil, SNR is typically improved for thin patients and comparable for large patients; however, the signal intensity across the image is usually far less uniform than that obtained from conventional circumferential transmit/receive coils (Fig. 9–14). With multicoil arrays such as these, results are usually best when the separate coil elements are close to each other.

Images acquired with multicoil arrays can be much improved if the signals detected by each of two or more coil components are processed separately, by separate radio receivers. Separate sets of raw data are generated for each local FOV and are then combined in the final stages of image reconstruction. Each set of raw data reflects the SNR of one local coil. Thus, the added anatomic coverage provided by the coil

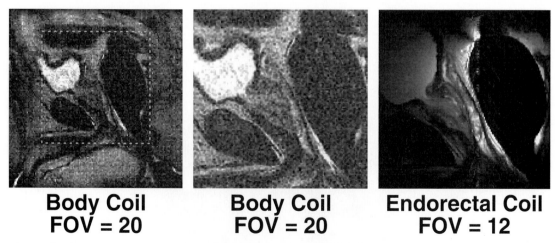

**Body Coil
FOV = 20**   **Body Coil
FOV = 20**   **Endorectal Coil
FOV = 12**

FIGURE 9–13. Sagittal fast spin echo T2-weighted images of the prostate, comparing body coil and endorectal coil techniques. The body coil image was acquired with field of view (FOV) of 20 cm and magnified in the center image to correspond anatomically with the endorectal coil image, which was acquired with FOV of 12 cm. Tissue near the prostate has higher SNR with the endorectal coil, even though the smaller FOV has resulted in smaller voxels. SNR decreases with increasing distance from the endorectal coil.

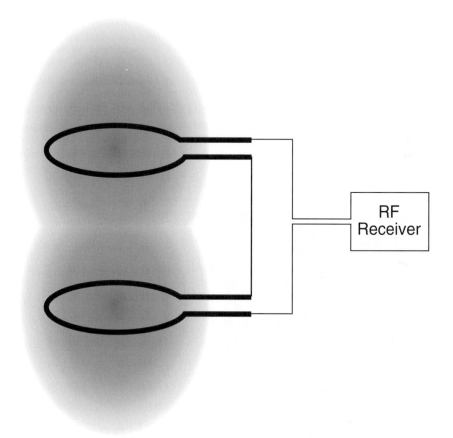

FIGURE 9–14. Helmholtz-type paired coil. Two paired loop coils detect signals, which are processed together by a single receiver. The effective size of the coil has been increased, so the volume of coil sensitivity has increased at the expense of signal sensitivity near the coil.

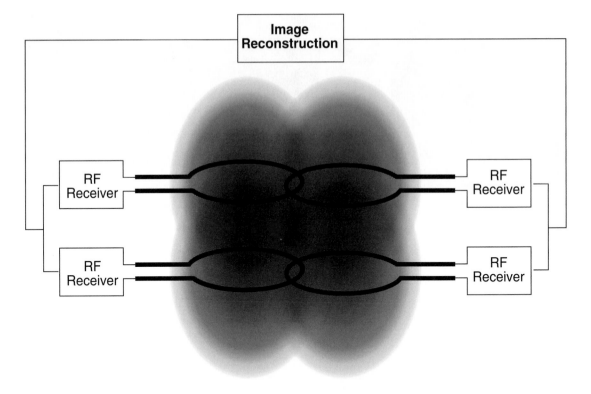

FIGURE 9-15. Four-element phased-array coil. Each coil detects signals, which are processed separately by four different RF receivers. Images are reconstructed by combining data from each receiver. Sensitivity near each element is not diminished as it was with the Helmholtz-type coil depicted in Figure 9-14.

array is not obtained at the expense of additional system noise. Multicoil arrays such as these are sometimes referred to as *phased-array coils* (Figs. 9-15 and 9-16).

Currently, phased-array coils are usually com-

posed of two or four components, each transmitting detected signals to separate receivers. Each component coil can be linear or quadrature, although the relative orientations of the coils need to be optimized for successful imple-

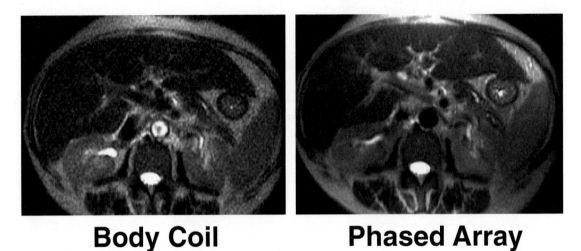

Body Coil   **Phased Array**

FIGURE 9-16. Comparison of single-shot fast spin echo images acquired using a standard-volume body coil *(left)* and a four-element multicoil phased-array coil *(right)*.

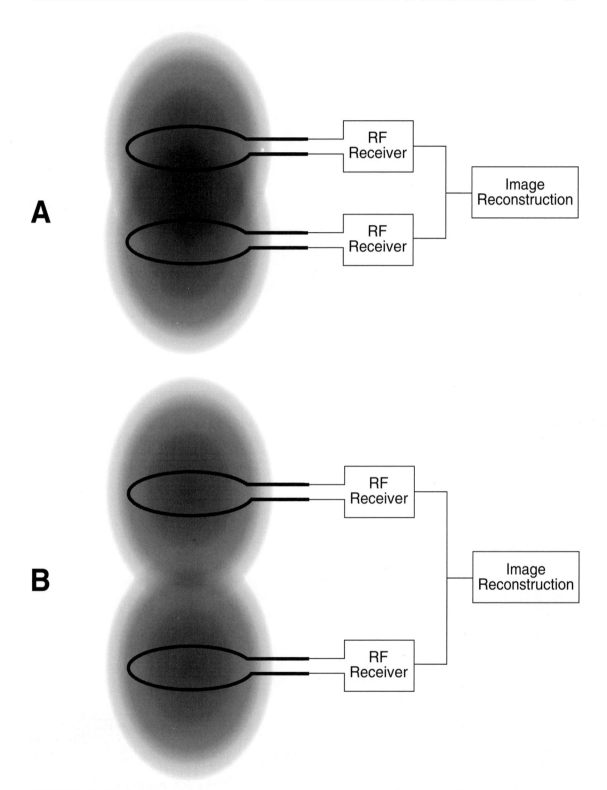

FIGURE 9–17. Effects of distance between coil elements for two-element phased-array coils. If the distance between the two elements is small *(A)*, as in thin patients or small body parts, SNR is satisfactory throughout the volume of interest. If, however, the two elements are far apart *(B)*, as in large patients or large body parts, SNR at the center of the volume of interest may be suboptimal.

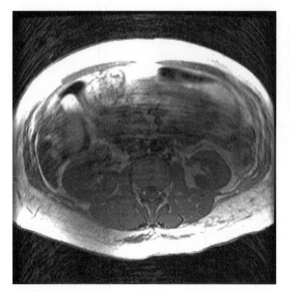 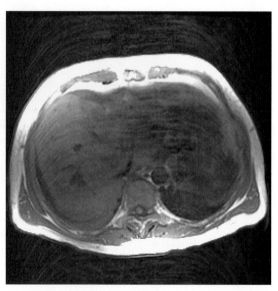

FIGURE 9–18. Image degradation due to anterior abdominal wall motion exacerbated by the use of a phased-array coil. T1-weighted spin echo 413/11 axial images acquired during respiration show high signal intensity of adipose tissue near the anterior and posterior components of the phased-array coil. The resulting artifact from anterior motion has produced high–signal intensity curvilinear bands throughout the image.

mentation of quadrature design. Like Helmholtz coils, phased-array multicoils are more useful for thin body parts than for thick ones (Fig. 9–17).

One significant disadvantage of a phased-array coil, as compared with a single circumferential transmit/receive coil, is that signal intensity is less uniform across the image. Generally, signal intensity is much greater at the surface of the coil than within deep tissues. Artifact originating from motion of a structure near one

coil can produce intense ghosts, which degrade the entire image (Fig. 9–18).

Nonuniformity of images acquired using phased-array coils can be reduced by image intensity–correction software. One form of image correction involves reducing intensity differences between neighboring regions of pixels, although this may have the undesired result of reducing image contrast (Fig. 9–19).

Another disadvantage of phased-array coils is the high cost associated with the need for two

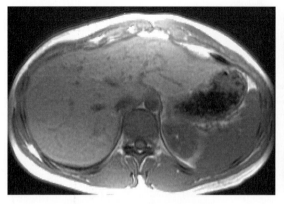 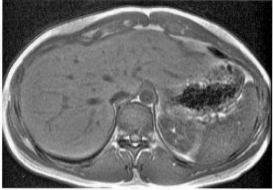

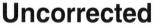
Uncorrected   **Corrected**

FIGURE 9–19. Image intensity correction. The T1-weighted gradient echo image at left has less signal intensity in the deep tissues than it does anteriorly or posteriorly. At right, image intensity correction has reduced the disparity, although tissue contrast has been degraded. Note the relative lack of contrast between liver and spleen in the corrected image *(right),* as compared with the uncorrected image *(left).*

or more separate sets of radio receivers and signal-processing hardware rather than the single set needed for other coils. Additionally, the number of separate signals that must be detected per unit of time and incorporated for image reconstruction increases in proportion to the number of radio receivers used. For example, a four-coil phased-array setup involves processing four times as much data. Additional system memory may be necessary, and image reconstruction typically takes four times as much time. Once an MRI unit is equipped with the phased-array capability, however, the price of additional coils should not be much more than the price of new conventional coils.

ESSENTIAL POINTS TO REMEMBER

1. SNR increases linearly with magnetic field strength, although other factors related to field strength cause the SNR benefit to be somewhat less.
2. Potential disadvantages of high magnetic field strength include higher costs, longer T1 relaxation times, and increased sensitivity to chemical shift, susceptibility, and motion artifacts.
3. The sampling bandwidth is the rate at which the analog MR signal is converted to digital data. A higher sampling bandwidth means faster sampling of the data for a shorter time.
4. If FOV is held constant, increased sampling bandwidth requires a stronger frequency-encoding gradient.
5. Increasing the sampling bandwidth decreases SNR.
6. Advantages of increased sampling bandwidth include faster data acquisition, reduced blurring of tissues with short T2 relaxation times, and reduced artifacts from chemical shift misregistration, magnetic field heterogeneity, and motion.
7. SNR can be increased by matching the size and configuration of the receiver coil with the body part of interest.
8. Circumferential transmit/receive coils provide uniform signal intensity throughout most of the enclosed volume.
9. Flat or curved receive-only coils produce a high SNR for tissues close to the coil but a lower SNR for deep tissues.
10. As the radius of a receive-only coil decreases, SNR close to the coil increases and SNR deep to the coil decreases.
11. Optimal SNR over a large region of interest can be obtained using a multicoil array in which signals from each coil component are processed by separate receivers (phased-array coils). This capability is expensive, and the data collection, processing, and reconstruction are more complicated.

CHAPTER

10 Motion-Induced Artifacts

The sensitivity of MRI to motion allows the modality to be used for noninvasive depiction of blood flow and other physiologic motion; however, this same sensitivity to motion complicates the process of data acquisition and results in many artifacts in the MR images themselves. The most successful method of avoiding motion artifact is preventing motion in the first place by having the patient suspend respiration and other voluntary motions during rapid image acquisition. Some images, however, cannot be acquired rapidly enough to allow suspended respiration, some patients cannot adequately control their movements, and cardiac-related motion cannot be suspended during image acquisition. Therefore, additional measures must be considered to limit the deleterious effects of motion on MR images.

An adequate understanding of the causes of motion artifacts allows a user to recognize them and to choose the best combination of methods for various clinical applications. Each method of mitigating motion artifacts addresses a specific aspect of motion; no method is a "magic button" that eliminates motion artifact entirely.

There are two basic categories of acquisition errors that lead to motion artifacts. Errors can occur during the acquisition of each echo, resulting in phase shifts within each view (within-view errors). Errors also occur when the strength (amplitude) of the MR signal varies from echo to echo (view-to-view errors). These two categories of errors are present to different degrees in different pulse sequences, and they are addressed by different artifact-reduction techniques. They are therefore addressed separately, along with corresponding techniques for artifact reduction.

GRADIENT-INDUCED (WITHIN-VIEW) PHASE CHANGES

Each MR echo sampled is referred to as a *view*. Each view is sampled during a finite period of time, during which the rephasing lobe of the frequency-encoding gradient (Gf) is applied. The echo is created by applying the rephasing lobe, which compensates for phase changes from the dephasing lobe of the gradient (see, Gradient Dephasing and Rephasing in Chapter 5). Similarly, the section-select gradient (Gs) has dephasing and rephasing lobes. The success of the rephasing components of frequency encoding and section-select gradients depends on the absence of any phase changes other than those caused by the imaging gradients themselves.

The dephasing and rephasing lobes of imaging gradients are each referred to as *unipolar gradients*. A pair of unipolar gradients such as these is designed to compensate for gradient-induced phase changes of *stationary tissue*; however, they cannot compensate for phase changes due to motion.

For example, consider the MRI signals that arise from blood flowing in a vessel. In this example, we assume that all blood within the vessel is flowing in the same direction at the same velocity (i.e., plug flow). During application of the dephasing lobe of frequency encoding or section-select gradients, the phases of signals from stationary tissue and from blood change, depending on their location along the axis of these gradients. For stationary tissue, these phase changes are reversed during application of the rephasing lobes of the gradients, so that, at the peak of the echo time (TE),

109

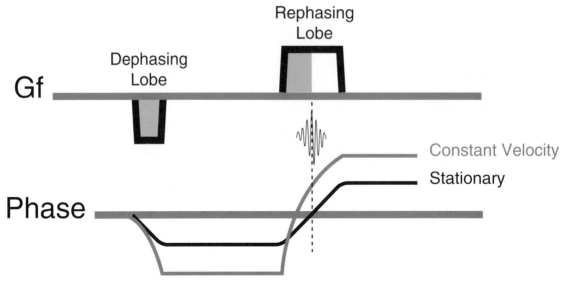

FIGURE 10–1. Phase changes for stationary and constant-velocity spins during the application of the dephasing and rephasing lobes of the frequency-encoding gradient (Gf). For stationary spins, dephasing caused by the dephasing gradient lobe is corrected for by exactly opposite phase changes that develop when the rephasing lobe is applied with reversed polarity. For moving spins, however, the phase changes during these two gradient lobes are not identical, so phase differences persist at the expected TE.

there are no phase differences. Flowing blood, however, moves between application of the dephasing and rephasing gradient lobes. Consequently, it experiences different gradient strengths during the dephasing and rephasing gradient lobes (Fig. 10-1).

If there were no phase-encoding gradient (Gp), the phases of all stationary MRI signals would be identical at the midpoint of the echo. The process of two-dimensional Fourier trans-

form image reconstruction depends on applying a phase-encoding gradient so that signals differ from one another, depending on their location along this gradient. If the phase of an MR signal is altered by something other than the phase-encoding gradient, phase-encoding errors result. Motion during and between applications of imaging gradients results in uncompensated phase shifts, which result in phase-encoding errors (Fig. 10-2).

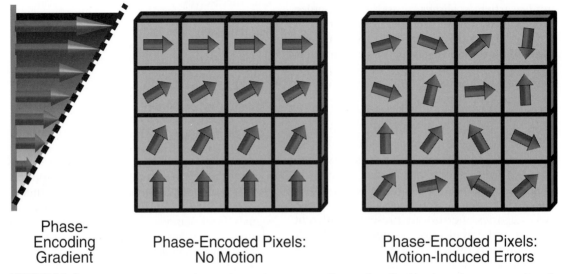

FIGURE 10–2. The phase-encoding gradient is designed to impart uniform and predictable phase changes across its axis, which are used to encode position. Additional phase changes produced by motion lead to incorrect phase encoding.

Appearance of Motion-Induced Artifact

Motion-induced phase-encoding errors manifest as artifact along the phase-encoding axis, regardless of the direction of the motion. This artifact is manifested as altered (usually increased) signal intensity, often accompanied by reduced signal intensity of the moving structure. For example, consider an abdominal image that contains a high–signal intensity gallbladder that is moving during respiration. The effect is as if some of the intensity of this gallbladder is misrepresented at various locations along the phase-encoding axis.

If motion is entirely random, the location within the image of the misrepresented signal intensity varies randomly. The artifacts in this case are smeared along the phase-encoding axis. Frequently, however, motion is repetitive and periodic, like motion due to respiration or cardiac activity. Artifact from periodic motion is more coherent and is located at regular intervals along the phase-encoding axis. The shape of these regularly spaced artifacts usually resembles that of the moving structure. Thus, artifacts that result from periodic motion during image acquisition are often referred to as *ghost artifacts* (Fig. 10-3).

The distance between ghost artifacts depends on the time between repetitive movements (TR) and the pattern of phase-encoding gradient changes. The distance between ghosts increases with the interval between movements and with TR. For example, the distance between ghosts from pulsatile flow increases as TR increases or as heart rate decreases (Fig. 10-4). When the TR is short enough so that a motion does not repeat, ghost artifact is not propagated throughout the entire phase-encoding axis. Rather, ghost artifacts on rapid images such as these may be manifested as edge blurring.

Intravoxel Phase Dispersion

When tissue or blood protons within a voxel are all moving at the same velocity, they undergo identical phase shifts. This is true whether or not their velocity is constant. If protons within a voxel all have identical velocities, the net intensity of the MR signals is strong, but there are motion-induced phase shifts that cause artifacts along the phase-encoding axis of the image.

When, however, protons within a voxel move at different velocities, there are several different phase shifts within the voxel. Thus, the coherence of the magnetization, and the resulting signal intensity, are reduced. In this case, signal intensity of the moving blood and of the ghost artifacts are less intense than if all phase shifts were identical. The loss of phase coherence, and the resulting loss of signal intensity, created when protons within a voxel move at different velocities or in different directions is referred to as *intravoxel phase dispersion*. Intravoxel phase dispersion is most common in blood vessels that have complex or turbulent flow or at the extreme periphery of a blood vessel adjacent to the vessel wall (Fig. 10-5).

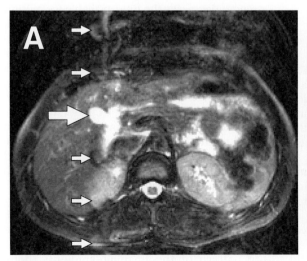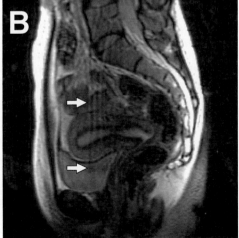

FIGURE 10-3. Examples of respiration-induced ghost artifacts on T2-weighted fast spin echo images. *(A)* Motion of the gallbladder *(large arrow)* during breathing has produced regularly spaced ghost images *(small arrows)*. *(B)* Motion of the anterior abdominal wall has produced several curved lines *(arrows)*.

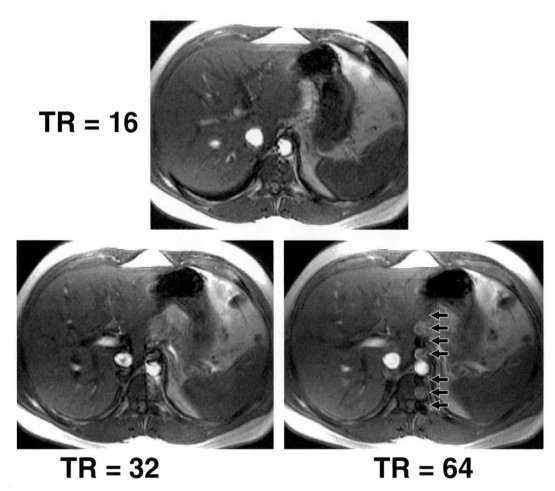

FIGURE 10–4. On single-section spoiled gradient echo images, the distance between the aorta and ghost artifacts *(arrows)* and the prominence of the artifacts increase with increasing repetition time (TR).

Factors That Affect Within-View Phase Errors

Within-view phase errors are especially severe for high-velocity motion. Phase error accumulates during the application of imaging gradients, so the magnitude of the error increases if the imaging gradients are strong and/or applied for long intervals. The phase error grows during the interval between signal excitation and the sampling of its echo, so these errors increase with longer TE.

As a single separate factor, stronger imaging gradients would increase the severity of motion artifact. In fact, however, the severity of motion artifact generally decreases as the strength of the frequency-encoding gradient is increased, because this is accompanied by an increase in the sampling bandwidth so long as the field of view is maintained. Increasing the sampling bandwidth decreases sampling time. Therefore,

increasing the frequency-encoding gradient strength decreases the time available for motion to occur. If imaging efficiency is maximized, increasing the sampling bandwidth allows reduced TE (or reduced time between echoes for pulse sequences where more than one echo is obtained per excitation radio pulse). The reduced TE (or interecho interval), in turn, further reduces the severity of motion artifact. Thus, increasing the sampling bandwidth is one useful method for reducing the severity of motion artifact. This beneficial effect of increased sampling bandwidth must, however, be considered along with its adverse effect on SNR.

Within-view phase errors are caused by phase momentum generated by imaging gradients, referred to as *gradient moments*. These gradient moments can be nulled by changing the pattern of the imaging gradients themselves, a strategy called *gradient moment nulling*.

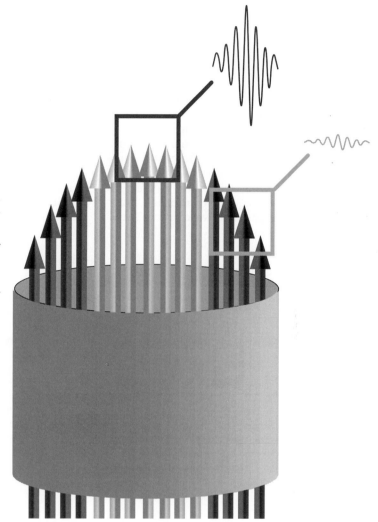

FIGURE 10-5. Intravoxel phase dispersion at the periphery of a blood vessel with laminar flow. Longer arrows represent faster flow. Flow velocity is high and nearly uniform at the center of the lumen, leading to little dephasing and therefore strong MR signals. Near the walls of the vessel, velocity decreases and there is a wider range of velocities with each voxel. This produces a wider range of phase changes in each voxel, leading to lower MR signals.

Gradient Moment Nulling

The phase shift that results from motion during and between the application of imaging gradients can be thought of as the building up of momentum due to gradients, or as a gradient moment. If the timing and duration of the gradients are altered appropriately, this gradient moment can be eliminated, or nulled. Techniques whereby within-view phase errors are eliminated or reduced are properly called *gradient moment nulling,* but vendor-specific synonyms include motion artifact suppression technique (MAST), gradient moment rephasing (GMR), flow compensation (FC), and flow-adjustable gradients (FLAG).

Gradient moment nulling involves increasing the complexity of the dephasing and rephasing components of the imaging gradients. With gra-dient moment nulling, phase shifts of signals from both stationary and moving tissue that occur during the dephasing portion of the imaging gradient are reversed during the rephasing portion of the imaging gradient and are therefore nulled at the time of the echo. The resulting pattern of imaging gradient applications, referred to as the *gradient waveform,* includes more lobes than the simple unipolar dephasing and rephasing lobes of the "non–motion-compensated" gradient waveform we have considered thus far.

The simplest form of gradient moment nulling, nulling of the gradient's first moment, consists of replacing the unipolar gradient lobes with bipolar gradients for both the dephasing and rephasing portions of the gradient waveform. The gradient's first moment is the gradient momentum produced by motion of constant velocity. Nulling of the gradient's first moment compensates for constant velocity motion that occurs between excitation and sampling of each echo (Figs. 10-6 and 10-7).

Higher orders of motion can be corrected by using increasingly complex gradient waveforms. The gradient's second moment refers to phase shifts that result from constantly changing velocity (acceleration), whereas the third moment refers to phase shifts from constantly changing acceleration (jerk). These higher orders of motion contribute less to the resulting phase shifts from complex motion. Correcting for them, however, requires increasingly complex and lengthy gradient waveforms. These

complex waveforms require more time, increasing the TE, which in turn increases the artifact that results from uncompensated motion. In practice, the best results are usually achieved by nulling the gradient's first moment and using the shortest possible TE or interecho interval. At best, the use of higher orders of gradient moment nulling yields marginal additional correction of motion artifact. In fact, if high sampling bandwidth and extremely short TEs (e.g., 2 msec or less) are used, the gradient moment may be so small that gradient moment nulling is not necessary.

Correction for constant velocity can reduce signal intensity loss from even highly pulsatile

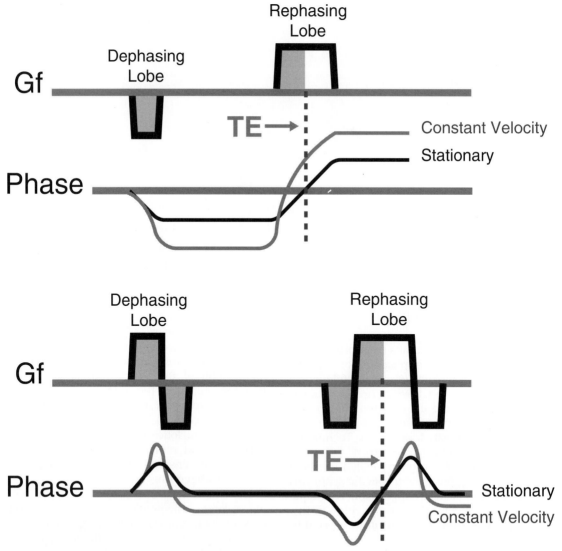

FIGURE 10–6. Phase changes for stationary and constant-velocity spins using simple bipolar gradients *(top)* and first moment nulling *(bottom)*. At the echo time (TE) *(dotted line)*, first moment nulling has eliminated phase changes for both stationary and moving spins.

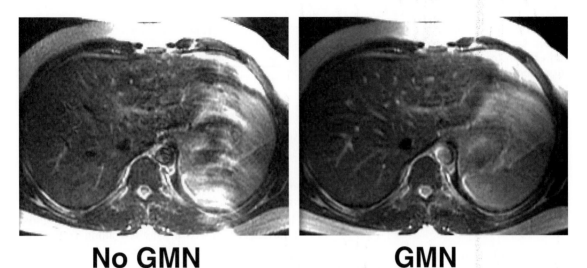

No GMN   GMN

FIGURE 10–7. Effects of gradient moment nulling (GMN) on T2-weighted spin echo 2000/80 image. Artifact is less with GMN. Note that aortic signal intensity is higher and there is less artifact from its pulsatile flow.

flow, such as that in the aorta or other arteries. This may seem surprising, since the flow velocity in these vessels is continually changing. Inspection of a typical arterial velocity waveform like that obtained by Doppler ultrasound or cardiac gated MR flow measurement techniques reveals that arterial flow is, in fact, never constant (Fig. 10–8). Flow in the aorta accelerates rapidly to a sharp peak during systole, decelerates, and is drastically reduced or disappears during most of diastole. Phase shifts from motion, however, occur *during the application of the dephasing and rephasing gradient lobes and the interval between them.* This brief pe-

riod of time is even less than the TE, a small fraction of a second. During this brief interval, constant-velocity flow is a reasonably close approximation. Thus, nulling the gradient's first moment compensates for most, but not all, of the phase shifts that occur between excitation and sampling of the resulting echo.

Even if all phase shifts resulting from motion were entirely eliminated, as by infinitely complex and precise gradient moment nulling or infinitely short TE, artifacts from pulsatile flow and other forms of rapidly changing motion would not be eliminated unless other methods of artifact correction were used. This is because

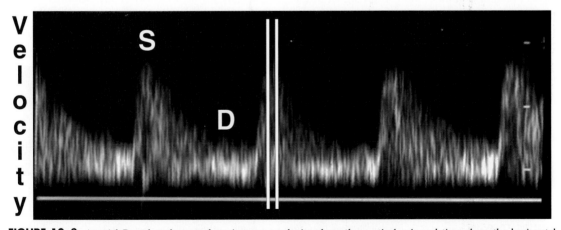

FIGURE 10–8. Arterial Doppler ultrasound tracing maps velocity along the vertical axis and time along the horizontal axis. Flow velocity varies from high during systole (S) to low during diastole (D). Velocity is not constant during any portion of the cardiac cycle; however, during intervals of a few milliseconds, as indicated by the paired vertical lines, there is little variation.

much of the artifact from inconstant motion results from view-to-view intensity changes rather than from within-view phase shifts. Gradient moment nulling is highly effective at reducing artifacts from within-view phase errors; however, some forms of motion, such as pulsatile flow, produce artifacts from view-to-view errors. Correction of view-to-view errors requires additional strategies.

TABLE 10–1. EFFECTS ON WITHIN-VIEW AND VIEW-TO-VIEW MOTION-INDUCED ERRORS OF DIFFERENT TYPES OF MOTION

Type of Motion	Within-View	View-to-View
Constant velocity motion	+ + +	–
Pulsatile flow	+ + +	+ + +
Complex motion	+ + +	+

VIEW-TO-VIEW INTENSITY ERRORS

As established in Chapter 5, the intensity of signals is greatest when weak phase-encoding gradients are applied (for gross tissue contrast) and least when strong phase-encoding gradients are applied (for fine image detail). Fourier transform image reconstruction includes the assumption that the amplitude (signal intensity) of each echo is changed only by variations of the value of the phase-encoding gradient.

If motion occurs during data acquisition, the intensity of signals arising from a particular site may vary from view to view (echo to echo). The process of phase encoding by Fourier transform reconstruction does not account for these variations, so phase-encoding errors result. The effect of such errors is artifact along the phase-encoding axis that is indistinguishable from those that result from within-view phase errors.

Let us consider, for example, view-to-view artifacts on an MR image of the abdomen that result from respiratory motion. During one view a particular voxel may contain hepatic tissue, resulting in moderately high signal intensity. During a later view, this same voxel may contain air, which has no signal intensity (Fig. 10–9). These variations in signal intensity result in phase-encoding mistakes, producing ghost artifacts that are distributed along the phase-encoding axis (Fig. 10–10).

As another example, let's consider high-velocity pulsatile flow. During systole, blood flows rapidly into the imaging volume, where it is excited by a radio pulse and an echo is sampled. Because this blood was outside the imaging volume during the previous excitation radio pulse, it entered the imaging volume completely unsaturated, with all of its longitudinal magnetization. During systole, therefore, blood has high signal intensity. During diastole, however, blood within the imaging volume is nearly stationary. It has been exposed to a series of excitation pulses, so that longitudinal magnetization has recovered partially rather than completely. Therefore, during diastole blood signal intensity is lower than it is during systole. The changing velocity of blood in the aorta leads to changing signal intensity, producing ghost artifacts from view-to-view intensity changes. These artifacts occur even if within-view phase errors are entirely eliminated. The effects of different forms of motion are summarized in Table 10–1.

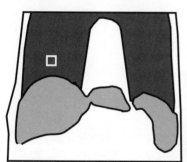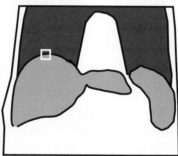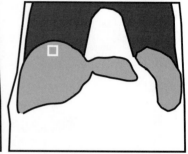

FIGURE 10–9. Diagram of view-to-view changes from breathing motion of the interface between liver and lung. Signals from a given position within the image can be from lung, liver, or both, producing varying echo amplitude and, thus, incorrect phase encoding.

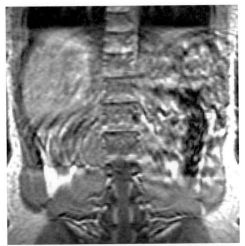 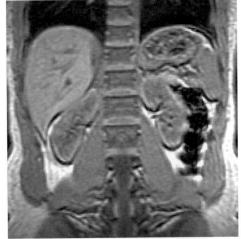

No Breath Hold   Breath Hold

FIGURE 10–10. Respiration-induced artifact on coronal T1-weighted spoiled gradient echo 100/1.8/80° images. Within-view errors are minimal because of the short echo time (TE). View-to-view changes during breathing produce ghost artifacts along the phase-encoding (left-to-right) axis, which obscure image detail. This can be corrected by breath holding *(right)*.

STRATEGIES FOR REDUCING MOTION-INDUCED ARTIFACTS

There are several strategies for reducing motion-induced artifacts. Some address artifacts due to both view-to-view intensity changes and within-view phase errors, whereas others are directed principally at one or the other of these basic causes. Strategies that reduce artifacts from both sources include averaging, cessation of motion (e.g., breath holding), reducing the signal intensity of the moving structures (e.g., suppressing the signal intensity of fat or of flowing blood), and reducing the time during which the center of k-space is filled (e.g., subsecond imaging). Gradient moment nulling is directed entirely toward reducing or eliminating artifact from within-view motion. Strategies that reduce artifact from view-to-view intensity changes include respiratory or cardiac monitoring (e.g., gating, triggering, or phase reordering).

Averaging

Averaging is a "brute force" method that decreases the conspicuousness of ghost artifacts without directly addressing the causes of either within-view or view-to-view artifacts. Averaging works simply by increasing the signal intensity of the tissues of interest more than the signal intensity of ghost artifacts, because real tissue has a more consistent location along the phase-encode axis than do the ghost artifacts (Fig. 10–11). Although body tissues may move 2 cm or more between views, this is far less than the changing position of ghosts, which may be located anywhere within the image along the phase-encode axis.

In most situations, averaging is accomplished by acquiring two or more echoes at each strength of the phase-encoding gradient before changing the strength of this gradient (Fig. 10–12). This results in each line of k-space being repeated two or more times before the next line is acquired.

This method of averaging is the simplest to implement, because it does not increase the number of times phase-encoding gradient strength is changed. The disadvantage of this method of averaging is that the signal intensity of a pixel tends to be similar in two sequential views. For example, little motion occurs during a 6.5-msec TR, so averaging two successive views at this TR has only a minimal effect on reducing motion artifacts. In fact, since the time between lines of k-space is increased from 6.5 to 13 msec, some forms of artifact may even be intensified (Fig. 10–13).

In general, motion artifact is best corrected by averaging when all lines of k-space are acquired before any is repeated (see Fig. 10–12C). This method of averaging is rarely used, how-

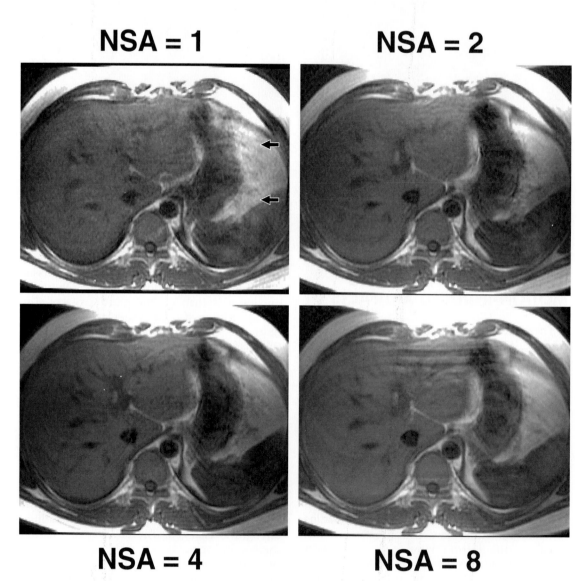

FIGURE 10–11. Effect of signal averaging on motion-induced artifact (SE 500/11). With no averaging *(top left)*, the image is degraded by artifact *(arrows)*. With increasing number of signals averaged (NSA) artifact is reduced and SNR is increased.

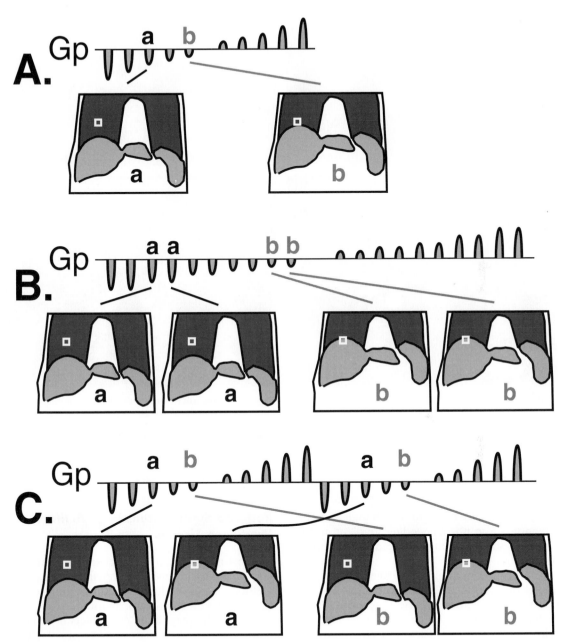

FIGURE 10-12. Effects of averaging on view-to-view errors in rapidly acquired images. Two different phase encoding gradient (Gp) strengths are labeled (*a* and *b*). *(A)* Without averaging, there is little change between views *a* and *b*. *(B)* If each phase-encoding gradient strength is repeated twice before changing, there is little change, so little is accomplished by averaging; however, more time elapses between *a* and *b*, increasing view-to-view errors. *(C)* If each phase-encoding gradient strength is applied once before any is repeated, the views being averaged are different from one another. In this example, the average of both *a* views is identical to the average of both *b* views.

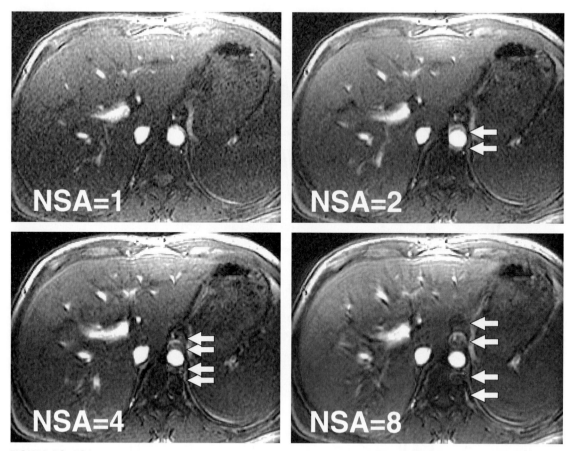

FIGURE 10-13. Effect of increasing the number of signals averaged (NSA) on artifact from pulsatile aortic flow *(arrows)* on axial gradient echo images with TR of 6.5 msec and TE of 1.5 msec. With one signal average *(top left)*, image acquisition is so rapid that there is little motion artifact. As NSA increases from one to eight, signal-to-noise ratio (SNR) improves but the time increases between changes of the phase-encoding gradient strength. This increases the severity of artifact and increases the distance between ghosts *(arrows)*.

ever, since it involves more changes of the strength of the phase-encoding gradient and is therefore somewhat more demanding to implement.

The major disadvantage of averaging is the longer time required. Thus, averaging is a viable option only for efficient pulse sequences. These include spin echo and gradient echo images with short TR, and T2-weighted images in which several echoes are obtained per excitation radio pulse (e.g., fast spin echo or turbo spin echo). Even with these techniques, other methods of artifact suppression are generally preferred when available, owing to their greater efficiency. Additionally, the longer time required for pulse sequences with averaging may, in fact, lead to increased motion during acquisition, and even to increased artifact.

Reduced Signal Intensity of Artifact-Producing Tissues

Ghost artifacts can be ameliorated by reducing the signal intensity of moving tissue. This method does not directly address the motion itself or the mechanism of motion artifact, but it reduces the magnitude of artifacts from both within-view and view-to-view errors. Artifact from flowing blood can be reduced by saturating the blood before it enters the volume of interest via a *spatially selective saturation pulse*. Such pulses reduce the signal intensity of both the blood within the vessel and ghost artifacts that arise from the blood (Figs. 10-14 to 10-16). Spatially selective saturation pulses can also be used to reduce or eliminate signal intensity from moving structures other than blood. For instance, a saturation pulse can be applied to the anterior abdominal wall to reduce artifact from moving adipose tissue (Fig. 10-17, *top*).

Another form of saturation pulse that is commonly used to reduce motion artifact is *fat saturation,* a form of *chemically selective saturation.* Here, a radio pulse is designed to match the frequency of methylene (CH_2) protons in adipose tissue rather than the various tissues at a given position along an imaging gradient. Reducing the signal intensity of adipose tissue decreases the severity of artifact generated by its motion (Fig. 10-17, *bottom*). Spatially and chemically selective saturation pulses are discussed further in Chapter 12.

Cardiac and Respiratory Monitoring

Most methods of motion artifact reduction that are based on monitoring of physiologic motion are directed principally toward view-to-view intensity changes. The cardiac cycle can be monitored either by electrocardiographic (ECG) or impedance plethysmographic (IPG) methods. ECG monitoring allows more accurate determination of the phase of the cardiac cycle throughout image acquisition. IPG methods are easier to implement and suffer less from artifacts due to extraneous cardiac or radiofrequency activity but do not allow any direct comparison between the phase of the cardiac cycle and the images themselves.

The respiratory cycle can be monitored by placing a bellows sensitive to respiratory motion around the upper abdomen. Other methods include spirometers or even the MR signal itself. Alternatively, patients can monitor their own breathing by signaling each breath to the MR technologist.

Gating and triggering techniques are used to ensure that the signal intensity in a given location is the same during each phase-encoding view of a particular image. These techniques reduce variations in view-to-view signal intensity. In some implementations, data is discarded during periods of active motion (e.g., cardiac systole or respiratory inspiration; Fig. 10-18). If this is done, actual motion during data acquisi-

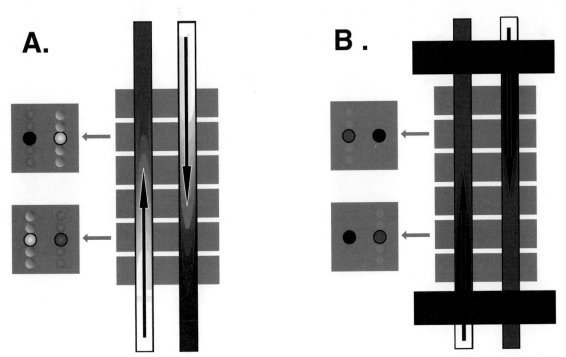

FIGURE 10-14. Spatial saturation pulses for reduction of flow-induced ghost artifacts in a 2D multisection acquisition. *(A)* Stationary tissue is partially saturated by repeated excitations; however, blood, which enters the imaged volume between excitations, is fully magnetized and thus can produce greater signal intensity. Ghost artifact and increased signal intensity are greatest at entry sections (i.e., the first sections in the stack encountered by fresh, fully magnetized blood). *(B)* With saturation pulses above and below the imaged volume, in-flowing blood has less magnetization, rather than more, relative to stationary tissue. The vascular lumen in the entry sections therefore has the lowest signal intensity and exhibits the least artifact.

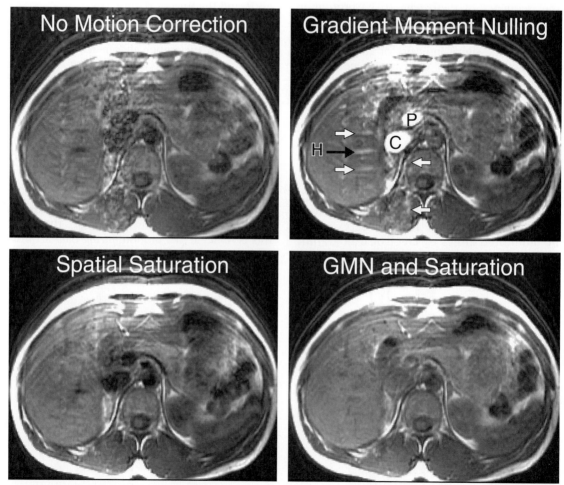

FIGURE 10–15. Effects of gradient moment nulling (GMN) and spatial saturation pulses on vascular ghost artifact in bottom sections of an axial SE 300/25 acquisition during quiet respiration. Without motion artifact correction *(top left)*, there is severe image degradation. With GMN *(top right)*, signal loss from within-view errors has been corrected, increasing the signal intensity of the inferior vena cava (C), portal vein (P), and hepatic vein (H). These vessels have the highest signal intensity, because this is the entry section for the inferosuperior flow direction of these vessels. There is still substantial artifact due to view-to-view changes from pulsatile flow in the inferior vena cava and hepatic veins *(white arrows)*, although there is less artifact from the nonpulsatile portal vein. With spatial saturation *(bottom left)*, the inferior vena cava and portal and hepatic veins are signal voids and artifact from these vessels has been reduced. With the combination of GMN and spatial saturation *(bottom right)*, signal intensity of the vessels has increased slightly.

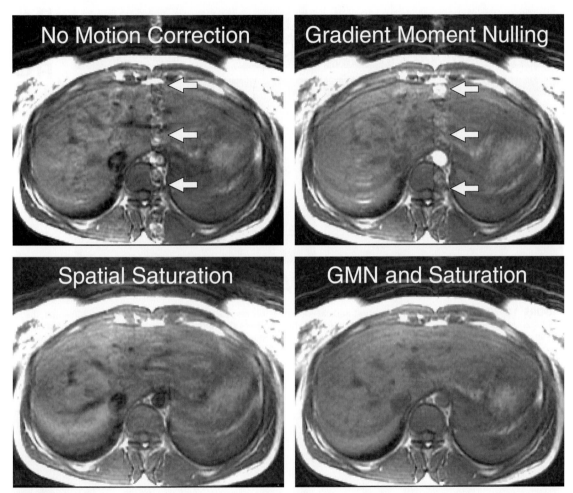

FIGURE 10-16. As in Figure 10-15, top sections. These are the entry sections for flow in the aorta, which produces severe artifact *(arrows)*. Gradient moment nulling (GMN) *(top right)* increases intraluminal signal intensity in the aorta but does not reduce ghost artifacts, which are caused primarily by view-to-view changes from pulsatile flow. Spatial saturation *(bottom left)* reduces the signal intensity of the aortic lumen as well as the artifacts. The combination of GMN and spatial saturation results in the least artifact, although vascular signal intensity is slightly higher.

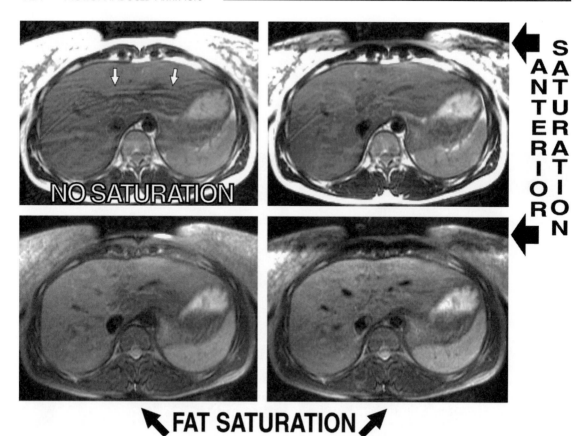

FIGURE 10–17. Effects of spatial saturation and fat saturation on respiration-induced ghost artifacts. T2-weighted FSE 2000/120 image acquired during quiet respiration shows ghost artifacts *(top left)* from motion of anterior adipose tissue. These artifacts are reduced by spatial saturation of the anterior abdominal wall *(top right)*, by chemical (fat) saturation of adipose tissue *(bottom left)*, or by combining the two methods *(bottom right)*.

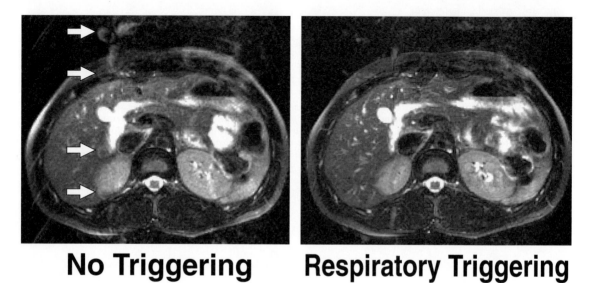

FIGURE 10–18. Respiration-induced T2-weighted FSE 3333/100 image shows artifact from motion of the gallbladder *(arrows)*, which is eliminated by triggering data acquisition to periods of minimal motion *(right)* by monitoring via respiratory bellows.

tion is reduced, minimizing both within-view and view-to-view errors; however, imaging time is prolonged when there are significant periods during which no data are acquired. A more efficient use of physiologic triggering involves obtaining different sections of a multisection acquisition during different phases of the physiologic cycle (Fig. 10-19). Alternatively, "cine" images can be obtained sequentially at a given location throughout the physiologic cycle (Fig. 10-20).

With the techniques described above, data acquisition is discontinuous, pauses generally occurring during the QRS complex. This can cause longitudinal magnetization to vary from view to view, introducing artifacts. One alternative involves continuous acquisition of data, using the R wave to trigger a change of phase-

encoding gradient strength (Fig. 10-21). These techniques, if implemented successfully, eliminate most view-to-view variations. The severity of artifact from within-view errors on a given image depends on the amount of motion that is occurring during that particular phase of the physiologic cycle.

Suspending Respiration

The best way to avoid artifact from respiratory motion is to avoid such motion during image acquisition. If image acquisition is short enough, the patient can voluntarily suspend respiration. With little effort, most patients can suspend respiration several times for 10 seconds or less. If the periods of suspended respi-

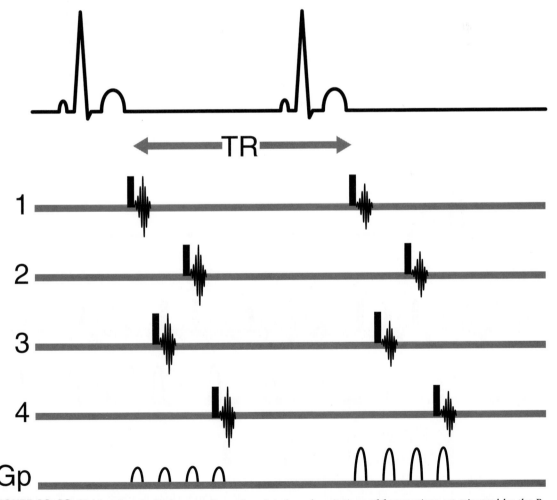

FIGURE 10-19. Multisection single-phase cardiac gating. Interleaved excitations of four sections are triggered by the R wave of an EKG signal. The value of the phase encoding gradient (Gp) is changed after the next R wave. For a given image section, all echoes occur during the same phase of the cardiac cycle. This minimizes artifacts from cardiac pulsations if the cardiac cycle is regular. Each section is acquired at a different cardiac phase.

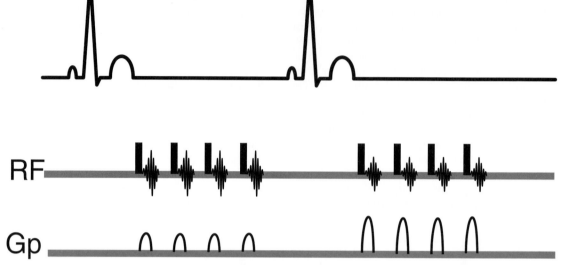

FIGURE 10–20. Single-section multiphase cardiac gating. Four excitations are obtained for each value of the phase encoding gradient (Gp), resulting in four images of the same physical site at four different phases of the cardiac cycle.

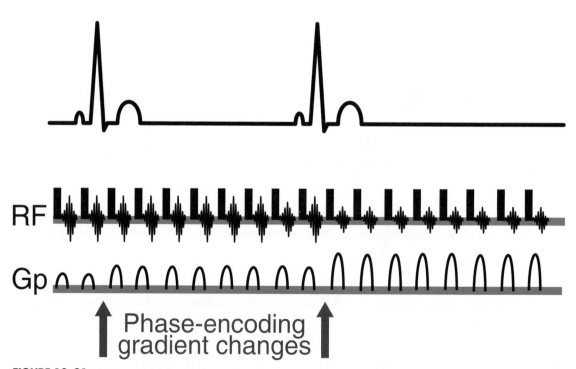

FIGURE 10–21. Continuous data acquisition with cardiac triggering. The TR is uniform throughout acquisition and is not related to the cardiac cycle. The value of the phase encoding gradient (Gp) is changed at each R wave. The number of cardiac phases encoded for is determined by the number of excitations that can occur during each cardiac cycle.

rations are few, most patients can suspend respiration for 20 seconds. With active coaching, rehearsal before the actual imaging, and encouragement during image acquisition, most patients can suspend respiration for as long as 30 seconds. If oxygen is administered via nasal cannula before breath holding, patients can suspend respiration even longer.

Suspension of respiration reduces artifacts from all abdominal contents, including bowel. In fact, ghost artifact from bowel is essentially eliminated by breath holding, because peristalsis is usually slow and of small magnitude; however, antiperistaltic agents such as glucagon are useful for increasing the clarity of bowel walls and for distending bowel lumens.

If satisfactory breath holding can be achieved, multisection acquisitions are usually ideal, since these techniques allow images with longer TR to be acquired efficiently. For T1-weighted images, the long TR allows the use of a flip angle of approximately 90°, which maximizes the transverse magnetization created for tissues with short T1 relaxation times and maximizes the saturation of tissues with long T1 relaxation times, thus maximizing SNR and T1 contrast. For T2-weighted breath hold images, maximal TR allows the most complete recovery of longitudinal magnetization between excitation radio pulses, maximizing SNR and reducing unwanted T1 contrast.

Most images with intermediate or long TR, however, are highly sensitive to motion, so artifacts occur if breath holding is not successful. Additionally, these images often have prominent ghosts from pulsatile flow. If a patient cannot successfully suspend respiration and other voluntary motion during image acquisition, artifact can be reduced by decreasing TR. If TR is decreased, flip angle should be smaller as well.

"Snapshot" Imaging

To reduce artifact from cardiac and vascular motion, from gross body or limb movement, or for patients who cannot suspend respiration, image acquisition must be faster than that for breath holding. Even though substantial motion may occur during a 1-second acquisition, motion artifact is severe only if the motion occurs during sampling of the center of k-space. The effects of various artifact-correction techniques on different components of motion-induced artifact are summarized in Table 10–2.

Special Consideration of Pulsatile Flow

Although the velocity of pulsatile flow changes throughout the cardiac cycle, nulling the gradient's first moment and using the shortest possible TE generally eliminate most gradient-induced artifacts. Most remaining artifacts are from view-to-view intensity changes. In other words, artifact from pulsatile flow on images with gradient moment nulling is due mostly to changing magnetization between systole and diastole.

During systole, high-velocity blood flow completely replaces blood between excitations, leading to high signal intensity. During diastole, however, slow or reversed flow leads to lower signal intensity. This changing signal intensity produces phase errors and, therefore, ghost artifacts. With this basic cause of artifacts from pulsatile flow in mind, we will now review several parameters and their effects on these artifacts:

Saturation Pulses. Ghost artifacts can be reduced, but not eliminated, by the use of saturation pulses. Saturation pulses are most effective for rapidly flowing blood. When there is no flow during diastole, for example, blood in an image section is not saturated by a saturation pulse. Thus, blood may exhibit more magnetization during diastole than during systole when saturation pulses are used. These view-to-view differences between systole and diastole cause artifacts.

TABLE 10–2. RELATIVE EFFECTIVENESS OF VARIOUS TECHNIQUES FOR MOTION ARTIFACT CORRECTION

Artifact-Correction Technique	Within-View	View-to-View	Blurring
Gradient moment nulling	+ + +	−	−
Minimal TE	+ + +	−	−
Minimal TR	−	+ + +	+
Increased sampling bandwidth	+	−	−
Averaging	+ + +	+ + +	−
Spatial saturation	+ + +	+ + +	−
Physiologic monitoring	−	+ + +	+ + +
Breath holding	+ + +	+ + +	+ + +
Reduced flip angle	−	+ + +	−

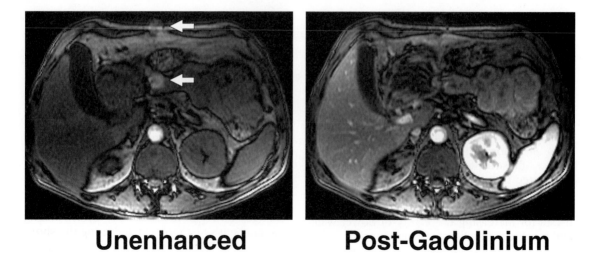

Unenhanced   Post-Gadolinium

FIGURE 10–22. Effect of gadolinium enhancement on pulsation artifacts in breath hold gradient echo T1-weighted images. Ghosts are prominent on the unenhanced image *(arrows)* but are less conspicuous "post-gadolinium," owing to decreased differences in systolic versus diastolic echo amplitudes.

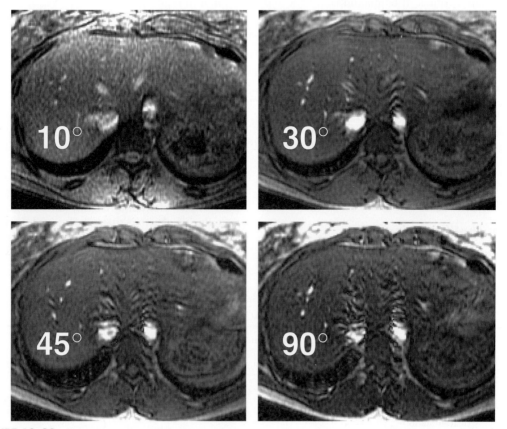

FIGURE 10–23. Effect of excitation flip angle on artifact from pulsatile flow, using single-section gradient echo images with TR–TE of 20/7. Artifact is increasingly severe as flip angle increases, owing to greater differences between systolic and diastolic echo amplitudes.

Contrast Enhancement. Gadolinium chelates and other T1-enhancing contrast agents reduce the T1 of blood, leading to faster recovery of magnetization after an excitation pulse. This increases the overall signal intensity of blood on T1-weighted images. In particular, the signal intensity of partially saturated blood during diastole is increased. The signal intensity of blood during systole does not change, however, since it is completely replaced between excitation pulses and thus is completely unsaturated. Therefore, T1 reduction decreases the difference between the signal intensity of blood during systole and during diastole. On images that have few within-view phase errors, such as rapid gradient echo images with TE less than 3 msec, gadolinium administration may therefore *decrease* the severity of ghost artifacts by decreasing view-to-view errors (Fig. 10–22).

Within-view artifacts are more severe after contrast enhancement, owing to the higher signal intensity of blood. Pulse sequences with longer TE or lower sampling bandwidth, especially those that do not include gradient moment nulling, generally have more vascular artifact after gadolinium administration.

Excitation Flip Angle. During systole, the use of a 90° flip angle produces maximal transverse magnetization and maximal signal intensity. At the time of the next excitation pulse, systolic blood in the image section is completely replaced, and thus unsaturated. During diastole, however, blood is partially saturated and thus has less longitudinal magnetization. The longitudinal magnetization of diastolic blood flow at the time of each excitation pulse can be increased by the use of a smaller flip angle, since this decreases the amount of saturation by each excitation pulse. A smaller flip angle reduces the amount of transverse magnetization formed from systolic blood flow. Thus, lower flip angle increases signal intensity of blood flowing during diastole and decreases signal intensity of blood flowing during systole, rendering them more similar to each other. This reduces the intensity of ghosts (Fig. 10–23).

Averaging. As described earlier, artifacts from pulsatile blood flow can actually increase in response to signal averaging, since the acquisition of data for the center of k-space is spread over a longer time. Artifact from pulsatile flow can be reduced by completing the acquisition of the center of k-space as rapidly as possible (fast imaging) by spatial presaturation or by cardiac gating, triggering, or reordering techniques.

ESSENTIAL POINTS TO REMEMBER

1. Simple bipolar gradients do not correct for motion that occurs between the dephasing and rephasing gradient lobes—within-view phase errors.
2. Variable phase changes within a voxel lead to intravoxel phase dispersion, which manifests as decreased signal intensity.
3. Motion can cause echo amplitude to vary from view to view. Phase-encoding errors from this mechanism are called view-to-view intensity errors.
4. Unanticipated phase changes from both within-view and view-to-view motion result in phase-encoding errors, which are manifested as artifacts along the phase-encoding axis.
5. Gradient moment nulling involves use of a more complicated gradient waveform that allows reduction of within-view phase errors. View-to-view errors are not affected.
6. View-to-view errors can be reduced by any measure that decreases view-to-view variation of signal amplitude from a given site within an image.
7. Methods for reducing view-to-view errors include arresting motion, applying spatial presaturation, gating or triggering data acquisition to the motion itself, or extremely rapid imaging.

11 Pulse Sequences: Gradient Echo and Spin Echo

Thus far, we have introduced most of the components that are combined to form the specific pulse sequences we use in daily MR practice. In this chapter, we describe the basic classifications of pulse sequences that are created from these building blocks.

A basic gradient echo pulse sequence consists of an excitation pulse followed by measurement of an echo. The echo is created by first dephasing the magnetization by applying the dephasing lobe of the frequency-encoding gradient (Gf) and then rephasing the magnetization by reapplying the gradient with reversed polarity. This results in a coherent echo.

UNSPOILED GRADIENT ECHO TECHNIQUES

Many gradient echo techniques achieve fast imaging times by using short repetition times (TRs). In fact, the TR is often comparable to or shorter than the T2 relaxation time of some of the tissues in the region of interest (Fig 11–1). The presence or absence of residual coherent transverse magnetization at the time of the next excitation pulse affects the signal-to-noise ratio (SNR) and tissue contrast of the resulting image.

First, let us consider a pulse sequence of short TR, where residual transverse magnetization is present at the time of each successive excitation pulse. With each pulse, the magnetization in rotated farther, until it has been rotated a full 360°. The residual transverse magnetization adds to the longitudinal magnetization that has recovered from previous excitations (Fig. 11–2).

With such a pulse sequence, once a steady state has been established after several excitation pulses, there are two basic sources of longitudinal magnetization. As with other pulse sequences, longitudinal magnetization recovers after an excitation pulse at a rate determined by the tissue's T1. If transverse magnetization is still present at the time of each excitation pulse, additional longitudinal magnetization is created by rotation back into the longitudinal plane of undecayed transverse magnetization. The amount of residual transverse magnetization present at the time of each excitation pulse is determined by the TR and by the T2 of the

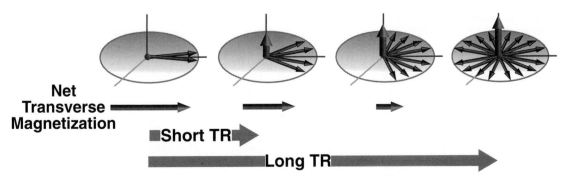

FIGURE 11–1. The relationship between persistent transverse magnetization and repetition time (TR). Transverse magnetization decays completely between excitations with long TR. With short TR, however, coherent magnetization may be persist at the time of the next excitation.

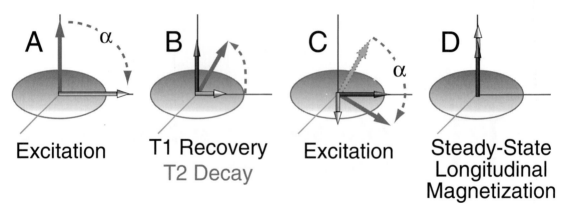

FIGURE 11-2. Rotation of persistent transverse magnetization into the longitudinal plane. *(A)* 90° excitation; *(B)* T1 (recovery) and T2 (decay) relaxation. With a sufficiently short TR, the next excitation *(C)* will rotate residual transverse magnetization *(light arrow)* into the longitudinal plane, as it rotates recovered longitudinal magnetization *(dark arrow)* into the transverse plane. Steady-state longitudinal magnetization *(D)* (and thus received MRI signal) therefore consists of contributions from both residual transverse *(light arrow)* and recovered longitudinal *(dark arrow)* magnetizations.

tissue. The shorter the time between excitations (short TR), the less time there is for the transverse magnetization to decay. The slower the decay of transverse magnetization (long T2), the more residual transverse magnetization will be present at the time of each excitation pulse.

Pulse sequences in which transverse magnetization is present at the time of excitation pulses are called *unspoiled gradient echo images.* Commercial implementations of unspoiled gradient echo techniques include fast imaging with steady-state precession (FISP) and gradient recalled acquisition in the steady state (GRASS). With these pulse sequences, the use of shorter TR both decreases the amount of recovered longitudinal magnetization and increases the amount of residual transverse magnetization. These effects tend to balance each other for tissues with long T2, so for such tissues signal intensity varies little with changes in TR (Fig. 11-3).

The echo time (TE) does not affect the amount of transverse magnetization present *at each excitation pulse.* The TE is the time between the creation of transverse magnetization and the measurement of its echo. TE determines the amount of transverse magnetization present *when the echo is measured;* however, after the echo is measured, transverse magnetization continues to decay, at a rate determined by the T2* (T2 plus the effects of magnetic field heterogeneity) of the tissue. The time available for decay is determined by the time between excitation pulses, the TR. The time during which transverse magnetization decays *between excitation pulses* is not affected by

whether the TE is immediately after the excitation pulse or immediately before the next excitation pulse. The amount of residual transverse magnetization present *at the time of an excitation pulse* is determined by the TR, not by the TE (Fig. 11-4).

In images where residual transverse magnetization is rotated back into the longitudinal plane, variable dephasing by the phase-encoding gradient (Gp) can cause artifacts. The strength of the phase-encoding gradient is changed after each excitation pulse, allowing determination of the position of spins along this axis. As the strength of the phase-encoding gradient increases, it causes more dephasing, which decreases the overall strength of the resulting echo. If it is not compensated for, this variable coherence of the transverse magnetization can produce artifacts.

The solution to this potential problem is similar to that for other imaging gradients. The phase-encoding gradient pulse can be considered a dephasing lobe. Just before each excitation pulse, a rephasing lobe is applied to undo the phase encoding. This rephasing lobe of the phase-encoding gradient is often referred to as a *rewinding gradient* (Fig. 11-5).

On unspoiled gradient echo images, signal intensity is a function of both the amount of longitudinal magnetization that has recovered between excitation pulses and the amount of transverse magnetization that persists between these pulses. The amount of recovered longitudinal magnetization is greater for tissues with short T1, and the amount of persistent magnetization is greater for tissues with long T2. Thus, short T1 and long T2 both contribute to in-

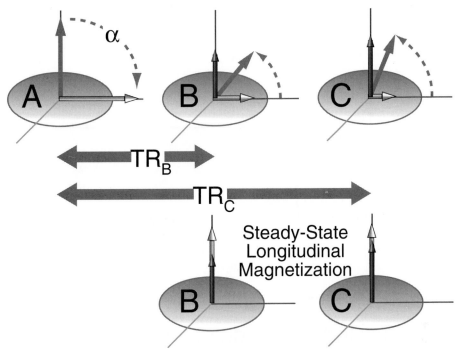

FIGURE 11–3. For unspoiled gradient echo techniques, the amount of equilibrium longitudinal may be similar at different TRs. *(A)* Transverse magnetization is created and longitudinal magnetization is saturated by a 90° pulse. With short TR *(B)*, there is abundant coherent transverse magnetization at the time of each excitation pulse, which is rotated back into the longitudinal plane. With longer TR *(C)* more longitudinal magnetization is recovered but less residual transverse magnetization persists.

creased signal intensity on unspoiled gradient echo images. These images can thus be considered to be *T2/T1 weighted* (Fig. 11–6).

For most tissues, T1 and T2 tend to parallel each other; that is, tissues with long T1 tend to have long T2. Therefore, T1 and T2 contrast tend to "compete" with each other, causing most tissues to have similar signal intensity on T2/T1-weighted unspoiled gradient echo images. For example, the liver has a short T1, which contributes to high signal intensity rela-

tive to most liver lesions; however, liver lesions and spleen usually have long T2, contributing to high signal intensity relative to the liver. The result of these two competing processes is relatively flat contrast and little differentiation between most tissues.

The tissues with the highest signal intensity on T2/T1-weighted gradient echo images are those in which T2 is as long, or almost as long, as T1. This is true of most fluids and lipids and causes fluid and adipose tissue to have

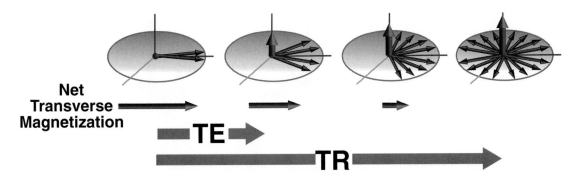

FIGURE 11–4. Decay of transverse magnetization after the echo time (TE). At the TE, coherent transverse magnetization is measured. During the remainder of the repetition time (TR), transverse magnetization continues to decay. The amount of transverse magnetization present during excitation is determined by the TR and by the T2 of the tissue.

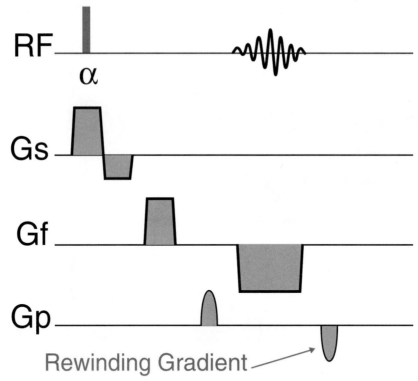

FIGURE 11-5. Rewinding gradient for reversing the effects of the phase-encoding gradient (Gp). Transverse magnetization is partially dephased by the phase-encoding gradient pulse. It is rephased by applying a rewinding gradient, which has identical magnitude but opposite polarity relative to the phase-encoding gradient.

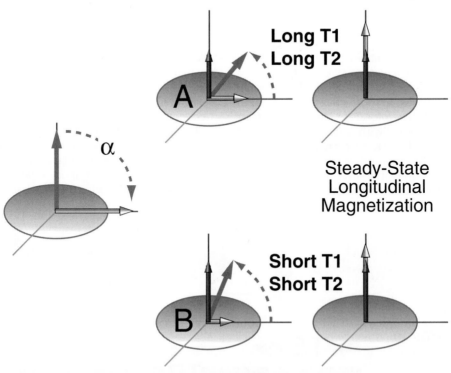

FIGURE 11-6. With unspoiled gradient echo techniques, tissues with long T1 and long T2 *(A)* may have signal intensity similar to that of tissues with short T1 and short T2 *(B)*, since they have similar T2/T1 ratios. Long T1 results in little recovery of longitudinal magnetization between excitations, but long T2 results in abundant persistent transverse magnetization, which gets rotated back into the longitudinal plane. In contrast, short T1 results in more recovery of longitudinal magnetization, while short T2 results in less persistent transverse magnetization.

Long T1
Long T2
(e.g., water)

Short T1
Short T2
(e.g., fat)

Long T1
Short T2
(e.g., muscle)

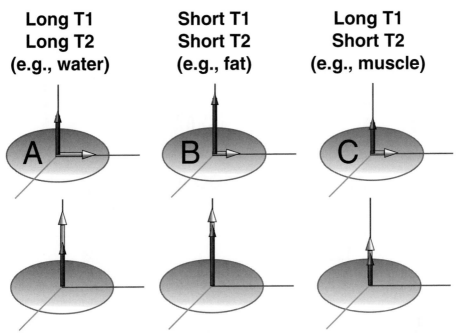

FIGURE 11-7. Effects of T2/T1 ratio on equilibrium longitudinal magnetization of unspoiled gradient echo images. Because both recovered longitudinal and persistent transverse magnetization contribute to equilibrium longitudinal magnetization, tissues with long T1 and long T2 (e.g., water) and short T1 and short T2 (e.g., fat) have similarly high T2/T1 ratios, and thus both have high signal intensity. Tissues with long T1 and short T2 (e.g., muscle and many other solid tissues) have lower T2/T1 ratios and, thus, lower signal intensity.

especially high signal intensity on T2/T1-weighted images. As discussed in Chapter 2, T1 is the upper limit for T2; a tissue's T2 cannot be longer than its T1. T1 and T2 are equal if T2 relaxation is simply a reconversion of transverse magnetization back into the longitudinal plane, as for pure water. Additional decay of transverse magnetization occurs in solid tissues because of exchange of energy between spins facilitated by association with nearby macromolecules. This causes T2 to be shorter than T1 for solid tissues, which in turn causes them to have low signal intensity on T2/T1-weighted gradient echo images (Fig. 11-7).

SPOILED GRADIENT ECHO TECHNIQUES

Effective T1 contrast can be achieved on images where signal intensity is principally a function of the amount of magnetization that has recovered between excitation pulses. Additional T2 weighting resulting from the rotation of persistent transverse magnetization into the longitudinal plane can obscure T1 contrast and is therefore undesirable if unambiguous T1

weighting is wanted. Thus, if T1 weighting is desired on simple gradient echo images, it is necessary to *spoil* the residual transverse magnetization before each excitation pulse. The residual transverse magnetization can be spoiled by applying a spoiling gradient that dephases the magnetization (Fig. 11-8). Spoiled gradient echo images generally have lower-equilibrium longitudinal magnetization, and thus lower SNR, than unspoiled gradient echo images (Fig. 11-9).

An alternative method for spoiling the transverse magnetization is *radiofrequency spoiling,* which involves the use of excitation pulses designed to render the magnetization incoherent at the time of the next excitation pulse. By either method, spoiled gradient echo images can be obtained in which residual transverse magnetization does not affect image contrast. When TR, TE, and flip angle are chosen appropriately, contrast can be heavily T1 weighted. Common examples of spoiled gradient echo techniques include fast low-angle shot (FLASH) and spoiled gradient recalled acquisition in the steady state (spoiled GRASS).

A comparison of spoiled and unspoiled gradient echo images with TRs of 10 and 120 msec is presented in Figure 11-10.

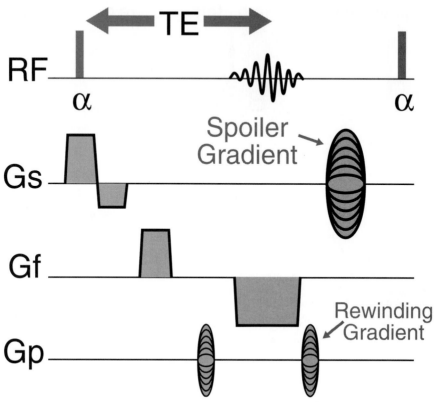

FIGURE 11-8. Spoiled gradient echo pulse sequence. Persistent transverse magnetization can be eliminated before each excitation by dephasing transverse magnetization via a spoiling gradient.

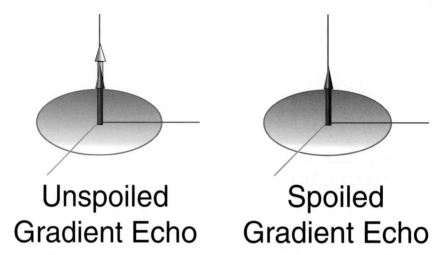

FIGURE 11-9. Equilibrium longitudinal magnetization on unspoiled and spoiled gradient echo images. Spoiled gradient echo images have lower signal intensity because there is no residual transverse magnetization to contribute to equilibrium longitudinal magnetization.

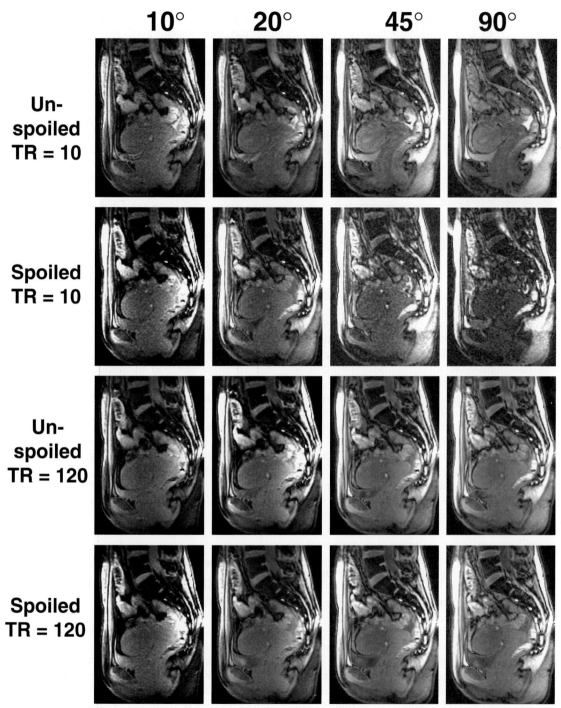

FIGURE 11-10. Sagittal gradient echo images of the pelvis with variable flip angle using unspoiled and spoiled technique, and repetition times (TRs) of 10 and 120 msec. With unspoiled technique and short TR, T2/T1 weighting increases with increasing flip angle, increasing the signal intensity of fluid. SNR does not change substantially with different flip angles. With spoiled technique, SNR decreases substantially with increased flip angles at TR of 10 msec. With the higher TR, the difference between unspoiled and spoiled images is less dramatic, because there is greater decay of transverse magnetization during the TR; however, T1 contrast is better with spoiled technique. (Note lower signal intensity of urine and CSF.)

Some tissues look similar on T1-weighted and T2/T1-weighted images. Adipose tissue, for example, has high signal intensity on both images, because 1/T1 (the relaxation rate) and T2/T1 are both high. Hemorrhagic and proteinaceous fluid may similarly have high signal intensity on both T1-weighted spoiled and T2/T1-weighted unspoiled gradient echo images. Simple fluid, however, has long T1 *and* T2 relaxation times, so 1/T1 is low whereas T2/T1 is high. Therefore, simple fluid has low signal intensity on T1-weighted spoiled gradient echo images and high signal intensity on T2/T1-weighted images.

REPETITION TIME AND FLIP ANGLE: EFFECTS ON TISSUE CONTRAST

TR is a major determinant of the acquisition time of unspoiled and spoiled gradient echo images, as for most other pulse sequences. As TR becomes shorter, acquisition time decreases. A shorter TR affords less time for recovery of longitudinal magnetization. To achieve adequate T1 weighting on a spoiled gradient echo image using a 90° excitation pulse, TR must be similar to or shorter than the tissue T1 relaxation times to be distinguished in the image.

If TR is *much* shorter than the T1 relaxation times, SNR may be reduced substantially unless the excitation flip angle is reduced along with TR. For a given TR and T1 relaxation time, there is an excitation flip angle for maximal SNR (Ernst angle). As TR is decreased, flip angle should generally be reduced if a comparable appearance is desired. Similarly, as flip angle is decreased, TR should generally be decreased as well.

TRs are short (less than 500 msec) for most currently used gradient echo techniques. Even a TR of 500 msec, however, is short enough to achieve heavy T1 weighting. Thus, the TR is generally not the principal determinant of tissue contrast on gradient echo sequences, although the choice of TR can affect image efficiency, SNR, or vulnerability to artifacts. For most gradient echo techniques, the excitation flip angle is a far more important determinant of image contrast than is TR.

To optimize contrast between tissues with different T1s, the excitation flip angle should be equal to or larger than the Ernst angle for the tissue with the shorter T1. In clinical practice, for a TR of 100 msec or more, an excitation flip angle of 60° to 90° produces useful T1 weighting. As TR is reduced below 100 msec, the flip angle should generally be less than 90°. As TR is reduced to 50 msec or less, for adequate T1-contrast and SNR the excitation flip angle should generally be held between 45° and 60°.

For spoiled gradient echo images, reducing the excitation flip angle below the Ernst angle for all tissue T1s of interest decreases the T1 weighting. For some applications this may be tolerable, or even desirable, if other contrast parameters (e.g., T2* or flow) are to be emphasized.

For unspoiled gradient echo images, changes in TR and flip angle have different effects on image contrast and SNR. As TR increases, less residual transverse magnetization remains at the time of each excitation pulse. In fact, with TRs longer than 200 msec, tissue contrast is similar on spoiled and unspoiled gradient echo images, except that on unspoiled images fluid has higher signal intensity. As TR is decreased and more transverse magnetization persists at the time of each excitation pulse, the difference between spoiled and unspoiled gradient echo images increases.

For spoiled gradient echo images, SNR decreases as TR does. The loss of signal intensity follows directly from the logarithmic T1 relaxation curve; a shorter TR can be thought of as moving earlier and earlier along this curve toward the origin. For unspoiled gradient echo techniques, however, the effect on SNR of reducing TR is less profound because residual transverse magnetization increases with shorter TR.

ECHO TIME: EFFECTS ON TISSUE CONTRAST

As TE increases, signal intensity on the resulting image decreases because of decay of transverse magnetization. Transverse magnetization decays fastest for tissues with short T2* relaxation time. Image contrast based on differences between tissues' rates of T2* decay is called *T2* contrast*. TE is the parameter of a gradient echo image that directly affects its T2* weighting.

If the purpose of a pulse sequence is to accentuate the T1 differences between tissues, the TE should be kept as short as possible, to minimize T2* contrast and artifacts from heterogeneous magnetic susceptibility. Another benefit of short TE is to minimize signal loss from flowing blood on "bright blood" flow pulse sequences; however, TE may be increased deliberately if T2* contrast is desired. T2*-weighted images may be useful to depict calcifications, iron, blood products, and tissues with especially short T2 (e.g., fibrous tissue).

STEADY-STATE FREE PRECESSION

Each radio pulse in a gradient echo pulse sequence is usually intended to be an excitation pulse. Thus, we are usually concerned principally with the effects of this pulse on longitudinal magnetization; however, each radio pulse also affects the transverse magnetization that has not decayed during the TR.

Earlier in this chapter we discussed unspoiled gradient echo techniques, in which residual transverse magnetization is rotated back into the longitudinal plane, augmenting the signal intensity of tissues with sufficiently long T2 relaxation time. Steady-state free precession techniques are also based on the effects of each radio pulse on transverse magnetization.

Each radio pulse, regardless of its flip angle, excites longitudinal magnetization and to some extent changes the rotational phase of transverse magnetization. This causes some refocusing of the transverse magnetization, although the extent of refocusing is less complete than with a 180° refocusing pulse in a typical spin echo pulse sequence. In other words, each of a series of radio pulses in a gradient echo pulse sequence creates transverse magnetization and refocuses transverse magnetization created by the preceding radio pulse. This echo, formed by the refocusing of transverse magnetization by a radio pulse, is a spin echo, similar to the spin echoes formed in typical spin echo pulse sequences.

Therefore, following a given radio pulse, a gradient echo is first formed by reapplying the frequency-encoding gradient with reversed polarity. Next, a spin echo is formed from the transverse magnetization created by the preceding radio pulse. The spin echo occurs at the time of the next radio pulse. The timing of the readout determines which of these two echoes contributes signal intensity to the resulting image.

A steady-state free precession image is created from the spin echoes produced by a series of successive radio pulses. As with conventional spin echo pulse sequences, the refocusing pulse occurs at the center of the TE, so the TE is double the time between the excitation and refocusing radio pulses. Thus, for steady-state free precession pulse sequences, the TE is actually twice as long as TR. For example, a typical steady-state free precession pulse sequence might have a TR of 30 msec and a TE of approximately 60 msec. These pulse sequences are thus T2-weighted.

One problem in designing a steady-state free precession pulse sequence is that at the time of the spin echo the section-select gradient and a radio pulse are both being applied. It is thus not possible to listen for an echo at the expected TE. One solution is periodically to miss an excitation pulse so that an echo can be sampled at the TE. More commonly, the echo is sampled before refocusing is complete (Fig. 11–11). The incomplete refocusing causes the image to be sensitive to T2* (susceptibility) contrast as well as to true T2 contrast. The sensitivity to susceptibility is based on the offset between the time of echo sampling and the time of complete refocusing of the spin echo, whereas the sensitivity to true T2 is based on the TE.

SPIN ECHO TECHNIQUES

The establishment during its first decade of MRI as an effective modality for clinical imaging was based principally on the success of spin echo pulse sequences for generating T1-weighted, T2-weighted, and intermediate pulse sequences. The spin echo pulse sequence is robust and very tolerant of imperfections in the main magnetic field, imaging gradients, and radio pulses.

A spin echo pulse sequence is virtually identical to a simple spoiled gradient echo pulse sequence, as described above, with the addition of a refocusing pulse at the center of the TE. Optimal refocusing is achieved with the use of a 180° pulse, but smaller pulses are occasionally used to reduce demands on the pulse amplifier or to reduce the radiofrequency exposure to the patient. Because the refocusing pulse reverses the phase differences between spins at either end of the frequency-encoding axis, the rephasing lobe of the frequency-encoding gradient is applied with the same polarity as that of the dephasing gradient rather than with reversed polarity, as with gradient echo techniques.

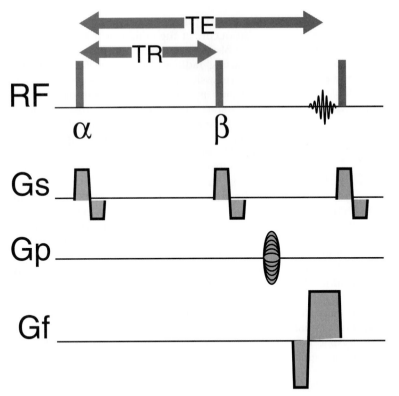

FIGURE 11-11. Steady-state free precession pulse sequence. Each radio pulse acts as an excitation pulse and as a refocusing pulse for transverse magnetization created by the preceding pulse. An echo is created by the readout gradient timed to occur in advance of the next radio pulse.

Spin echo techniques are generally more tolerant of system imperfections than are corresponding gradient echo pulse sequence. Refocusing radio pulses not only eliminate phase differences caused by the frequency-encoding gradient itself but also correct for imperfections in the main magnetic field and for microscopic magnetic field gradients caused by heterogeneous magnetic susceptibility in the patient. The principal disadvantage of spin echo pulse sequences is the time required for application of the refocusing radio pulse and its accompanying section-select gradient (Fig. 11-12). The suitability of the pulse sequences discussed in this chapter for providing T1, T2, T2*, and T2/T1 contrast is summarized in Table 11-1.

ESSENTIAL POINTS TO REMEMBER

1. Gradient echo images involve applying an excitation radio pulse and then forming an echo by reapplying the frequency-encoding gradient with direction reversed.
2. With some gradient echo techniques, tissues with T2 similar to or longer than the TR may have persistent transverse magnetization at the end of the TR. This unspoiled transverse magnetization is rotated back to the longitudinal plane by subsequent excitation pulses, and it thus contributes to image signal intensity. These pulse sequences are referred to as unspoiled gradient echo techniques.
3. For unspoiled gradient echo images, short T1 and long T2 relaxation times both contribute to increased signal intensity. These images are therefore T2/T1 weighted.

TABLE 11-1. POTENTIAL OF VARIOUS PULSE SEQUENCES FOR ACHIEVING T1, T2, T2*, OR T2/T1 CONTRAST*

Pulse Sequence	Contrast Mechanisms		
	T1	T2 or T2*	T2/T1
Unspoiled GRE–90°	−	T2*	+ + +
Unspoiled GRE–10°	−	T2*	−
Spoiled GRE–90°	+ + +	T2*	−
Spoiled GRE–10°	−	T2*	−
Steady-state free precession	−	T2 and T2*	−
Spin echo	+ + +	T2	−

Examples of 90° and 10° flip angles are used to illustrate high and low angles for the gradient echo pulse sequences. The amount of T2 or T2 contrast with any of these pulse sequences is generally determined by the TE. Adequate T1 contrast with spoiled GRE or SE techniques depends on the use of a TR that is similar to or less than the T1 relaxation times of the tissues of interest.

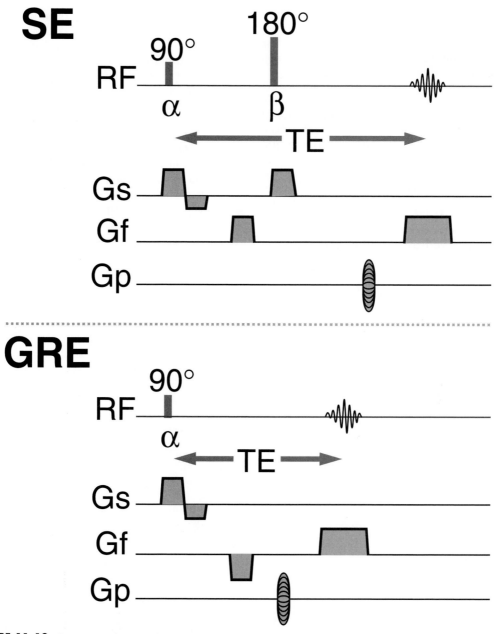

FIGURE 11–12. Comparison between spin echo (SE) *(above)* and gradient echo (GRE) *(below)* pulse sequences. The GRE pulse sequence does not include a 180° refocusing pulse or its accompanying section-select gradient, so TE can be shorter than for SE sequences.

4. In unspoiled gradient echo images, fluid and fat tend to have high signal intensity and most other tissues have intermediate signal intensity.

5. Spoiled gradient echo images are T1 weighted, because residual transverse magnetization is dephased at the end of each TR, before the next excitation pulse.

6. With longer TR or shorter tissue T2, residual transverse magnetization becomes less important, as does the difference between spoiled and unspoiled techniques.

7. Artifacts from residual transverse magnetization due to the varying strengths of the phase-encoding gradient can be reduced by applying a rewinding gradient, which is a repetition of the phase-encoding gradient with reversed polarity.

8. For short-TR techniques, SNR can be low if a 90° excitation pulse is used, since there is little time for T1 recovery. SNR can be improved if the flip angle is smaller. As TR is increased, comparable contrast can be achieved by increasing the excitation flip angle.

9. On gradient echo images, decay of transverse magnetization is due to both T2 relaxation and local magnetic field heterogeneity. The combined contrast mechanism is T2* contrast. As TE increases in gradient echo images, contrast due to T2* differences increases.

10. In steady-state free precession techniques, each radio pulse serves both as an excitation pulse and as a refocusing pulse for the previous excitation. The resulting images are T2-weighted. TE is longer than TR.

11. Spin echo techniques are similar to gradient echo techniques, except that a 180° refocusing pulse is applied at the midpoint of the TE (to correct for heterogeneous magnetic field and chemical shift effects), and the rephasing lobe of the frequency-encoding gradient has the same polarity as the dephasing lobe, rather than the opposite.

12 Preparatory Pulses

Repetition time (TR), echo time (TE), and excitation flip angle can be manipulated to alter T1, T2, or T2* contrast on gradient echo and spin echo images, as described earlier. Additional radio pulses applied before a gradient echo or spin echo pulse sequence affect contrast in a variety of ways. These additional pulses are called *preparatory pulses* (Fig. 12-1).

INVERSION RECOVERY

A 180° inversion pulse before one or more excitation pulses imparts strong T1 contrast. This T1 contrast is in addition to the tissue contrast that results from the remainder of the

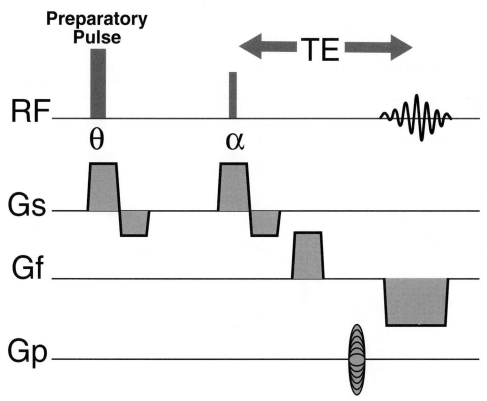

FIGURE 12–1. A preparatory pulse (θ) precedes the excitation pulse (α). A section-select gradient (Gs) is applied, so the effects of the preparatory pulse are restricted to the desired image section.

143

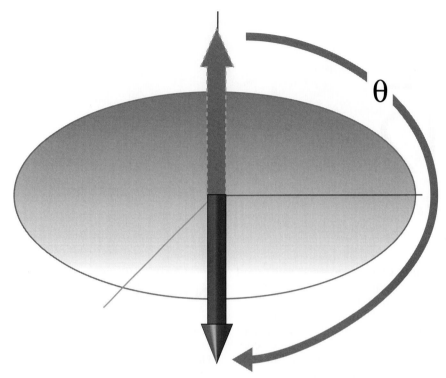

FIGURE 12-2. A 180° inversion pulse rotating equilibrium longitudinal magnetization from the positive to the negative longitudinal plane.

pulse sequence itself. Ideally, no transverse magnetization results from the inversion pulse. Rather, the 180° pulse only *inverts* the longitudinal magnetization, converting it from positive to negative (Fig. 12-2).

Once inverted, the negative magnetization begins to recover, initially toward zero and then toward its equilibrium positive value. The rate at which the longitudinal magnetization recovers is determined by its T1; that is, the rate of

recovery following a 180° inversion pulse is 1/T1 (Fig. 12-3).

During the course of this recovery, an excitation radio pulse is transmitted, creating transverse magnetization. The amount of transverse magnetization depends on the amount of longitudinal magnetization that had recovered after the inversion pulse. The time between the inversion and excitation pulses is defined as the *inversion time* (TI). Figure 12-4 is a diagram of

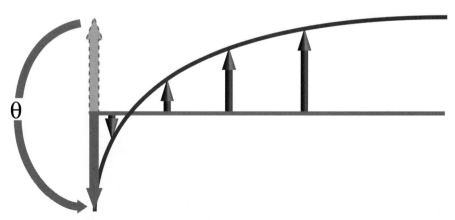

FIGURE 12-3. Following inversion by a 180° inversion pulse, longitudinal magnetization recovers logarithmically toward zero, then toward its original positive equilibrium level.

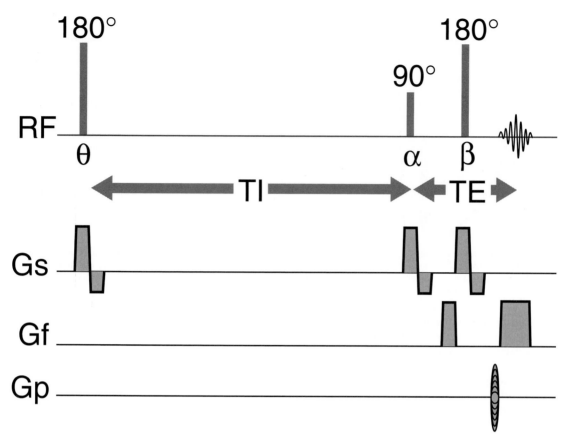

FIGURE 12–4. Spin echo inversion recovery pulse sequence. Each excitation pulse (α) is preceded by an inversion pulse (θ). The time between the inversion and excitation pulses is the inversion time (TI).

the components of a basic spin echo inversion recovery pulse sequence.

The amplitude of the MR signal is determined by the magnitude of the transverse magnetization created by the excitation radio pulse, which in turn is determined by the absolute value of the longitudinal magnetization immediately before the excitation pulse. That is, negative and positive longitudinal magnetization both give rise to transverse magnetization with positive polarity (Fig. 12-5).

The amplitude of the positive longitudinal magnetization at the time of each inversion pulse is determined by the amount of T1 recovery since the previous excitation pulse. This is maximal when the TR is long, so inversion recovery pulse sequences usually utilize a long TR. The principal determinant of tissue contrast on most inversion recovery pulse sequences is the TI. Figure 12–6 shows the contrast behavior for two representative tissues.

When the TI is long enough (i.e., at least 1 second or longer), the longitudinal magnetization of nearly all protons has time to recover

beyond zero. Contrast on inversion recovery images with sufficiently long TI resembles that of T1-weighted spin echo or spoiled gradient echo images, in that tissues with short T1 relaxation times have higher signal intensity than tissues with long T1 relaxation times.

Contrast between any two tissues with different T1 relaxation times can be optimized on inversion recovery images by choosing a TI such that the longitudinal magnetization of one of the tissues will have recovered to zero, but not beyond. On such an image, this target tissue has no signal intensity. The signal intensity of this tissue is said to have been *nulled,* and the TI needed to null the signal intensity from a given tissue is called the *null point* for that tissue. For example, an inversion recovery pulse sequence with a TI of approximately 600 msec allows time for signal intensity from spleen and many tumors to recover toward zero at 1.5 T, nulling their signal intensity on these images and producing effective contrast for detecting focal liver lesions. Similar contrast can be obtained at 0.5 T using an inversion recovery

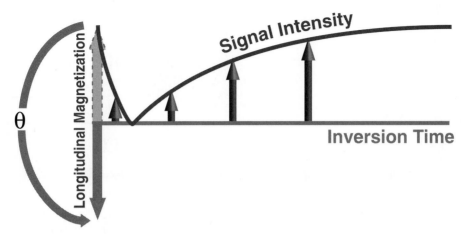

FIGURE 12–5. Transverse magnetization is created by excitation of either negative or positive longitudinal magnetization. Similar signal intensity can therefore result from excitation of either negative or positive longitudinal magnetization. The signal intensity on an image reflects the *absolute value* of longitudinal magnetization at the time of the excitation pulse.

pulse sequence with a 400-msec TI. Figure 12–7 illustrates tissue contrast at various TIs.

On many inversion recovery pulse sequences, signal intensity can be ambiguous. That is, longitudinal magnetization of tissues with short T1 may have recovered beyond zero to achieve positive longitudinal magnetization, whereas tissues with longer T1 may have merely recovered to lower magnitudes of negative longitudinal magnetization. The amount of transverse magnetization created by the excitation pulse is determined by the *magnitude* of the longitudinal magnetization, without regard to its *polarity;* that is, without regard to

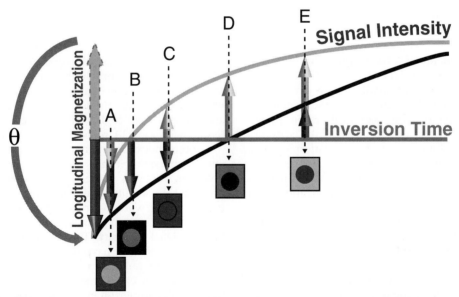

FIGURE 12–6. Inversion recovery tissue contrast at different TIs. The light gray line and arrows indicate short T1 (e.g., solid tissue) while the dark line and arrows indicate a tissue with long T1 (e.g., simple fluid). At the bottom, solid tissue is represented by the boxes and fluid by the circles within them. With short TI (A), solid tissue *(dark box)* has recovered farther toward zero and, therefore, has lower signal intensity than does fluid *(light circle)*. With slightly longer TI (B), solid tissue *(black box)* has relaxed to zero, and, therefore, is a signal void. With further prolongation of TI (C), the magnitude of the negative longitudinal magnetization of fluid is equal to that of the positive magnetization of solid tissue, so they will be isointense except for a cancellation void at their interfaces. With longer TI (D), fluid *(black circle)* will have relaxed to zero, depicted in the image as a signal void. With longer TI, both tissues will have positive longitudinal magnetization, which will be greater for solid tissue.

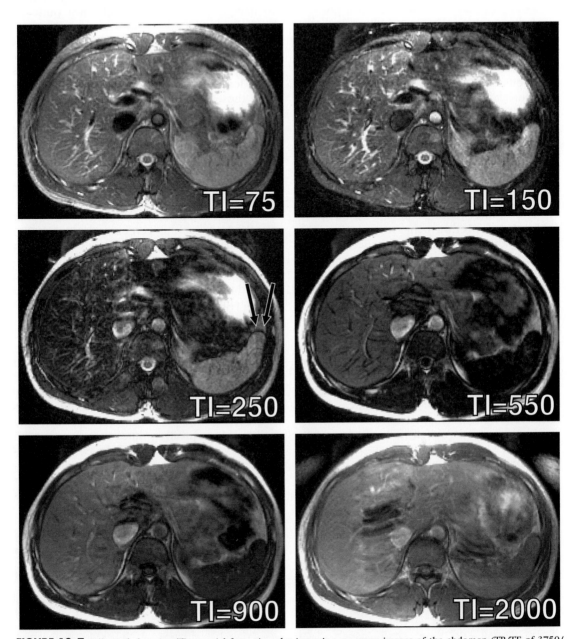

FIGURE 12–7. Effect of changing TI on axial fast spin echo inversion recovery images of the abdomen (TR/TE of 3750/30 msec). With TI of 75 msec, longitudinal magnetization of all tissues is negative; tissues such as the spleen, gastric fluid, and CSF have long T1 and therefore higher negative longitudinal magnetization than tissues with shorter T1, which have relaxed closer to zero. With TI of 150 msec, adipose tissue has relaxed to zero, while tissues with longer T1 still have negative longitudinal magnetization. With TI of 250 msec, adipose tissue has positive longitudinal magnetization, having relaxed past the null point, while spleen and fluid have negative longitudinal magnetization. Note the bounce-point artifact at the interface between the positive and negative longitudinal magnetization of, respectively, adipose tissue and the spleen *(arrows)*. At this TI (250 msec), liver longitudinal magnetization is nulled. With TI of 550 msec, splenic magnetization is nulled. With TI of 900 msec, most magnetization is positive, and contrast resembles that of a spin echo T1-weighted image. With TI of 2000 msec, longitudinal magnetization of CSF is near zero, while all other magnetization is positive.

whether the longitudinal magnetization is positive or negative. Thus, at a given TI, a tissue with short T1 may have an amount of positive longitudinal magnetization equal to the amount of negative magnetization of a tissue with longer T1. These two tissues have identical signal intensity, although their T1s may be considerably different.

Fortunately, two tissues with different T1s but identical signal intensities on an inversion recovery image may be distinguished from each other if they share a border, because this border is depicted as a signal void. This signal void between two tissues on opposite sides of the null point on an inversion recovery image is referred to as a *bounce-point artifact* (Fig. 12–8). The bounce-point artifact may be quite useful for depicting otherwise isointense lesions within a tissue, as in liver lesions with a long T1.

Inversion recovery images with short TI have become popular for many applications. This particular form of inversion recovery pulse sequence has even received its own acronym, STIR (short tau [TI] inversion recovery). The TI in STIR pulse sequences is usually chosen so that the longitudinal magnetization of adipose tissue is nulled. Adipose tissue therefore has little if any signal intensity on these images, even in the absence of any chemical shift–selective technique (e.g., fat saturation). At 1.5 T, adipose tissue is nulled if TI approximates 150 msec, whereas at 0.5 T the appropriate TI is approximately 100 msec.

STIR images are also particularly attractive because T1 contrast and T2 contrast tend to be additive, rather than destructive, for most tissues; that is, most tissues with long T1 tend to have long T2 as well. With most pulse sequences, long T1 leads to low signal intensity and long T2 to high signal intensity. On STIR images, however, long T1 causes less recovery toward zero than does short T1, causing tissues with long T1 to have higher signal intensity than those with short T1. As in other images, long T2 contributes to high signal intensity. Thus, long T1 and long T2, which tend to occur together in tissues, both contribute to high signal intensity on STIR images.

On the opposite end of the spectrum of specialized inversion recovery pulse sequences are those in which TI is quite long (approximately 2 seconds). A TI such as this is chosen so that simple fluid, such as cerebrospinal fluid (CSF) is nulled. These pulse sequences have been referred to as fluid-attenuated inversion recovery (FLAIR). Typically, FLAIR images have a long TE and are thus T2-weighted, although CSF and other simple fluids have no signal intensity (Fig. 12–9).

Inversion recovery techniques are among the most powerful and flexible available for generating T1 contrast, with or without additive T2 contrast; however, except for STIR and FLAIR, inversion recovery images are not commonly used in clinical practice. This is because inversion recovery images have lower signal intensity and longer acquisition times than do comparable images without inversion pulses. Signal intensity is lower because the additional T1 contrast on inversion recovery images is based on variable rates of decay during the TI; all tissues

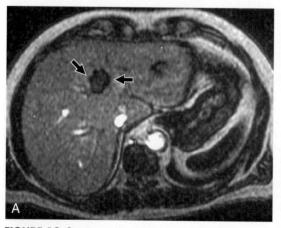
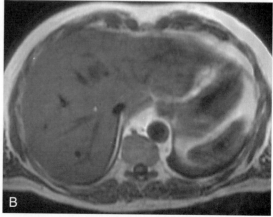

FIGURE 12–8. Bounce-point artifact on inversion recovery images. *(A)* Magnetization prepared gradient echo image with TI of 550 msec. Spleen signal has been nulled. Liver magnetization has recovered past zero, while the magnetization of a cavernous hemangioma *(arrows)* is negative. The liver and hemangioma are nearly isointense although their magnetizations are opposite, causing a signal cancellation artifact at their interface. *(B)* T1-weighted spin echo image, showing absence of a signal void surrounding the hemangioma.

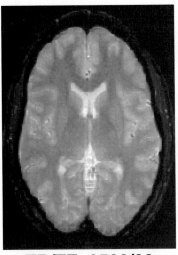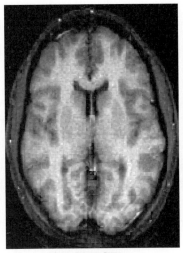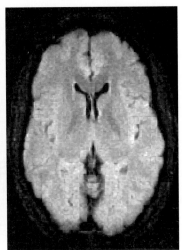

TR/TE=2500/80   TR/TE/TI =   TR/TE/TI =
                       2000/20/800   10,000/100/2200

FIGURE 12–9. Multishot echo planar imaging comparing T2-weighting *(left)* with two different echo planar methods for producing low–signal intensity cerebrospinal fluid CSF. With a short TE and an 800-msec TI, there is substantial T1 contrast between gray and white matter and the positive longitudinal magnetization of these tissues is greater than the value of the negative longitudinal magnetization of CSF. With longer TR, TE, and TI *(right)*, contrast between gray and white matter is T2-weighted, while signal intensity of CSF has been nulled. This image is an example of FLAIR.

lose signal intensity during this time, but at different rates. Acquisition time is often longer for a given number of sections because during the TI additional image sections could have been acquired. Inversion recovery thus involves spending more time to achieve lower SNR.

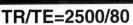

SPATIALLY SELECTIVE SATURATION

One popular form of preparatory pulse is a *spatially selective saturation pulse,* which saturates the magnetization from a certain region of tissue from which signal intensity is not desired. This is done by selectively exciting this region and then applying a dephasing gradient to spoil the transverse magnetization (Fig. 12–10). The magnetization in the unwanted region is now saturated. A subsequent excitation pulse, targeted to the section of interest, produces signal intensity only from the desired tissue. Commonly, there is one saturation pulse before each excitation pulse (Fig. 12–11), although some fast imaging techniques include several excitation pulses per saturation pulse.

The most common application of spatially selective saturation pulses is to saturate magnetization from flowing blood or moving tissue

(see Chapter 10, Reduced Signal Intensity of Artifact-Producing Tissue). These saturation pulses are usually targeted outside the volume of interest. The magnetization of blood is thus reduced substantially before it enters the image section, so that it has less signal intensity than it would otherwise. The excitation radio pulses delivered to tissue within the image section thus generate more signal intensity from the stationary tissue than from the saturated blood that flows into the image section. The blood vessels in the section of interest thus have lower signal intensity and produce less artifact than on comparable images without spatial saturation pulses. Saturation pulses may also be targeted in an image section, to reduce unwanted signal intensity arising from blood vessels in the image section itself or from moving adipose tissue.

CHEMICALLY SELECTIVE SATURATION

Saturation pulses may be targeted to certain chemical shifts rather than to spatial regions. Currently, most chemical shift saturation pulses are nonselective; that is, they are applied in the absence of imaging gradients. For example, a

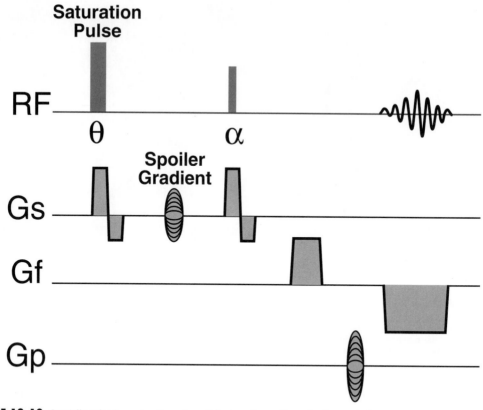

FIGURE 12–10. Spatially selective saturation. A spatial saturation radio pulse is targeted to a particular volume of tissue by simultaneously applying a section-select gradient. The transverse magnetization created by this radio pulse is then dephased by a spoiler gradient.

radio pulse with a narrow range of frequencies corresponding to the resonant frequency of methylene (CH_2) protons within adipose tissue excites these protons but has little effect on water protons (Fig. 12-12). Next, a spoiler gradient dephases the transverse magnetization created by the CH_2-selective excitation pulse (Fig. 12-13). After such a *fat saturation pulse* and the subsequent spoiler gradient, an excitation pulse creates transverse magnetization principally from water, so that signal intensity in the resulting image is mostly from water.

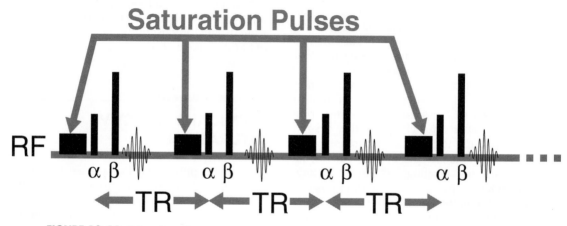

FIGURE 12–11. Spin echo pulse sequence with one saturation pulse prior to each excitation (α) pulse.

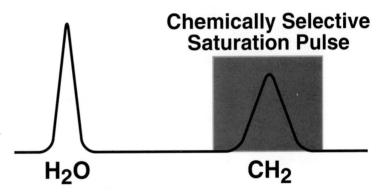

Chemically Selective Saturation Pulse

H₂O

CH₂

FIGURE 12-12. Chemically selective saturation. A chemically selective radio pulse with a frequency that matches that of the undesired protons is applied to the entire volume of tissue, without a section-select gradient. In this example, CH_2 protons are saturated (fat suppression).

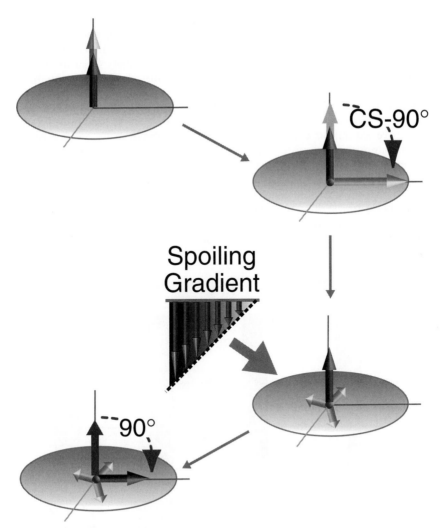

FIGURE 12-13. Fat saturation. A chemically selective pulse excites CH_2 magnetization *(light arrows)*. The resulting transverse magnetization is then dephased by a spoiler gradient. Next, an excitation pulse excites the remaining water longitudinal magnetization *(dark arrows)*, generating signal primarily from water protons.

With most current techniques, imaging gradients are turned off during application of chemically selective pulses. Therefore, chemical saturation is reapplied each time a section is excited, affecting all sections each time (Fig. 12-14).

The excitation flip angle of a fat saturation pulse should optimally be larger than 90° because of the short T1 of CH_2 protons in adipose tissue. Following a fat saturation pulse, longitudinal magnetization recovers so rapidly that, by the time the excitation pulse occurs, there is substantial recovery of lipid longitudinal magnetization. The lipid longitudinal magnetization that recovers during the time between the saturation and excitation pulses can produce substantial lipid signal intensity on the resulting image. A saturation pulse greater than 90°, however, rotates longitudinal magnetization more than 90°, so that recovery to zero may occur by the time the excitation pulse is applied. In this way, lipid magnetization can be minimized. The exact optimal fat saturation flip angle varies, depending on the interval between the saturation and excitation pulses, but typically it is between 100° and 130° (Fig. 12-15).

Chemically selective saturation can be combined with other magnetization preparation techniques. For example, inversion recovery and chemically selective preparatory pulses can be combined to produce silicone-only images in patients with prosthetic breast implants. STIR technique can be used to null signal from adipose tissue, and chemically selective saturation

can be used to suppress signal from water. The only remaining signal is from silicone, which has a chemical shift different from that of CH_2 or water (Fig. 12-16).

MAGNETIZATION TRANSFER

In Chapter 7 we discussed how magnetization from macromolecular protons is saturated by radio pulses that do not correspond to the resonant frequency of water and lipid protons in an image section. The saturated magnetization is then transferred to water protons near these macromolecules, producing decreased signal intensity from tissues that contain bound water. This process, referred to as *magnetization transfer* (MT), does not affect protons in free water or lipid molecules.

If signal intensity from tissues rich in bound water is not desired, it can be reduced by applying saturation pulses targeted to macromolecular protons. These MT saturation pulses may consist of strong pulses targeted to frequencies above or below that of the water and lipid protons in the desired image section (Fig. 12-17).

Alternatively, a series of pulses may be targeted to the section of interest that imparts a total of 0° or 360° of rotation to free water and lipid but dephases magnetization from macromolecular protons (Fig. 12-18).

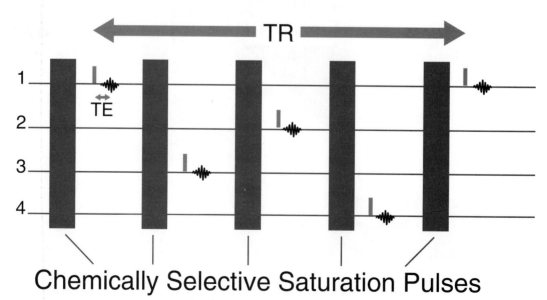

FIGURE 12-14. Multisection fat saturation. There is no section-select gradient during application of the fat saturation pulses. CH_2 magnetization throughout all image sections is therefore saturated before each excitation for each image section.

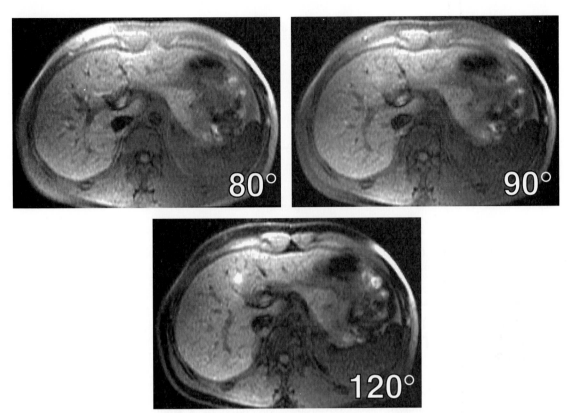

FIGURE 12-15. T1-weighted spin echo images showing improved fat suppression as the flip angle of the fat saturation pulse increases to 120°. Nonuniform magnetic field has caused suboptimal fat suppression, especially at the left anterior superficial region.

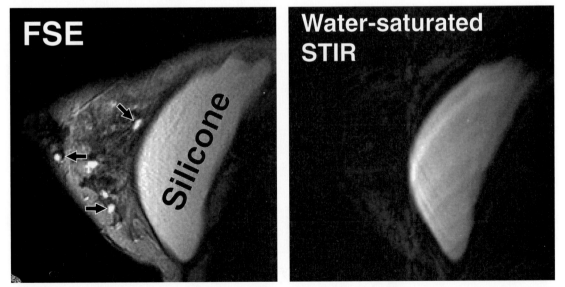

FIGURE 12-16. Silicone-only image obtained by combination of short T1 inversion recovery (STIR) and chemically selective water saturation. T2-weighted fast spin echo (FSE) image *(left)* depicts adipose tissue, cysts *(arrows)*, and silicone in a breast prosthesis as having high signal intensity. With a combination of water saturation and STIR techniques, signal intensity from water and fat are both suppressed, leaving only silicone signal in the image.

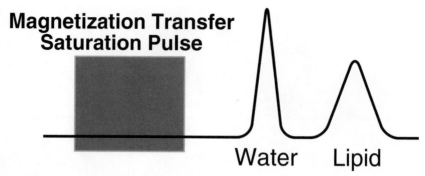

FIGURE 12-17. Magnetization transfer saturation pulse is applied at a frequency different from that of water or lipid, exciting the short T2 protons of macromolecules such as proteins.

MT pulses decrease the signal intensity of tissues that contain bound water (Fig. 12-19).

MAGNETIZATION-PREPARED RAPID GRADIENT ECHO TECHNIQUES

The preparatory pulses described thus far have been applied once before each excitation pulse. Applying these preparatory pulses and associated gradients takes time. If each excitation pulse is preceded by a preparatory pulse, the number of image sections that can be acquired during a given TR decreases. The decrease in number of sections per TR or increase in acquisition time may be particularly severe for inversion recovery techniques, since data often are not acquired during the TI.

The efficiency of magnetization-prepared pulse sequences can be improved greatly if each preparatory pulse can prepare the magnetization for more than one excitation pulse.

This is generally feasible only if the TR is short, as for gradient echo techniques with TR no longer than 10 msec.

Because of the very short TR, small flip angles (usually 30° or less) are necessary. Without preparatory pulses, these images have very little tissue contrast. In fact, tissue contrast on these images is determined principally by the preparation pulse. As an extreme case, a rapid gradient echo image with TR less than 10 msec can be acquired in approximately 1 second, preceded by a single preparatory pulse (Fig. 12-20). This is currently most common with inversion recovery preparatory pulses, allowing acquisition of heavily T1-weighted images in less than 2 seconds. Examples of rapid inversion recovery–prepared gradient echo images are shown in Figure 12-21. The appearance of rapid gradient echo images can also be changed by preceding them with spatial, chemical shift, or MT presaturation pulses.

T2-weighted gradient echo images can be acquired by applying a preparatory *series* of pulses. This series typically begins with a 90° excitation pulse, which creates transverse mag-

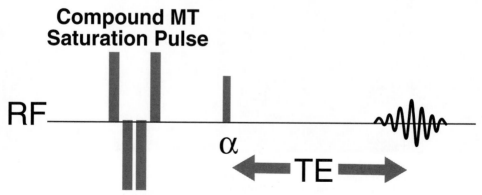

FIGURE 12-18. A series of pulses imparts a total of 0° rotation to water and lipid protons. The rotation of macromolecular protons is less precise, so their magnetization is partially saturated.

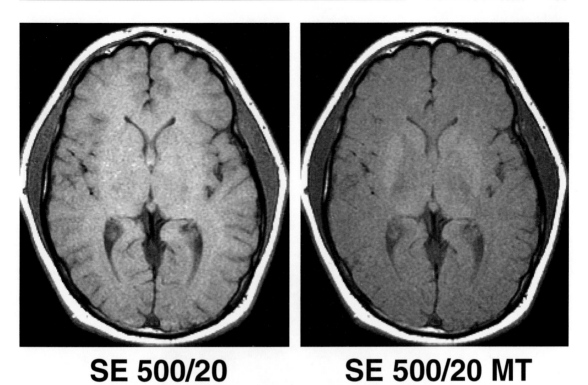

SE 500/20   SE 500/20 MT

FIGURE 12–19. Effect of magnetization transfer (MT) preparatory pulse on SE 500/20 image of the brain. With the MT saturation pulse, brain parenchymal signal intensity is reduced, especially from white matter.

netization. This is followed by a 180° refocusing pulse, which refocuses the transverse magnetization. Finally, a second 90° pulse returns the residual transverse magnetization to the longitudinal plane. The amount of transverse magnetization that is returned to the longitudinal plane depends on the T2 of the tissue. The time between the two 90° pulses is equivalent to the TE of a standard spin echo pulse sequence (Fig. 12–22).

Because contrast on the ensuing rapid gradient echo pulse sequence is affected by T2 differences among the tissues, these images are T2-weighted. T2-weighted magnetization-prepared gradient echo images have not become popular, because rapid T2-weighted images obtained by other techniques (see Chapter 13) generally have better image quality.

The increased efficiency afforded by using only a single preparatory pulse for magnetiza-

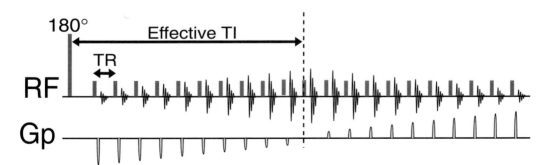

FIGURE 12–20. Inversion recovery-prepared rapid gradient echo pulse sequence. There is a single preparatory 180° inversion pulse before the remainder of the pulse sequence. Without this preparatory pulse there would be little tissue contrast. The inversion pulse generates T1 contrast, based on the time between the inversion pulse and the weak phase-encoding gradients. This is the *effective* inversion time (TI), since the echoes that result from these weak phase-encoding gradients are used to fill the center of k-space.

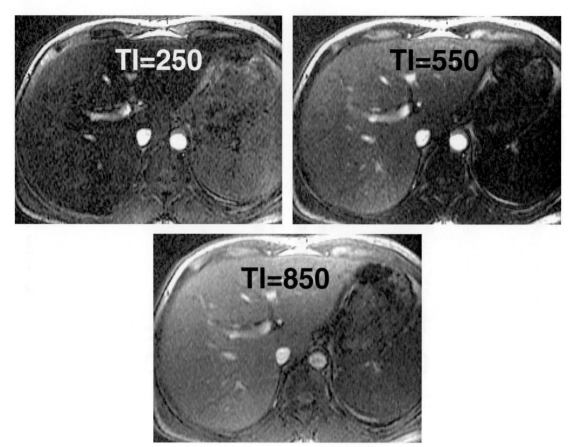

FIGURE 12-21. Inversion recovery–prepared rapid gradient echo images with TI varying between 250 and 850 msec. TR/TE/flip angle are 6.5/1.5/30°. For each image there is only one inversion pulse.

tion-prepared gradient echo images is not without cost. Throughout the acquisition of the rapid gradient echo, which usually takes about 1 second, longitudinal magnetization recovers toward its baseline equilibrium value. Therefore, echoes acquired at the beginning and the end of the sequence have significantly different contrast. For example, consider an inversion recovery magnetization–prepared gradient echo sequence with a TI of 250 msec. The TI for the first echo is 250 msec and that for the last echo is greater than 1000 msec. This causes

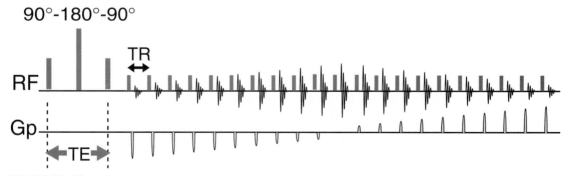

FIGURE 12-22. T2-weighted magnetization-prepared gradient echo pulse sequence. The initial 90° pulse creates transverse magnetization, which decays according to its T2. A 180° refocusing pulse corrects for magnetic field and chemical shift heterogeneity. A second 90° pulse rotates the persistent transverse magnetization back into the longitudinal plane. The magnetization available for the rapid gradient echo pulse sequence is therefore that of the tissues with long T2, so the image is T2-weighted.

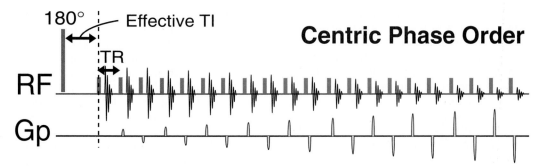

FIGURE 12–23. Inversion recovery–prepared gradient echo sequence with centric view order. The first echoes, with weakest phase encoding, are the strongest and, therefore, determine tissue contrast.

significant edge artifacts and image blurring and increases the importance of the order in which the phase-encoding gradient (Gp) strengths are changed.

As discussed in Chapter 6, image contrast is determined by the echoes with the weakest phase-encoding gradients. The timing relative to the preparatory pulse is therefore most important for the echoes with weakest phase-encoding gradients. One way to ensure that the expected contrast is achieved is to obtain the echoes with weak phase-encoding gradients, that is, the central lines of k-space, first. This order of filling k-space is referred to as *centric view order.* This is distinguished from the standard order used for conventional gradient echo and spin echo pulse sequences, *sequential order,* whereby phase-encoding gradient strength proceeds from the strongest negative one, through zero, and ends with the strongest positive one. Figure 12–20 shows the rapid inversion recovery–prepared gradient echo pulse sequence with sequential phase order; Figure 12-23 shows a comparable pulse sequence with centric view order.

Tissue contrast can be controlled most effectively, and edge artifacts minimized, when more than one preparatory pulse is used. In a segmented variation of magnetization-prepared gradient echo technique, several preparatory pulses are applied, each before a segment of the excitation pulses. With this modification, only a segment of the total number of views is acquired after each of several preparatory pulses. The variability of longitudinal magnetization among echoes is therefore decreased substantially. With such segmenting of the acquisition, the time that elapses during acquisition of each image is increased severalfold. Overall imaging efficiency is maintained by exciting additional sections during the intervals between a given section's data acquisition and

its next inversion pulse; however, the much longer acquisition time leads to greatly increased sensitivity to motion.

ESSENTIAL POINTS TO REMEMBER

1. Preparatory pulses are applied before an excitation pulse to alter tissue contrast or reduce signal intensity of undesired tissues.

2. Examples of preparatory pulse are inversion, spatial saturation, chemical shift saturation, and MT saturation pulses.

3. A preparatory pulse can occur before every excitation pulse, before some pulses, or only once, before a rapid gradient echo pulse sequence (i.e., magnetization-prepared gradient echo techniques).

4. An inversion pulse rotates longitudinal magnetization 180°, converting it into negative longitudinal magnetization. Spins recover according to their T1, initially toward zero and then toward equilibrium positive magnetization. The time between the inversion and excitation pulses is the TI.

5. Following an inversion pulse and subsequent excitation pulse, the transverse magnetization created will be positive, regardless of whether the longitudinal magnetization was positive or negative. Thus, the farther the positive or negative longitudinal magnetization is from zero, the greater will be the resulting transverse magnetization.

6. Inversion recovery techniques can be used to null specific tissues based on their T1s, by choosing a TI so that the inverted longitudinal magnetization has recovered to zero at the time of the excitation pulse.

7. Inversion recovery images where the TI is short enough to null the signal intensity of adipose tissue are called STIR images. On these images, signal intensity is greatest for tissues with long T1, since the longitudinal magnetization of these tissues is farthest from zero.

8. On STIR images, long T1 and long T2 both contribute to high signal intensity, rendering T1 and T2 contrast additive for most tissues.

9. Inversion recovery images with intermediate TI can be heavily T1-weighted, depicting tissues with long T1 as low signal intensity.

10. On inversion recovery images with TI of about 2000 msec, free water magnetization has relaxed to zero and is therefore nulled. These FLAIR images depict free fluid as low signal intensity, even if they are T2-weighted owing to long TE.

11. Spatially selective saturation pulses can be used to saturate flowing blood before it enters an image section or to saturate moving tissue to reduce its generation of artifacts.

12. Chemically selective saturation pulses have a narrow frequency range targeted to a specific population of protons (e.g., CH_2 protons in fat). The selectively excited spins are then spoiled, so that there is little magnetization from these undesired protons at the time of the excitation pulse.

13. MT saturation pulses are targeted at frequencies other than those of water or CH_2. Macromolecular protons have extremely short T2 and resonate over an extremely wide bandwidth, so that they are saturated by these off-resonance pulses. This saturation is transferred to nearby water molecules.

14. With magnetization-prepared gradient echo techniques, contrast is determined by the *effective TI,* which is the time between the preparatory pulse and the acquisition of the center of k-space (using the lowest phase-encoding values).

15. Sequential phase-encoding order refers to beginning with strong negative phase-encoding values, progressing through zero toward high positive values.

16. *Centric phase-encoding order* refers to beginning with the weak phase-encoding values (center of k-space). With centric phase encoding, the effective TI corresponds to the delay between the preparatory pulse and the onset of the rapid gradient echo pulse sequence.

13 Multiecho Techniques

Thus far, we have considered pulse sequences in which each excitation pulse creates one echo. With such sequences, for example, 256 excitation pulses are needed to produce 256 echoes. A variety of multiecho techniques acquire more than one echo with each excitation pulse.

IMAGES WITH MULTIPLE IMAGE CONTRAST

Multiecho techniques were first used to produce multiple images with different image contrast within a single series without increasing acquisition time. For instance, consider a spin echo pulse sequence with repetition time (TR) of 1800 msec and echo time (TE) of 120 msec. The phase-encoding gradient is pulsed briefly during the 120-msec interval between the excitation pulse and the echo, but most of this time is otherwise wasted, as no image data are obtained. However, a 180° refocusing pulse can be applied at 30 msec, followed by application of the rephasing lobe of the frequency-encoding gradient (Gf) at 60 msec, forming an echo. A second 180° refocusing pulse may be applied at 90 msec, followed by a second rephasing lobe of the Gf and a second echo at 120 msec (Fig. 13-1). These two echoes, one obtained with a TE of 60 msec and the other with a TE of 120 msec, each contribute one view (one line of k-space) to one of two separate images from the same site, with TEs of 60 and 120 msec. The process is then repeated after an additional excitation pulse, using a different value for the phase-encoding gradient.

Double echo pulse sequences, in which the second echo has a TE twice that of the first TE, are referred to as *symmetric double echo pulse sequences*. Techniques in which the first echo has a TE that is less than half the TE of the second echo are referred to as *asymmetric double echo pulse sequences* (Fig. 13-2). For example, 180° refocusing pulses may be applied at 4.5 msec and at 64.5 msec after the excitation pulse, producing echoes with TEs of 9 and 120 msec (64.5 msec after the excitation pulse corresponds to half the time between TEs of 9 and 120 msec). Symmetric double echo techniques tend to have less motion artifact, because gradient moment errors accumulated during the first half of the TE are compensated for by reapplication of the gradients for the second echo, which results in nulling of the gradients' first moment (see Chapter 10). Figure 13-3 illustrates images of the pelvis acquired with asymmetric and symmetric techniques.

MULTIECHO CONJUGATE TECHNIQUES

Multiecho techniques can be used to decrease acquisition time, rather than to generate images with different tissue contrast. With such techniques, different values of the phase-encoding gradient are applied for each of the multiple echoes, so that each echo fills a different line of k-space in the same image.

First, some new terminology must be introduced. Each set of echoes that follows an excitation pulse is referred to as an *echo train*. The amount of time during which these echoes are acquired is the *echo train duration,* and the number of echoes in the echo train is the *echo train length*.

Throughout the echo train duration, transverse magnetization decays. That is, the signal intensity of a given tissue is different at the beginning of the echo train than at the end. In

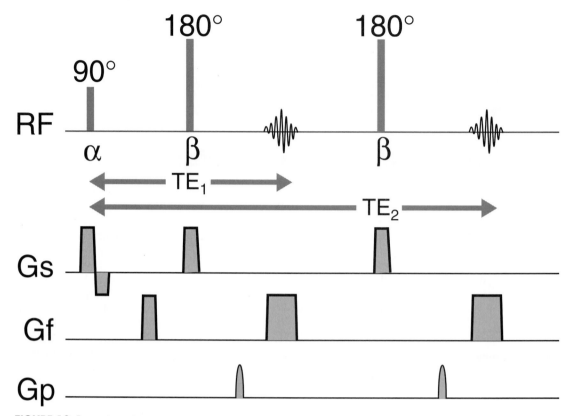

FIGURE 13–1. Double echo spin echo pulse sequence. Following excitation, two echoes, each refocused by a 180° pulse, are created by applying rephasing lobes of the frequency-encoding gradient (Gf) twice. The value of the phase-encoding pulse is identical for both. These two echoes are applied to different images with different TEs.

fact, each echo is acquired using a different TE. This imparts a great degree of flexibility in tissue contrast for these techniques but also gives rise to some unique artifacts and sources of image degradation. Understanding this allows one to achieve greater appreciation of the differences between single-echo and multiecho techniques.

As discussed previously, tissue contrast, as well as most signal intensity in an image, is defined by the echoes acquired using the weakest phase-encoding gradients (the central lines of k-space). These lines of k-space can be assigned to any position in the echo train by using the weakest phase-encoding gradients at this time. Thus, for a given echo train, consisting of multiple TEs, the image contrast can be defined by any of the included TEs. The TE of the echo that is acquired using a phase-encoding gradient strength of zero, representing the center of k-space, is defined as the *effective TE* (TE_{ef}) (Fig. 13–4). The other echoes contribute less to image contrast and more to edge detail, as the strength of the phase-encod-

ing gradient increases. The TE_{ef} (zero phase-encoding gradient) can be assigned to any echo in the echo train, including one at its beginning, middle, or end. Thus, for a multiecho technique with a given echo train, there is a remarkable degree of flexibility in image contrast (Fig. 13–5). This flexibility is limited somewhat, however, by artifact that arises from abrupt changes in signal intensity between adjacent lines of k-space.

The presence of echoes with several TEs introduces a variety of artifacts. Surprisingly, gross tissue contrast, at least for large objects, is not markedly altered. The most significant artifacts of multiecho techniques are those that involve edge detail, including blurring of edges and ghost artifacts. For similar acquisition parameters and matrix, multiecho images are blurrier than their single-echo counterparts.

Blurring of multiecho images is caused by decay of transverse magnetization during the echo train. Thus, blurring is most severe for tissues with short T2, because the transverse magnetization of these tissues varies most dur-

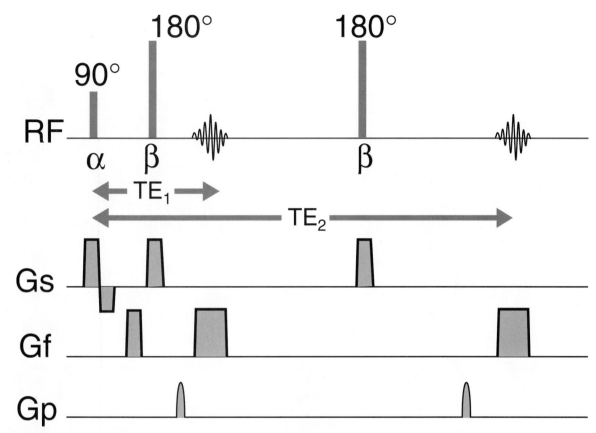

FIGURE 13–2. Asymmetric double echo spin echo pulse sequences. The first TE is less than half the second TE. The second 180° refocusing pulse occurs halfway between the two echoes.

ing the echo train. Generally, images are blurriest, and ghost artifacts most severe, when the effective TE is near the beginning of the echo train, that is, when the TE_{ef} is short.

ECHO PLANAR TECHNIQUES

Echo planar techniques acquire multiple gradient echoes per excitation. The most extreme versions of such multiecho techniques are single-shot techniques in which all the echoes used to form an image are obtained after a single excitation pulse. This is accomplished by oscillating the Gf rapidly, producing numerous gradient echoes (Fig. 13–6). In echo planar techniques, the strength of the phase-encoding gradient pulses is changed for each echo to impart different values of phase encoding for each of these echoes (Fig. 13–7).

Single-shot echo planar images are among the most rapidly acquired MR images, usually requiring less than 100 msec for complete acquisition; however, these images require ex-

tremely rapid switching of gradients, which is not possible with most MR units in clinical use as we write this. Even with extremely rapid gradient switching, a finite interval is necessary to sample each echo, resulting in a long echo train duration. During this time, transverse magnetization decays owing to T2* relaxation, including decay secondary to imperfections of the main and local magnetic fields and to imperfections of the magnetic gradients themselves. Additionally, transverse magnetization oscillates because of different chemical shifts, producing severe artifacts unless CH_2 magnetization is suppressed. Even with the best imaging systems available, spatial resolution of single shot echo planar images is limited by the necessarily long echo train duration, also referred to as the *acquisition window.* Single-shot echo planar images can be extremely T2- or T2*-weighted, since there is effectively no TR; the excitation is not repeated. This is sometimes referred to as *infinite TR.*

Signal-to-noise ratio (SNR), spatial resolution, and artifact reduction can be improved by using multishot echo planar techniques, in which the

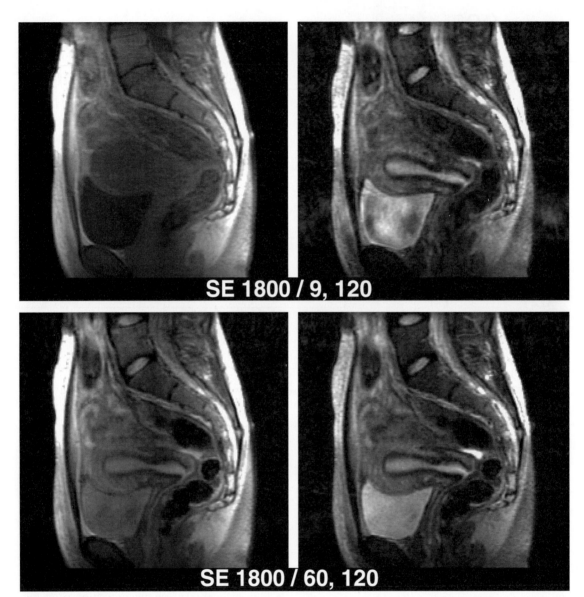

FIGURE 13-3. Double echo spin echo (SE) sagittal images of the pelvis using asymmetric and symmetric techniques. With the asymmetric technique *(top)*, short TE of 9 msec for the first echo minimizes T2-weighting (note the low signal intensity of urine). With symmetric technique *(bottom)*, both images are T2-weighted. Note that motion-induced artifact is worse with the asymmetric technique because of the longer time between echoes.

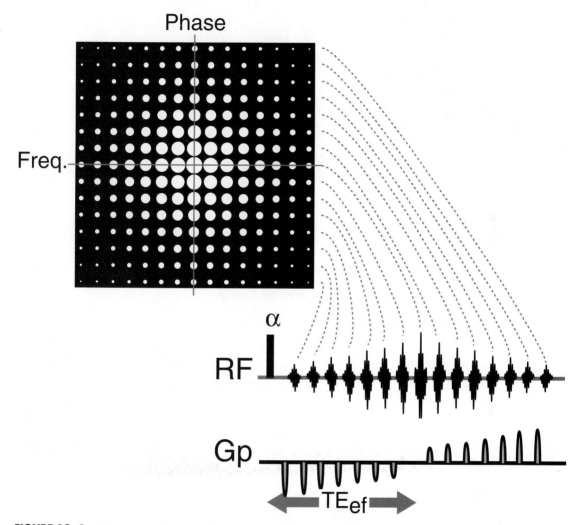

FIGURE 13-4. Filling of k-space for a single-shot multiecho technique. Each echo has a different phase-encoding gradient (Gp) strength. The strong phase-encoding gradients produce weak echoes, which fill the peripheral lines of k-space for fine detail, while the weak phase-encoding gradients produce strong echoes that fill the central lines of k-space and define the effective TE (TE$_{ef}$).

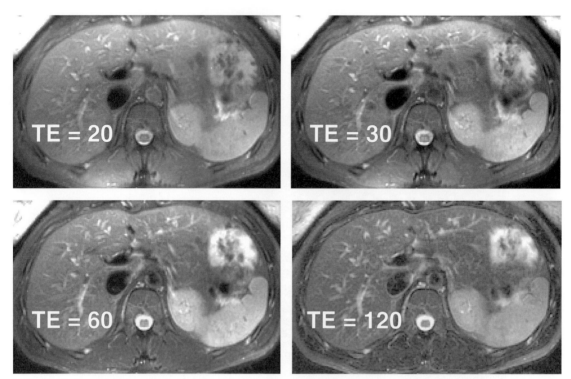

FIGURE 13–5. Axial fast spin echo images of the abdomen using TR of 3000 msec and an echo train of 16. For each of these images, the timing of each of the 16 echoes in the echo train is identical but the order of phase encoding is changed so that the effective TE (TE_{ef}) varies from 20 to 120 msec, increasing T2-weighting.

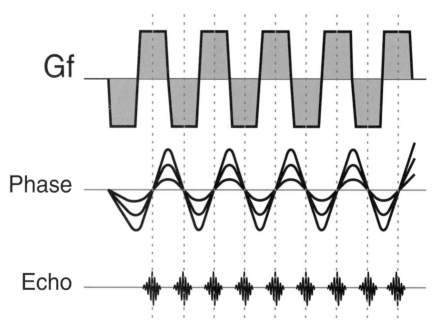

FIGURE 13–6. Creation of multiple echoes for echo planar by oscillating the Gf. At the center of each lobe of this gradient, the transverse magnetization is refocused, producing the echo.

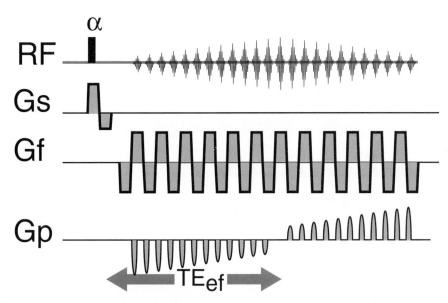

FIGURE 13–7. Echo planar pulse sequence, showing multiple echoes created for a single excitation pulse (α). The TE_{ef} corresponds to the weakest Gp strength.

echo train can be any number of echoes. After each excitation pulse, several, but not all, echoes are obtained (Figs. 13–8 and 13–9). Thus, in contrast to single-shot techniques, there is a TR. By reducing the echo train duration, blurring and other artifacts can be reduced. SNR can also be increased by obtaining two or more echoes for each value of the phase-encoding gradient. Multishot images are far more sensitive to motion, however, since acquisition time is longer.

T2* contrast and artifacts from heterogeneous magnetic susceptibility can be reduced by refocusing transverse magnetization during acquisition of the central lines of k-space, when the weakest phase-encoding gradients are used. This is accomplished via a single 180° refocusing pulse timed so that the maximum refocusing occurs at the effective echo time (TE_{ef}; Fig. 13–10). The gross contrast on these images is principally T2-weighted, rather than T2*-weighted, although susceptibility artifacts cannot be avoided entirely.

FAST SPIN ECHO (RAPID ACQUISITION WITH RELAXATION ENHANCEMENT, TURBO SPIN ECHO)

Rapid acquisition with relaxation enhancement (RARE) is the spin echo analog of echo planar. Vendor-introduced terms for RARE include *fast spin echo* and *turbo spin echo*. Because of wide familiarity with the term, *fast spin echo* has become an acceptable generic alternative to the less familiar term *multishot RARE*.

With fast spin echo, each echo is preceded by a refocusing pulse, usually of 180°. Thus, while echo planar consists of the acquisition of multiple gradient echoes per excitation pulse, fast spin echo consists of the acquisition of multiple spin echoes per excitation pulse. The refocusing pulses correct for magnetic field and chemical shift heterogeneity, eliminating many of the artifacts and sources of image degradation that plague echo planar; however, the refocusing pulses and the section-select gradient (Gs) pulses that accompany them add considerably to the duration of the echo train (Fig. 13–11).

Like echo planar, fast spin echo allows single-shot techniques. With the initial versions of fast spin echo, the long echo train took so much time that only simple fluid was depicted. While there were some signals from tissues with shorter T2 relaxation times, blurring was so severe that their margins were unidentifiable. However, single-shot fast spin echo images such as these were able to depict fluid structures such as cysts, bile ducts, urinary collecting structures, and cerebrospinal fluid (CSF).

Recently, there has been renewed interest in modifications of single-shot fast spin echo, us-

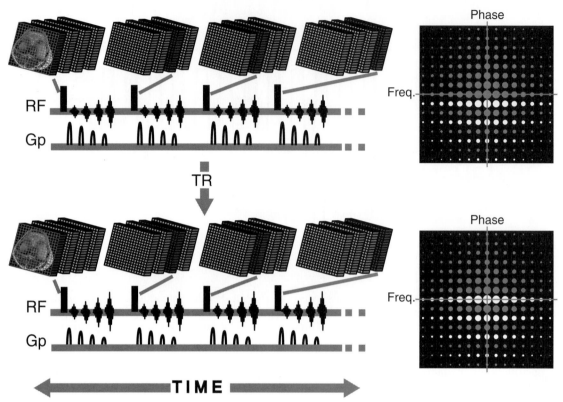

FIGURE 13–8. Filling of k-space in multisection, multishot echo planar techniques. In this example, four echoes follow each excitation pulse, filling four lines of k-space for a given section. After each section has been excited once, filling four lines of k-space for each, the sections are excited for a second time, at the TR, filling four additional lines of k-space.

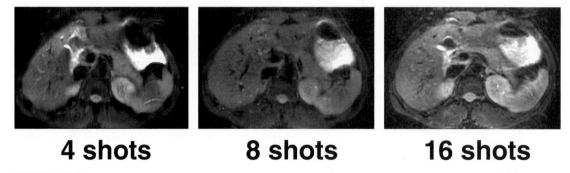

4 shots   8 shots   16 shots

FIGURE 13–9. Effect of number of shots on axial echo planar images with TR/TE_{ef} of 2500/60 msec. With four shots of 24 echoes each *(left)* there is substantial blurring and other artifact. Image quality improves as the acquisition is divided into a larger number of shots, such as 16 shots of six echoes each *(right)*.

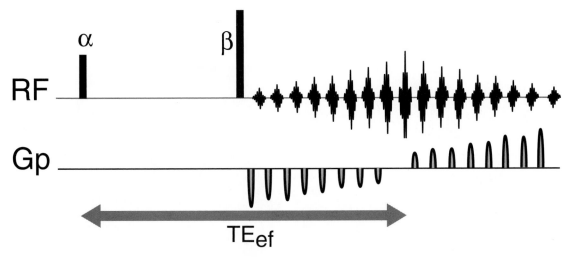

FIGURE 13–10. Spin echo–echo planar imaging (SE-EPI) pulse sequence. The 180° refocusing pulse (β) occurs at half the TE$_{ef}$, refocusing the echo at this TE. Refocusing of other echoes is less complete at greater distances from the TE$_{ef}$.

ing high-speed imaging gradients and partial-Fourier techniques. Examples include half-Fourier acquisition single-shot turbo spin echo (HASTE) and single-shot fast spin echo (SSFSE). With SSFSE technique, every echo is refocused, resulting in relative insensitivity to susceptibility artifact (Fig. 13–12). These images can be obtained in less than one-half second and are nearly free from visible motion-induced artifact (Fig. 13–13). Multi shot fast spin echo techniques are far more common (Fig. 13–14). In fact, these techniques have virtually replaced single-echo spin echo techniques for acquisition of T2-weighted images in many practices.

Fast spin echo images contain several excitation pulses, each of which is followed by a train of refocusing pulses that in turn generate a train of spin echoes. Each of these echoes is usually free of degradation due to magnetic field and chemical shift heterogeneity. These images can have high spatial resolution and high SNR. Although fast spin echo images are subject to blurring and edge artifacts, these can be minimized by the use of high acquisition matrix and judicious choice of echo train length and TE$_{ef}$ (Fig. 13–15). Generally, edge definition is sharpest with high acquisition matrix, short echo train length, short echo train duration, and long

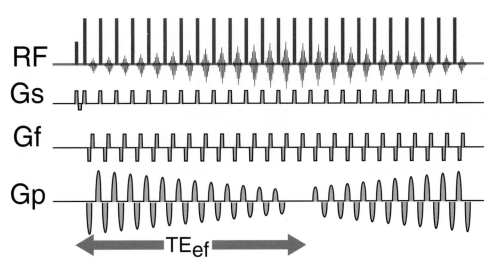

FIGURE 13–11. Fast spin echo pulse sequence. As with single-shot echo planar, all echoes are created following a single excitation pulse as the value of the phase-encoding gradient is changed. However, each echo is a spin echo refocused by a 180° refocusing pulse.

Single-Shot FSE; TE = 96 msec

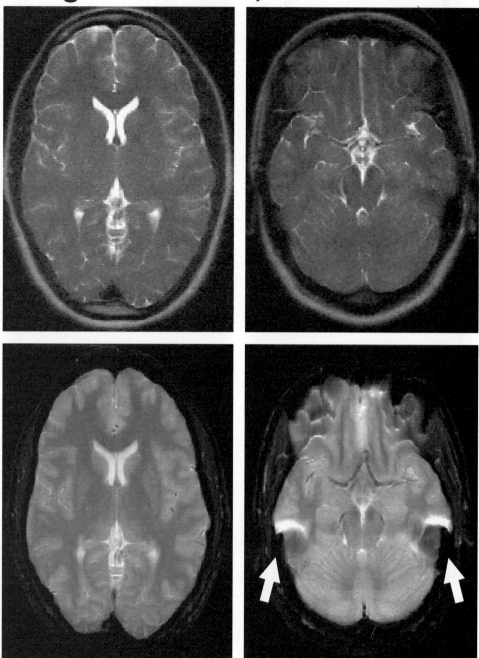

Multishot EPI; TR/TE = 3400/80

FIGURE 13–12. Comparison of T2-weighted multiecho images of the brain. The multishot echo planar images (EPI; *bottom*) show mild blurring and susceptibility artifacts near the petrous air spaces *(arrows)*. The images at top were acquired using a single-shot fast spin echo technique, where every echo is refocused, whereas only the central echo of each echo train is refocused for echo planar. Contrast between gray and white matter is better with echo planar, owing to the near absence of magnetization transfer effects.

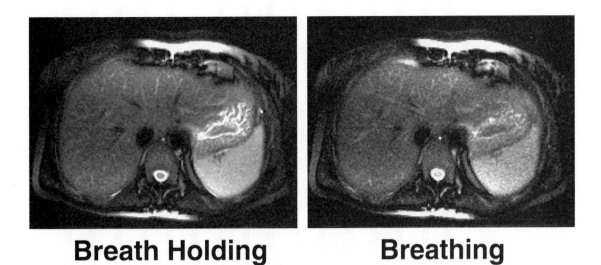

Breath Holding

Breathing

FIGURE 13-13. Single-shot fast spin echo images with TE of 100 msec, acquired during breath holding *(left)* and during quiet breathing *(right)*, show negligible artifact even with motion.

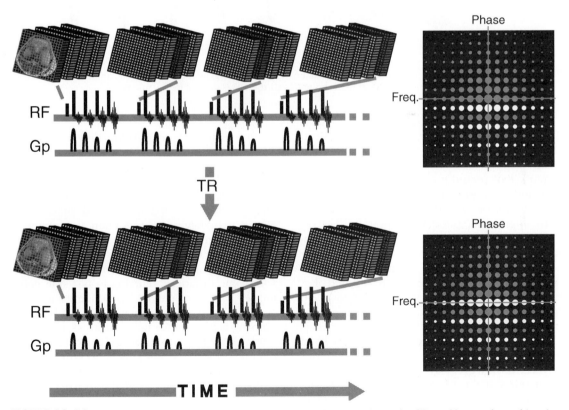

FIGURE 13-14. Filling of k-space by multisection fast spin echo. This is similar to the filling of k-space by multisection echo planar (see Fig. 13-8).

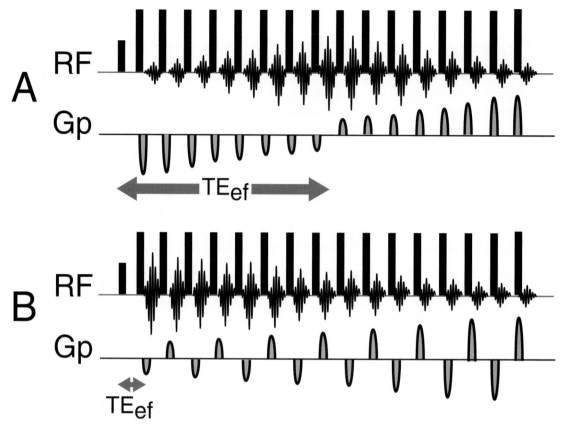

FIGURE 13–15. For a given echo train, the TE$_{ef}$ can be varied by changing the order of the phase-encoding steps. *(A)* The TE$_{ef}$ is defined by the middle echo in the echo train; *(B)* the TE$_{ef}$ is defined by the first echo.

TE$_{ef}$ (Fig. 13–16). For best edge definition, the TE$_{ef}$ should be near the end of the echo train.

With FSE techniques, most time is spent applying refocusing pulses and sampling echoes. The major gain of efficiency, as compared with single-echo spin echo techniques, is that, during a given TE, multiple echoes are obtained. This increases efficiency by a factor equal to the number of echoes that can be obtained by the time the TE$_{ef}$ is reached. For example, if six echoes can be obtained in 90 msec, a fast spin echo technique with an echo train of 6 and a TE$_{ef}$ of 90 msec is six times as efficient as a single-echo technique with a TE of 90 msec. When the echo train length increases beyond 6, however, fewer image sections can be acquired if the TR remains constant. To obtain the same number of image sections while using a longer echo train, it is necessary to increase TR (Fig. 13–17). Thus, efficiency is not substantially improved once the echo train becomes longer than the TE$_{ef}$. Echoes acquired after the TE$_{ef}$ contribute to image blurring but

do not reduce the acquisition time of a multi-section stack of images (Fig. 13–18).

There are certain situations in which the echo train should increase beyond the TE$_{ef}$, even though this could increase artifacts. These include situations in which the desired TR is longer than necessary to obtain the required number of image sections (e.g., sagittal imaging of the spine) or in which short acquisition time is essential (e.g., breath hold imaging).

In some instances, blurring in fast spin echo images can, paradoxically, produce an appearance of edge enhancement. This is because blurring is greatest for tissues with short T2 but minimal for those with long T2. For example, fluid has crisp edges on long echo train images. Tissues with short T2, however, have blurred edges, causing some signal intensity to be mapped in adjacent pixels, increasing their apparent signal intensity. At the interface between fluid and tissues with short T2, the short-T2 tissue's signal intensity is smeared, overlapping the signal intensity of adjacent fluid. This produces artifactual edge enhancement because

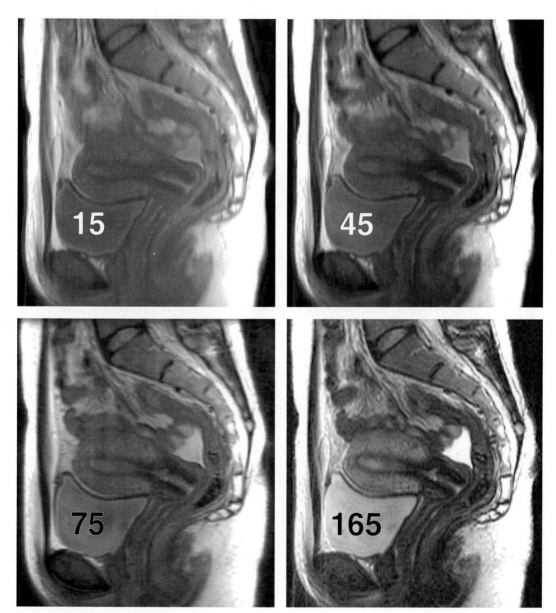

FIGURE 13–16. Effect of increasing TE_{ef} on sagittal fast spin echo images of the pelvis using TR of 3000 msec and an echo train of 16. For each of these images, the timing of each of the 16 echoes in the train is identical, but the order of phase encoding is changed. Note that image blurring decreases, and T2-weighted increases, as TE_{ef} increases.

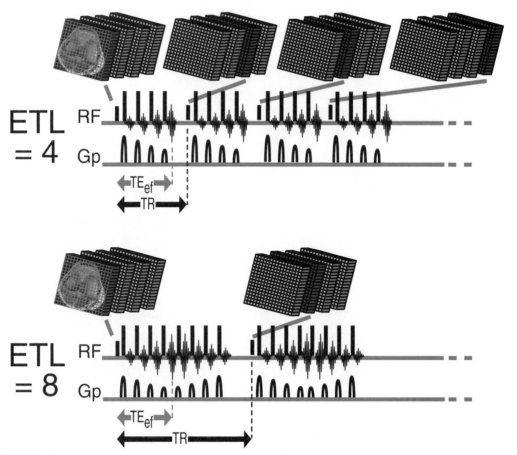

FIGURE 13–17. With multisection fast spin echo, acquisition efficiency is not necessarily improved by increasing the echo train length (ETL) beyond that needed for a given TE_{ef}. In this example, with ETL of 4, the TE_{ef} is defined by the last echo. With ETL of 8, TE_{ef} is unchanged but only half as many image sections can be obtained during a given interval. To obtain the same number of image sections with double the ETL, the TR must be approximately doubled.

the periphery of the short-T2 tissue has decreased signal intensity, whereas the margins of the long-T2 tissue has increased signal intensity (Figs. 13–19 and 13–20).

One major determinant of efficiency with fast spin echo techniques is echo spacing (i.e., the time between echoes). If echoes are obtained more rapidly, echo train length can be longer for a given echo train duration, decreasing the number of excitations that must be repeated (Fig. 13–21). Most fast spin echo pulse sequences are implemented so that echo spacing is minimized by default; however, changes in bandwidth affect the duration of echo sampling and thus have a substantial effect on echo spacing. As bandwidth increases, echo spacing decreases (Fig. 13–22). For this reason, sampling bandwidth should be as high as possible with fast spin echo techniques unless it is limited by system hardware or SNR. (Larger bandwidth reduces SNR.)

The principal differences between contrast on fast spin echo images and conventional spin echo images with comparable TR and TE are that adipose tissue is brighter relative to simple fluid and solid tissues are darker (Fig. 13–23). Both differences are the result of the more frequent application of refocusing radio pulses with fast spin echo as compared with standard spin echo techniques.

The signal intensity of adipose tissue on standard spin echo T2-weighted images is lower than would be predicted from its true T2 relaxation time. This is because adipose tissue has multiple proton environments that produce many different chemical shift resonances. This leads to a phenomenon known as *J coupling*, in which signal loss is due to interaction between different lipid resonances during the gaps between refocusing radio pulses. These gaps are large in conventional spin echo T2-weighted imaging, typically 40 msec or more; with fast

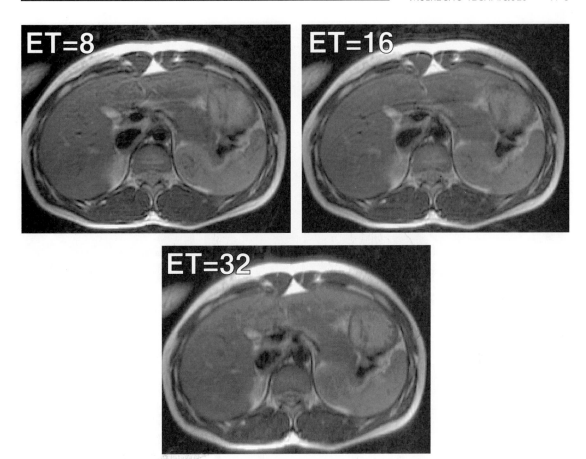

FIGURE 13–18. Increased blurring with increasing echo train (ET) length on axial images of the abdomen with TR/TE$_{ef}$ of 3000/100 msec.

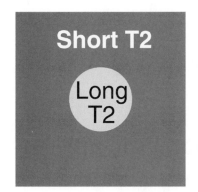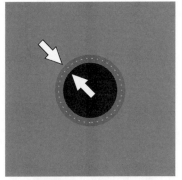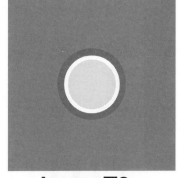

Blurring of Short T2 Edges   **Long T2 + Short T2**

FIGURE 13–19. Paradoxical edge enhancement due to blurring of short T2 tissue (e.g., brain) on fast spin echo images with long echo train. Blurring of brain tissue causes decreased signal intensity at its margins that extends into the area occupied by a tissue with longer T2 (e.g., fluid). The middle image depicts brain tissue with fluid omitted. The dotted line represents the true margin of brain tissue; the arrows indicate its blurred boundary. The image at right depicts brain and fluid, showing decreased signal intensity adjacent to the fluid and increased signal intensity at the edge of the fluid, the result of summation of signal intensity from fluid and the blurred brain edge.

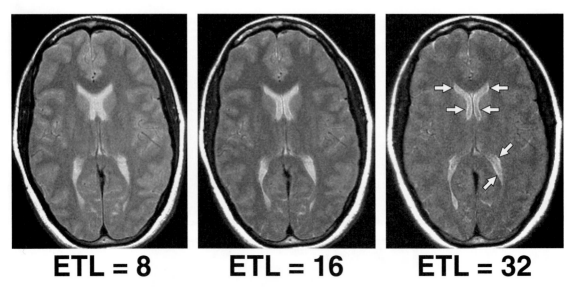

FIGURE 13-20. Blurring of contrast between gray and white matter, and artifactual edge enhancement of the cerebral ventricles, with increasing echo train length (ETL) *(arrows)*.

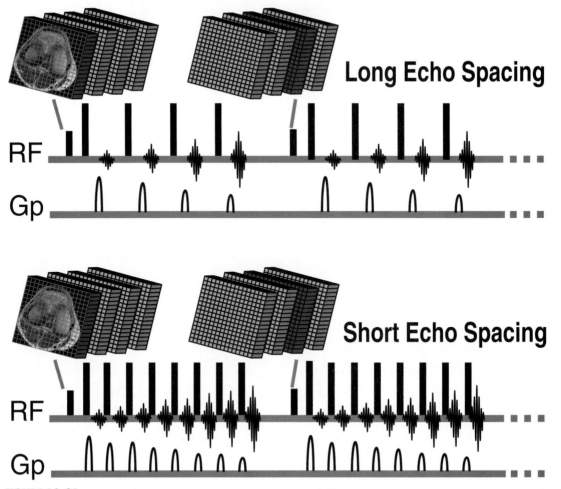

FIGURE 13-21. Effect of echo spacing on acquisition efficiency. With shorter echo spacing, the echo train length can be increased without reducing the number of image sections obtained at a given TR.

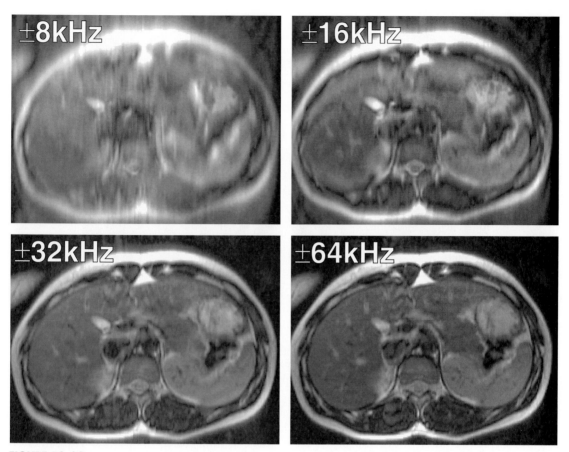

FIGURE 13–22. Effects of increasing sampling bandwidth on fast spin echo 3000/100 images with echo train of 16. With low bandwidth, blurring artifact is severe, owing to the longer echo spacing and echo train duration. Detail increases with higher bandwidth.

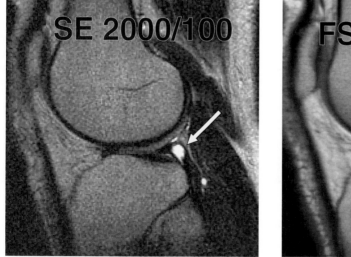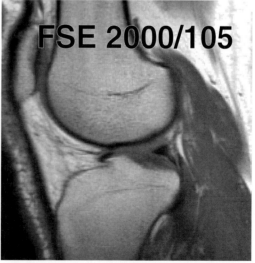

FIGURE 13–23. Comparison of conventional spin echo (SE) *(left)* and fast spin echo (FSE) *(right)* T2-weighted images with similar parameters. With FSE adipose tissue and bone marrow have higher relative signal intensity because of the higher signal intensity of lipid. Overall SNR and detail are higher with FSE, but fluid *(arrow)* is more conspicuous with SE. To depict fluid on FSE with comparable conspicuity, longer TE, longer TR, and/or fat suppression is necessary.

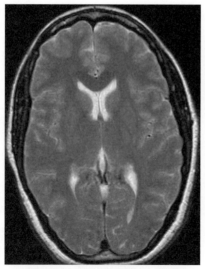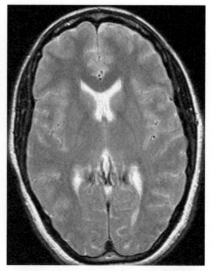

Multisection 100% Gaps   Single-Section

FIGURE 13–24. Effects of MT on multisection axial fast spin echo images of the brain (TR/TE$_{ef}$ is 2000/105 msec). The images on the left were acquired using 100% gaps to eliminate cross-talk, but signal intensity is decreased because of MT effects. MT contrast is eliminated by the use of a single-section technique *(right)*. Note higher signal intensity of brain parenchyma, especially of white matter, with single-section technique.

spin echo techniques, however, refocusing radio pulses occur much more rapidly (currently 10 to 20 msec apart), allowing less time for signal loss due to J coupling. Thus, on fast spin echo images adipose tissue has high signal intensity, because the images reflect the T2 relaxation of adipose tissue more accurately than do standard spin echo T2-weighted techniques.

Solid tissues have lower signal intensity on fast spin echo images than on standard spin echo T2-weighted images because magnetization transfer (MT) saturation is greater with fast spin echo. MT (see Chapter 7, Magnetization Transfer) involves saturation of the longitudinal

magnetization of macromolecular protons like those within protein molecules. The saturated magnetization of these macromolecular protons is transferred to water protons, which are closely associated with these macromolecules. Thus, MT reduces the signal intensity of solid tissues, because of their large concentrations of macromolecules. With multisection fast spin echo techniques, each 180° refocusing radio pulse targeted to a particular image section has the added effect of partially saturating macromolecular protons in the other imaging sections, since macromolecular protons are saturated by a larger range of radio frequencies (Fig. 13–24).

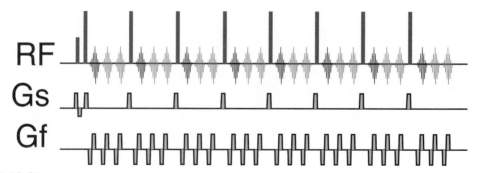

FIGURE 13–25. GRASE pulse sequence. In this example, there is one 180° refocusing pulse for every three echoes, producing complete refocusing for one third of the echoes and only partial refocusing for all other echoes.

GRE-EPI

SE-EPI

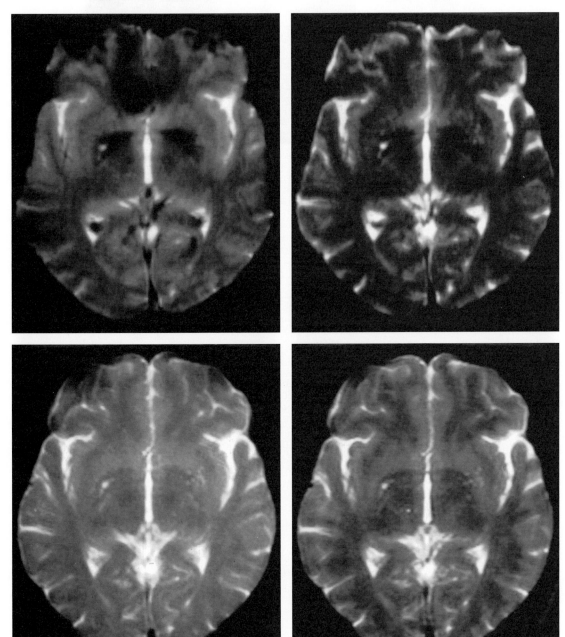

FSE

GRASE

FIGURE 13–26. Comparison between axial single-shot GRASE and other methods of single-shot T2-weighted images of the brain. With gradient echo–echo planar technique (GRE-EPI) *(top left)*, susceptibility artifact from nearby bone and air has degraded image quality. This is reduced somewhat by refocusing the echo at the center of k-space via spin echo–echo planar technique (SE-EPI) *(top right)*. Artifact is nearly eliminated by refocusing every echo, using fast spin echo (FSE) technique *(bottom left)*, although magnetization transfer has reduced tissue contrast. With GRASE technique *(bottom right)*, artifact is minimal and soft tissue contrast is preserved. (Courtesy of David A. Feinberg, M.D., Ph.D.)

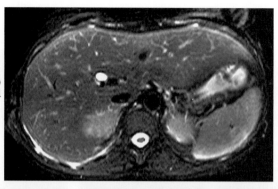

FSE-STIR

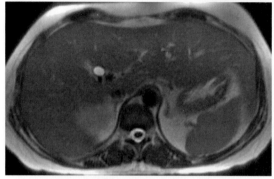

Single Shot FSE

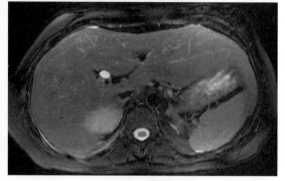

GRASE

FIGURE 13-27. Comparison between axial multishot GRASE and other methods of breath hold T2-weighted images of the abdomen. With FSE-STIR technique *(top)*, additive effects of T1 and T2 differences produce strong image contrast between liver and spleen. With single-shot FSE *(bottom left)*, MT contrast and unsuppressed fat have reduced the conspicuousness of this contrast. With fat-suppressed GRASE *(bottom right)*, there is less effect from MT and contrast is improved. (Courtesy of Neil M. Rofsky, M.D.)

GRADIENT RECALLED AND SPIN ECHO TECHNIQUES

Gradient recalled and spin echo (GRASE) techniques represent a hybrid between echo planar and fast spin echo techniques. With echo planar, all echoes are gradient refocused. With fast spin echo all echoes are refocused spin echoes. With GRASE, some echoes are spin echoes and others, gradient echoes (Fig. 13-25). GRASE images thus have some of the artifacts present with echo planar but ameliorated with fast spin echo, and are more efficient than fast spin echo but less efficient than echo planar (Figs. 13-26 and 13-27). Less MT contrast is present in GRASE than in fast spin echo.

The major limitations of echo planar techniques relate to the length of the nonrefocused echo trains. The long acquisition windows necessary to acquire the echo trains of echo planar render these images subject to degradation from heterogeneous magnetic field and chemical shift. Such artifacts can be corrected by application of 180° refocusing radio pulses. If the number of refocusing pulses is less than the number of echoes, some echoes are refocused and others only partially refocused. The ratio of gradient echoes to spin echoes has been referred to as the *GRASE factor.*

At the time of this writing, clinical applications for GRASE have not been established, nor have the best methods of varying phase-encoding gradient strength to minimize artifacts. GRASE promises to offer an extremely flexible platform of fast and efficient imaging, trading off efficiency for completeness of refocusing. GRASE can potentially be implemented as a flexible spectrum, varying echo train from one (conventional gradient echo or spin echo) to the total number of echoes (single-shot echo techniques) and varying the GRASE factor from zero (fast spin echo) to infinity (echo planar).

ESSENTIAL POINTS TO REMEMBER

1. Two or more echoes can be acquired after each excitation pulse. If each echo is acquired using the same phase-encoding pulse, each echo may be used to provide one view in two or more separate images with different TE.
2. Two or more echoes can be acquired after each excitation pulse using different values of the phase-encoding gradient. These echoes can be used to fill different portions of k-space within the same image, to reduce acquisition time.
3. Images in which two or more gradient echoes are obtained per excitation pulse are referred to as *echo planar images*.
4. Images in which two or more spin echoes are obtained per excitation pulse are referred to as *fast spin echo* images, or as RARE or turbo spin echo images.
5. Compared with fast spin echo images, echo planar images are faster but have more artifacts and lower spatial resolution.
6. Images in which a combination of two or more gradient echoes and spin echoes are obtained per excitation pulse are referred to as *GRASE images*.
7. Echo planar, fast spin echo, or GRASE images can be obtained using single-shot techniques (only one excitation pulse), or as multishot techniques (two or more excitation pulses, each followed by acquisition of several echoes).
8. Image contrast on multiecho techniques is determined by the timing within the echo train of the echoes with weak phase-encoding value (center of k-space).
9. With multiecho techniques, artifacts can often be reduced by minimizing the time between echoes (the interecho intervals).

CHAPTER

14 **T1-Weighted Pulse Sequences**

Most applications of MRI involve obtaining at least one set of T1-weighted images. Many methods are currently available for accomplishing this. In this chapter, some of the basic T1-weighted techniques introduced in the previous few chapters are reconsidered and put into perspective relative to one another.

SPIN ECHO

Conventional spin echo technique (Fig. 14–1) has throughout the past decade been the most common method for acquiring T1-weighted images for most applications of MRI, although other techniques have gained favor recently. Using optimized spin echo technique, high-quality images with moderate T1-weighting can be obtained within a few minutes, with few artifacts for most parts of the body. Of all techniques, T1-weighted spin echo images are perhaps the most robust—and the most forgiving of hardware limitations.

Generally, repetition time (TR) is 600 msec or less. As field strength decreases, lower TRs should be used. One limitation of the use of short TRs is that only a few image sections can be acquired per TR. With modern software, however, this limitation is not significant, because several sets of images can be programmed simultaneously and acquired sequentially. For example, two sets of images with TR of 300 msec can be acquired as simply and as rapidly as one set of images with TR of 600 msec, whereas the T1 contrast of the former is superior (Fig. 14–2).

Echo time (TE) is at least as critical a factor as TR for optimizing contrast in T1-weighted SE images, although it is perhaps easier to understand. Quite simply: the shorter, the better. During the TE, transverse magnetization decays de-

pending on T2, reducing signal-to-noise ratio (SNR) but more important introducing T2 contrast. Since T2 contrast is usually opposite to T1 contrast for most tissue comparisons, T2 contrast is generally undesirable on T1-weighted images. T2 contrast can be minimized by using the shortest possible TE (Fig. 14–3).

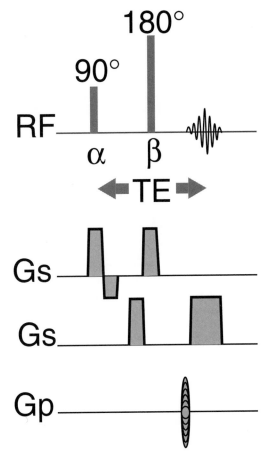

FIGURE 14–1. Standard spin echo pulse sequence for T1-weighted spin echo images.

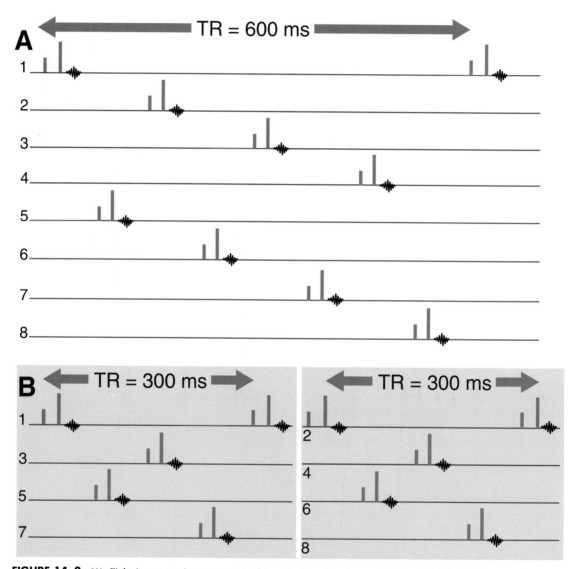

FIGURE 14–2. *(A)*, Eight image sections are acquired in a single spin echo acquisition with TR of 600 msec. *(B)*, Four images are acquired in each of two interleaved spin echo acquisitions with TR of 300 msec, each of which is acquired in half the time owing to the shorter TR. The end result is improved T1-weighting without increased total acquisition time.

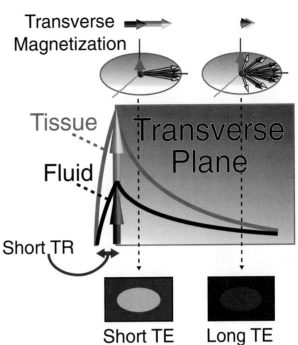

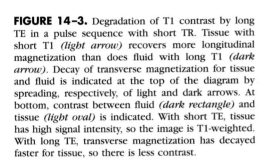

FIGURE 14–3. Degradation of T1 contrast by long TE in a pulse sequence with short TR. Tissue with short T1 *(light arrow)* recovers more longitudinal magnetization than does fluid with long T1 *(dark arrow)*. Decay of transverse magnetization for tissue and fluid is indicated at the top of the diagram by spreading, respectively, of light and dark arrows. At bottom, contrast between fluid *(dark rectangle)* and tissue *(light oval)* is indicated. With short TE, tissue has high signal intensity, so the image is T1-weighted. With long TE, transverse magnetization has decayed faster for tissue, so there is less contrast.

Because a certain amount of time is required to produce a refocusing pulse and its associated imaging gradients, spin echo techniques require longer TE than comparable gradient echo techniques. This introduces additional T2 contrast and permits fewer image sections per TR. Thus, the two major limitations of spin echo technique for acquisition of T1-weighted images are contamination by inclusion of T2 contrast and long acquisition time. For both of these reasons, gradient echo images with minimized TE are becoming more popular for T1-weighted imaging.

INVERSION RECOVERY

Inversion recovery techniques can be used to achieve stronger and more flexible T1 contrast on spin echo images that can be achieved using conventional spin echo technique. As discussed in Chapter 12, spin echo inversion recovery images are acquired by preceding each excitation pulse with an inversion pulse (Fig. 14–4).

To obtain heavily T1-weighted images where tissues with short T1 are depicted as having high signal intensity, the excitation pulse is applied at a time after inversion (T1) so that one tissue is nulled while tissues with shorter T1

relaxation time have higher signal intensity because they have passed their null point. The use of an inversion pulse does not decrease the contribution of T2 contrast due to the TE; rather, it improves the dynamic range of T1 contrast and thus exaggerates depiction of T1 contrast beyond that depicted on standard spin echo T1-weighted images.

Inversion recovery spin echo images have stronger T1-weighted contrast than do comparable conventional spin echo images, but acquisition time is increased considerably and SNR is usually lower. Given the wide choice of currently available techniques, a technique with lower SNR and longer acquisition time is rarely preferred. Therefore, inversion recovery technique is rarely used to obtain spin echo images with "conventional" T1 contrast (short T1 depicted as high signal intensity). Spin echo inversion recovery technique is often used for short TI inversion recovery (STIR) images, however, particularly at low or midfield as a substitute for T2-weighted images.

MULTISECTION SPOILED GRADIENT ECHO

Multisection spoiled gradient echo images are acquired in a similar manner as multisection

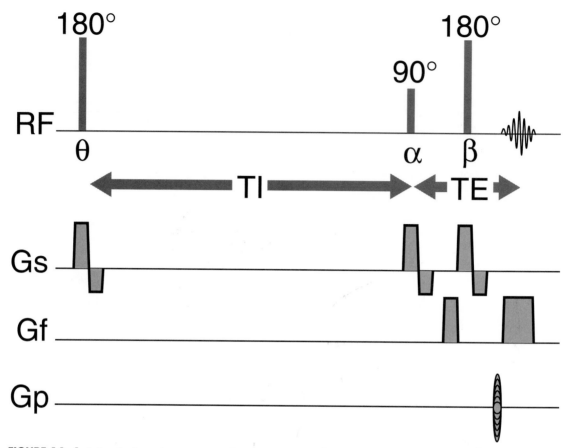

FIGURE 14-4. Spin echo inversion recovery pulse sequence. A 180° inversion radio pulse inverts magnetization for the selected section, defined by Gs. Following TI, a 90° excitation pulse creates transverse magnetization, which is refocused by a 180° refocusing pulse and detected at TE.

spin echo images, but without the refocusing pulses and their associated imaging gradients. The greater simplicity of gradient echo, as compared with spin echo techniques, results in greater efficiency, leading to shorter TEs and more image sections for any TR. Therefore, with appropriate hardware and software these images can have equivalent T1 contrast and higher SNR per unit time than comparable spin echo images. The reduced acquisition time can be used to allow breath holding or dynamic scanning after the injection of contrast material (Fig. 14-5).

Whereas gradient echo images can be limited by sensitivity to magnetic field heterogeneity, generally this is not a significant problem with gradient echo images optimized for T1 contrast because of their short TEs and high sampling bandwidth.

The clinical use of spoiled gradient echo technique for obtaining T1-weighted images is complicated somewhat by chemical shift oscil-

lations as TE is changed (see T1-Weighted Chemical Shift Pulse Sequences). Depending on the application, fat-water in-phase or opposed-phase images may be preferred, and tissue contrast can be significantly different. Fat-water effects must be carefully considered when choosing the TE for T1-weighted gradient echo images.

SINGLE-SECTION SPOILED GRADIENT ECHO

Single-section spoiled gradient echo images can be acquired in 1 second or less, but acquisition of these images is not more *efficient* than is acquisition of multisection images with longer TR but comparable TE. That is because, for a given number of image sections, the same number of excitation pulses is applied and the same number of echoes is sampled. The princi-

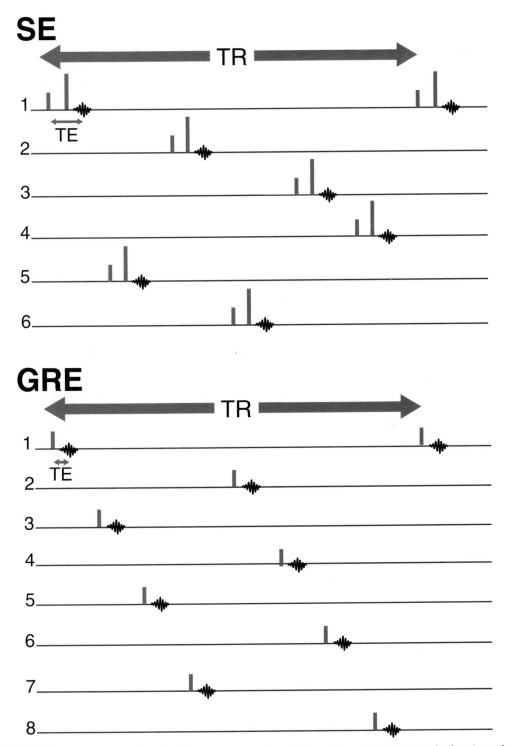

FIGURE 14-5. Comparison of spin echo (SE) and gradient echo (GRE) techniques. The absence of refocusing pulses in gradient echo techniques allows the use of shorter TE than with spin echo techniques and thus allows the acquisition of more image sections during a given TR.

pal difference between multisection and single-section techniques is that with the former a stack of several sections is acquired in an interleaved manner during a particular interval, whereas with the latter several images are acquired separately and sequentially over the same interval (Fig. 14–6).

If the goal is to acquire a set of images during a specified interval, the multisection technique is generally preferred. Multisection techniques allow a longer TR and larger flip angle, producing greater SNR per unit of time; however, if the goal is to obtain images rapidly with little motion artifact or to obtain images rapidly during several different phases of a physiologic event (e.g., dynamic motion or perfusion with a contrast agent), the single-section technique is preferred. Although overall efficiency is comparable with the two techniques, temporal resolution is much better with single-section methods.

MAGNETIZATION-PREPARED GRADIENT ECHO

Inversion recovery–prepared gradient echo techniques (see Chapter 12, Magnetization-Prepared Rapid Gradient Echo Techniques) generate rapid images with heavy T1-weighting. SNR of magnetization-prepared gradient echo images is less than that of multisection spoiled gradient echo techniques. Factors that contribute to low SNR in these sequences include the reduced signal intensity inherent in all inversion recovery techniques (see Chapter 11, Unspoiled Gradient Echo Techniques), as well as the short TR and small flip angles of rapid gradient echo images. The strong and flexible T1-weighted

contrast obtainable makes these techniques interesting, however, in situations in which acceptable SNR is possible, as with large voxel sizes or the use of specialized local receiver coils.

T1-WEIGHTED CHEMICAL SHIFT PULSE SEQUENCES

Because of the short T1 of methylene (CH_2) protons, most biologic lipids contribute more signal intensity on T1-weighted images than would be expected from their proton density alone. As a result, T1-weighted images are sensitive to the presence of lipids owing to their short T1. Thus, chemical shift techniques usually have greater impact on T1-weighted images than on other images. This is true of both fat-saturated images and fat-water opposed-phase images.

Fat saturation can be used to reduce artifacts and optimize dynamic range on T1-weighted images for special applications. Perhaps the greatest use of fat suppression on T1-weighted images is for improving the conspicuousness of enhancing tissue after administration of gadolinium chelates. If surrounding adipose tissue has high signal intensity, mild enhancement may be subtle. Fat suppression can also increase the conspicuousness of hemorrhage or of subtle contrast in musculoskeletal structures (e.g., menisci) or within hepatic or pancreatic parenchyma.

Even if fat-suppressed T1-weighted images are obtained, additional T1-weighted images without fat suppression are often important. It is on these images that fat planes and fatty bone

TABLE 14–1. COMPARISON OF T1-WEIGHTED PULSE SEQUENCES*

Pulse Sequence	Attributes for T1 Weighting			
	Contrast	*SNR*	*Efficiency*	*Artifact-Free*
Spin echo	+ +	+	+	+ + +
Fast spin echo	+	+ +	+ +	+ +
Inversion recovery	+ + + +	−	−	+
Single-section spoiled gradient echo	−	−	+ + +	+
Multisection spoiled gradient echo	+ + +	+ + +	+ + +	+ + +
3D–Fourier transform spoiled gradient echo	+ +	+ + + +	+ + +	+ +
Inversion recovery–prepared gradient echo	+ + + +	−	+	+

*Relative advantages of various T1-weighted pulse sequences regarding T1 contrast, SNR, efficiency, and freedom from artifacts. The best contrast can be achieved with spin echo or gradient echo inversion recovery techniques, but other attributes are less desirable. SNR is highest for 3D-FT or 2D-multisection techniques, and lowest for single section techniques. Gradient echo techniques are more efficient than spin echo or magnetization-prepared techniques.

Multisection GRE

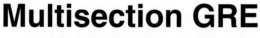

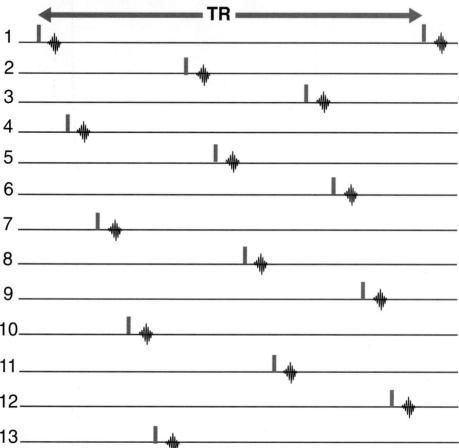

Single-Section GRE

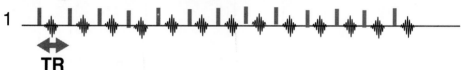

FIGURE 14–6. Comparison of multisection and single-section gradient echo techniques. In this example, 13 sections are obtained during a comparable interval with each technique; however, acquisitions are interleaved with the multisection technique and sequential with the single-section technique, and TR is much longer with the multisection technique.

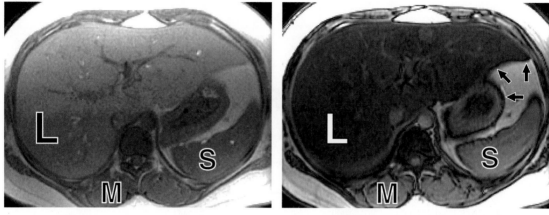

TE = 4.2 msec   TE = 2.1 msec

FIGURE 14-7. Fatty infiltration of the liver depicted using gradient echo in-phase (TE = 4.2 msec) and opposed-phase (TE = 2.1 msec) images at 1.5 T. On the in-phase image *(left)*, liver (L) has higher signal intensity than spleen (S) or skeletal muscle (M). With opposed-phase technique, liver has markedly low signal intensity owing to destructive interference between comparable amounts of water and lipid magnetization. There has been little change in the signal intensity of adipose tissue, most of which is from lipid magnetization. The small black arrows *(right)* indicate signal voids at fat-water interfaces secondary to inclusion within these voxels of water and lipid.

marrow are depicted with the greatest clarity, providing important anatomic detail of many body parts.

In addition to improving the intensity of contrast between certain tissues, chemical shift techniques are useful for sensitive and specific identification of lipid in tissues. Definitive identification of lipid is accomplished best by comparing in-phase T1-weighted images with either fat-suppressed images or opposed-phase im-

ages. The choice between these latter two techniques depends on the relative tissue concentration of lipid.

For tissues whose MR signal originates principally from lipid, the high signal intensity of fat must be distinguished from other high-signal intensity sources (e.g., hemorrhage, flow, contrast enhancement). The high signal intensity of fat on T1-weighted images can be changed most dramatically by using fat satura-

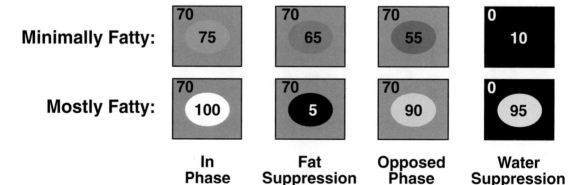

FIGURE 14-8. Contrast between water *(boxes)* and minimally fatty *(top ovals;* 65 signal units from water and 10 from fat) or mostly fatty *(bottom ovals;* five signal units from water and 95 from fat) tissues on T1-weighted images with a variety of chemical shift techniques. Numbers indicate arbitrary signal intensity units. Mostly fatty tissues *(bottom)* have short T1 and, therefore, more signal intensity on in-phase T1-weighted images. With fat suppression, signal intensity is markedly reduced for mostly fatty tissues but only minimally affected for minimally fatty tissues *(top)*. On opposed-phase images, the signal intensity reduction is greater for minimally fatty tissues but less for mostly fatty tissues, as compared with that from fat suppression. With water suppression, all remaining signal intensity is from fat, which is much greater for mostly fatty tissues.

tion techniques, which convert it to low signal intensity.

In contrast, the effect of fat saturation pulses on tissues with minimal fat, such as mildly fatty liver, may be barely noticeable. For definitive identification of small quantities of lipid, comparison of in-phase and opposed-phase images is best (Fig. 14–7). This is because a small quantity of lipid signal interferes destructively with and removes from the image an equivalent amount of water signal. The opposed-phase effect is therefore double the effect of fat saturation on tissues with small amounts of lipid. Water suppression can also be effective; if water is completely saturated, any visible signal indicates lipid. In clinical practice, however, water suppression techniques are particularly vulnerable to artifact; it may be difficult to distinguish minimally fatty tissue from artifactual signal. Figure 14–8 is a diagram explaining the effects on relative signal intensity of partially fatty tissues of various chemical shift techniques.

ESSENTIAL POINTS TO REMEMBER

1. Spin echo technique is useful for obtaining images with moderate T1 contrast and less artifact than many other techniques. There is more experience with spin echo than with any other technique for obtaining T1 contrast.
2. For T1-weighting, regardless of method, T1 contrast is optimal if TE is minimized.
3. Inversion recovery spin echo techniques can be used to achieve strong and flexible T1 contrast, but acquisition time is long and SNR per unit of time is low.
4. Multisection spoiled gradient echo techniques allow acquisition of moderately T1-weighted images with high efficiency and high SNR per unit of time. It is important to recognize that the phases of fat and water magnetizations are commonly opposed to each other on these images.
5. Single-section spoiled gradient echo techniques have efficiency similar to that of multisection techniques but with lower SNR and contrast; however, they are less sensitive to motion and have greater temporal resolution.
6. Inversion recovery magnetization–prepared gradient echo images have strong and flexible T1 contrast but low SNR and spatial resolution.
7. Because of the high signal intensity of fat on T1-weighted images, chemical shift techniques are usually most useful when applied with T1-weighted pulse sequences.
8. T1-weighted images without fat suppression are most useful for depicting anatomy based on the high signal intensity of fat planes or fatty marrow.
9. Fat saturation is useful for decreasing artifacts from fat and for improving the conspicuousness of subtle changes in nonfatty high-signal tissues.
10. Definitive identification of tissue lipid is accomplished best by comparing in-phase T1-weighted images with either fat-suppressed or opposed-phase images.
11. Fat suppression is most useful for identifying tissues that contain principally fat, whereas fat-water opposed-phase images are most useful for depicting small quantities of lipid.

15 T2-Weighted Pulse Sequences

Nearly all clinical imaging protocols involve obtaining at least one T2-weighted pulse sequence. In this chapter we review some of the techniques that are used to depict T2 differences between tissues and to consider their relative advantages and disadvantages.

SPIN ECHO TECHNIQUES

Like T1-weighted images, T2-weighted images have been obtained principally via spin echo technique during the past decade. T2-weighted spin echo images provide acceptable T2 contrast for most tissues. Signal-to-noise (SNR) per unit time is much lower for T2-weighted than for T1-weighted spin echo images, however. Although strong T2 weighting with conventional spin echo technique is possible, the number of image sections that can be acquired per repetition time (TR), and therefore acquisition time for a stack of images, increases with longer echo time (TE). Therefore, there is a practical limit to the TE that can be tolerated in clinical practice before unacceptably low anatomic coverage and long acquisition times are reached (Fig. 15–1).

One benefit of conventional spin echo technique for obtaining T2-weighted images is that one or more additional echoes can be obtained to generate other images with identical TR but lower TE, without taking any more time. These two images, acquired during the same period of time using double-echo spin echo technique, can be used to calculate T2 values or T2 images. In clinical practice, these images are usually compared visually to gain an impression of a tissue's T2 (Fig. 15–2). Until recently, the principal reason for the long survival of T2-weighted spin echo images in clinical practice, in spite of their relative inefficiency, was the lack of acceptable alternatives.

GRADIENT ECHO TECHNIQUES

Gradient echo images with moderate TE depict (T2*) contrast. In some situations, such as certain spine or musculoskeletal applications, these images resemble T2-weighted ones; however, gradient echo images with long TE are less efficient and have lower SNR and more artifacts than gradient echo images with short TE. In clinical practice it is often difficult to obtain sufficient T2* contrast without introducing unacceptable levels of image degradation (Fig. 15–3).

For some applications, T2*-weighted images can be quite useful. These images can have short TR, allowing thin section acquisition by 3D–Fourier transform technique. The signal intensity loss near bone trabeculae helps depict bone (Fig. 15–4). *Bone marrow* is obscured on T2*-weighted images; spin echo or fast spin echo images, or gradient echo images with short TE, are needed to evaluate bone marrow. T2*-weighted images also depict iron sensitively (Fig. 15–5).

STEADY-STATE FREE PRECESSION

By sampling the spin echoes, rather than the gradient echoes, that result from repeated application of radio pulses, heavily T2-weighted gradient echo images can be obtained (see Chapter 11, Steady-State Free Precession). On these images, TE is approximately twice TR. There is some T2* contrast in addition to T2 contrast, however, since the echo must be sampled at a

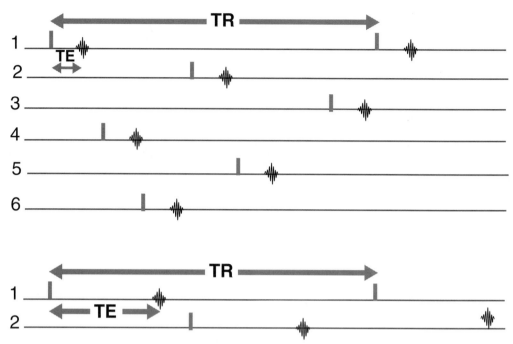

FIGURE 15–1. Effect of TE on efficiency. With short-TE spin echo techniques *(top)*, more sections can be acquired for a given TR than with long-TE spin echo techniques *(bottom)*.

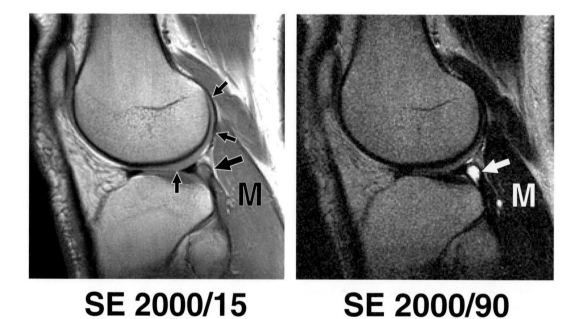

SE 2000/15   SE 2000/90

FIGURE 15–2. Comparison of first and second echo images for inference of tissue T2. With spin echo 2000/15 technique *(left)*, articular cartilage *(small arrows)*, synovial fluid *(large arrow)*, and muscle (M) are all isointense. By comparing these two images, it becomes clear that articular cartilage has a T2 intermediate between the high T2 of synovial fluid and the low T2 of muscle.

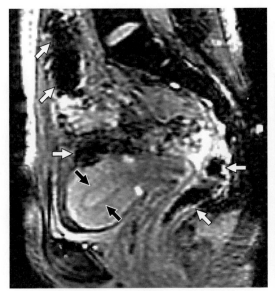 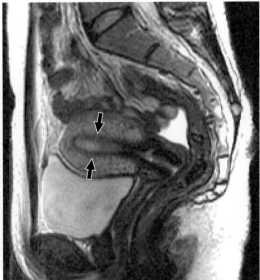

GRE 80/34/20°   FSE 3000/165

FIGURE 15–3. Comparison between T2* and T2 contrast. With gradient echo (GRE) 80/34/20° technique *(left)*, there is moderate contrast between uterine zones *(black arrows)*, but T2* contrast has caused prominent loss of signal intensity near bowel gas *(white arrows)* and in bone marrow. With fast spin echo (FSE) 3000/165 technique, there is more contrast between uterine zones and better image quality.

time when it is not completely refocused. This is because the time of complete refocusing of the spin echo occurs during the next excitation pulse. Owing to short TR, small flip angle, and degradation from magnetic field heterogeneity, steady-state free precession images tend to have low SNR and significant artifacts (Fig. 15–6). SNR is increased and artifacts decreased, however, if 3D acquisition is used. Although not used by most MR clinicians, 3D steady-state free precession techniques have aroused some interest as a way of rapidly obtaining 3D T2-weighted images. In fact, this technique might have become more popular had not fast spin echo been introduced into clinical practice just as steady-state free precession techniques were being developed.

MULTISHOT FAST SPIN ECHO TECHNIQUES

Only a few years after its introduction into clinical practice multishot fast spin echo has become the method of choice for T2-weighted imaging of most body parts. It is a modified spin echo technique that corrects the most glaring

drawback of conventional spin echo imaging for generating T2 contrast: inefficiency.

Conventional spin echo technique is inefficient for generating T2 contrast because the echo time (approximately 100 msec for most applications) is essentially unproductive dead time, except for the generation of a second, less heavily T2-weighted image. Fast spin echo improves efficiency by acquiring data throughout the effective TE (TE_{ef}). If the echoes are acquired rapidly enough (i.e., if echo spacing is minimized) and the echo train is just long enough to allow acquisition of enough echoes to fill the TE_{ef}, fast spin echo images resemble spin echo images. For a given acquisition matrix, fast spin echo images are blurrier than comparable spin echo images; however, the added efficiency of multishot fast spin echo permits the use of a higher acquisition matrix, allowing the generation of images with crisp edge definition (Fig. 15–7).

For most applications, fast spin echo is preferable to standard spin echo for T2-weighted images because of its greater efficiency and flexibility. There are more user-selectable options with fast spin echo techniques, however, and these must be selected carefully for optimal clinical effectiveness. Perhaps the most fundamental difference between these two classes of

FSE 2000/29

FSE 2000/87

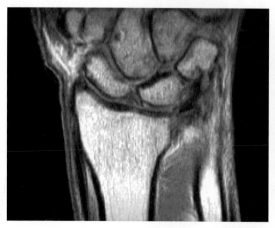

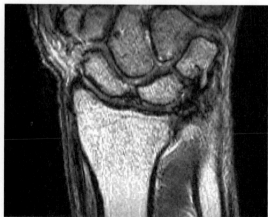

GRE
40/12/45°

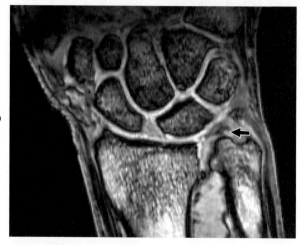

FIGURE 15–4. Comparison of fast spin echo (FSE) and 3D Fourier transform gradient echo (GRE) 40/12/45° images. The 3D gradient echo technique allows acquisition of contiguous 1.2-mm sections, less than half the thickness of the fast spin echo images. Additionally, bone structures are defined more clearly, as is the triangular fibrocartilage complex *(arrow)*.

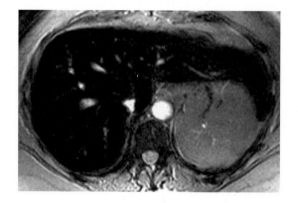

FIGURE 15–5. Gradient echo 20/7/45° image shows markedly decreased signal intensity of the liver relative to spleen, muscle, and other tissues, owing to hepatic iron overload in a patient with preclinical idiopathic hemochromatosis.

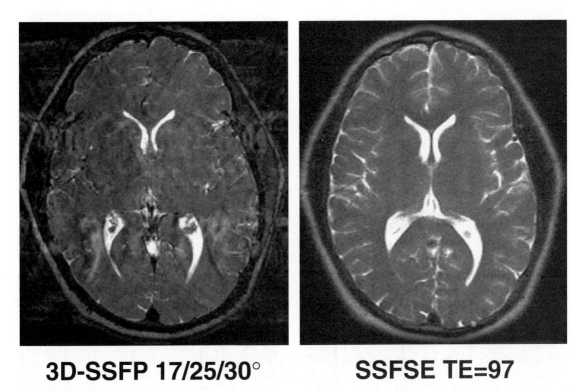

3D-SSFP 17/25/30°   SSFSE TE=97

FIGURE 15-6. Three-dimensional steady-state free precession (3D-SSFP) 17/25/30° technique allows rapid acquisition of T2-weighted images *(left)*, although image quality may be poor. Single-shot fast spin echo image is shown at right for comparison.

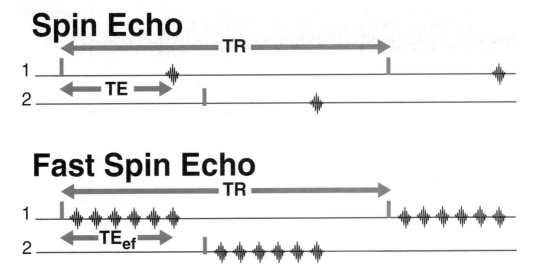

FIGURE 15-7. Fast spin echo techniques reduce acquisition time dramatically as compared with conventional spin echo by acquiring several echoes during the effective TE.

T2-weighted techniques is that with standard T2-weighted images, a second set of images of identical TR and shorter TE can be obtained without increasing acquisition time. With fast spin echo, a subset of the echo train can be designated toward creating a first echo image, but this increases acquisition time in direct proportion to the number of echoes that are not used to form the T2-weighted images. Thus, the use of a dual-echo technique is a virtual "free lunch" with standard spin echo techniques, but not with fast spin echo.

The first step toward choosing a fast spin echo protocol for clinical imaging is to decide whether an image with long TR and short TE_{ef} is necessary. If not, fast spin echo acquisition time can be reduced significantly by designating all echoes toward a single T2-weighted image. For most applications outside the central nervous and musculoskeletal systems, images with long TR and short TE have little clinical importance and can be eliminated safely.

If an image with long TR and short TE_{ef} is considered important, the next step is to decide whether both this image and its corresponding T2-weighted image can be optimized within the constraints of a dual-echo fast spin echo pulse sequence. For most currently available implementations of fast spin echo TR, acquisition matrix, and number of signal averages must be identical between the two pulse sequences. In many situations, images with long TR and short TE can best be optimized by a second separate acquisition rather than as a component accompanying the T2-weighted images. Images with long TR and short TE (commonly referred to as *proton density-weighted,* or more appropriately as *intermediate-weighted images*) are considered in greater detail in Chapter 16.

Fast spin echo allows a greater range of practical choices than does standard spin echo with regard to the familiar parameters of TR and TE_{ef}. With standard spin echo, TR is usually set as the minimum needed to ensure acquisition of sufficient image sections. Increasing TR beyond this length increases acquisition time proportionally. Increasing TE decreases the time during which additional image sections can be excited, decreasing the number of image sections that can be acquired during a given TR. Thus, increasing TE often leads to an increased TR and therefore to an increased acquisition time. Choices of TR and TE on standard spin echo images are often a compromise between the desired tissue contrast and constraints on acquisition time.

With fast spin echo, both TR and TE_{ef} can be increased without increasing acquisition time by making appropriate increases in the number of echoes in the echo train (echo train length). For example, an echo train length of 32 allows one to choose a TE as long as 350 msec or longer with available techniques, without imposing any penalty of acquisition time. Heavily T2-weighted images, with parameters such as TR greater than 10,000 msec and TE_{ef} greater than 200 msec, can therefore be obtained within a few minutes with fast spin echo, but not with standard spin echo. As echo train length increases, the time available for additional image sections per TR decreases, as it does when TE increases with standard spin echo techniques. In contrast to standard spin echo techniques, however, the longer time required for longer TR is balanced by the smaller number of excitation radio pulses needed; because each echo train is longer, fewer trains are needed. In practice, acquisition time changes little, if at all, as TR increases along with echo train length in order that the same number of image sections be acquired (Fig. 15-8).

Once the desired TE_{ef} is chosen for multishot fast spin echo, many other parameters become easier to chose. Generally, the echo train length should be as short as possible, so long as the desired TE_{ef} is one of these echoes. Increasing the echo train length beyond what is needed to accommodate the desired TE_{ef} has little or no effect on acquisition time but leads to increased image blurring and other artifacts. TR is generally chosen as the shortest one necessary to accommodate the echo train length and number of image sections needed. Blurring and artifacts are minimized if the acquisition matrix is high, preferably at least 256×256, and if the field of view is kept as small as possible, within the constraints of SNR and anatomic coverage.

The increased signal intensity of adipose tissue on fast spin echo images can be an advantage or a disadvantage, depending on the clinical application. High signal intensity of adipose tissue, comparable with that typically present on T1-weighted spin echo images, allows clear depiction of anatomic detail delineated by fat planes; however, high–signal intensity lesions, such as bone marrow edema, may become less conspicuous, and artifacts from moving fat increase when adipose tissue has increased signal intensity (Fig. 15-9). The signal intensity of moving fat can be reduced by preceding each radio excitation pulse with a fat-saturation pulse, or with an inversion pulse and short inversion time (TI) chosen to null the signal intensity of adipose tissue.

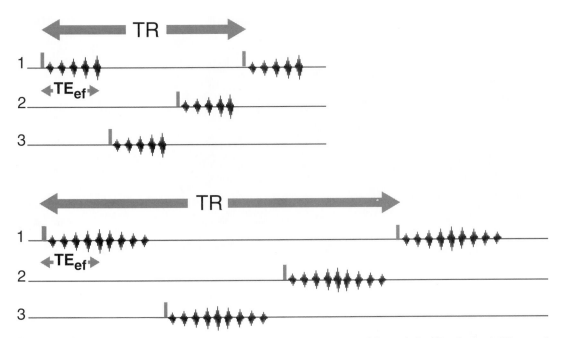

FIGURE 15–8. Relationship of TR and echo train. If echo train is increased beyond the TE_{ef} *(bottom)*, TR must be increased to allow sufficient time for acquisition of a given number of image sections. Overall acquisition time for a given number of image sections is not necessarily changed by increasing the echo train beyond the TE_{ef}.

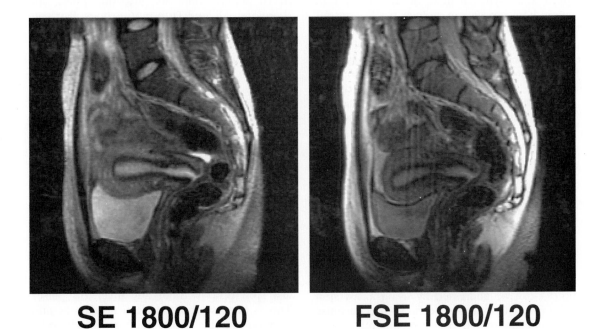

FIGURE 15–9. Effect of high signal intensity of adipose tissue on motion-induced artifact. Sagittal T2-weighted images of the pelvis without fat suppression, using identical TR and TE. The increased signal intensity of adipose tissue with fast spin echo *(right)* has led to increased motion artifact and decreased conspicuousness of the high signal intensity of urine, endometrium, and peritoneal fluid posterior to the cervix.

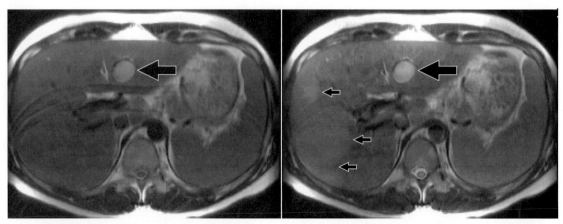

Multi-section FSE   Single-section FSE

FIGURE 15–10. MT effects in multisection fast spin echo *(left)* have obscured liver metastases. A simple cyst *(large arrow)* is very conspicuous. At right, the identical pulse sequence was repeated, but with acquisition of only one image. The conspicuousness of the cyst is unchanged, but the metastases are now visible *(small arrows).*

Reduced signal intensity of solid tissue relative to fat or fluid as a result of magnetization transfer (MT) is a more refractory alteration of contrast on multishot fast spin echo images. MT is helpful for depicting fluids, such as cerebrospinal fluid, synovial fluid, or that in cysts or ducts; however, it can reduce tissue contrast between solid tissues (e.g., between hepatic parenchyma and solid malignant tumor; Fig. 15–10). The decreased contrast is often more than compensated for by increased spatial resolution and SNR, which is possible because of the added efficiency of fast spin echo, leading to more signal averaging and higher acquisition matrix.

FAST SPIN ECHO–INVERSION RECOVERY

Attractive features of short TI inversion recovery (STIR) include nulling of fat signal and synergistic T1 and T2 contrast. The major deficiencies of STIR—low SNR and long acquisition times—can be addressed by using a fast spin echo rather than a single-echo spin echo pulse sequence, following the inversion pulse (Fig. 15–11).

Fast spin echo-STIR techniques involve inverting longitudinal magnetization using a 180° inversion pulse and waiting a delay (i.e., the TI) before the 90° excitation pulse, just as with conventional spin echo STIR. However, with fast spin echo-STIR, a train of echoes follows

each excitation pulse. Just as fast spin echo requires fewer TRs than spin echo to acquire a given amount of data, fast spin echo-STIR requires fewer TIs as well. For example, a fast spin echo-STIR technique with an echo train of 16 requires only one inversion pulse, and therefore only one TI, per 16 echoes. Fast spin echo-STIR is thus far more efficient than conventional spin echo-STIR.

Spin echo-STIR techniques usually use relatively short TEs (e.g., 30 msec or less), because long TEs decrease SNR and decrease the number of image sections that can be acquired per TR. With fast spin echo-STIR, however, longer TE_{ef} are practical. SNR can be maintained because the increased efficiency of fast spin echo–STIR allows more signal averages. Additionally, there is no time penalty to the use of longer TE_{ef} with fast spin echo techniques, including fast spin echo-STIR, as long as the echo train is long enough to cover the TE_{ef}. If long TE_{ef} is used, fast spin echo-STIR images are truly T2-weighted, in addition to the T1 contrast inherent in STIR techniques.

Fast spin echo-STIR is less efficient than is fast spin echo without any inversion pulses. This is because there is often no data acquisition during the TI. As with spin echo-STIR techniques, the TI involves more time during which longitudinal magnetization is recovering toward zero, so that signal magnitude is decreasing. As discussed in Chapter 12 Inversion Recovery, decreasing the TI below the optimal level for nulling of fat signal may increase SNR and increase the number of sections that can

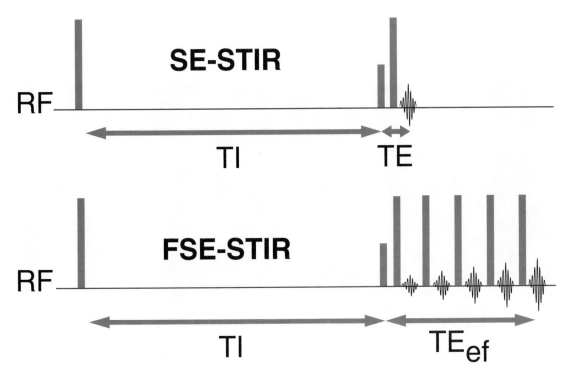

FIGURE 15–11. Compared with conventional spin echo-short TI inversion recovery (SE-STIR) technique *(top)*, more echoes are obtained per inversion pulse with fast spin echo (FSE-STIR) *(bottom)*. Fewer inversion pulses are therefore necessary.

be acquired per TR. The increased efficiency of fast spin echo techniques also renders practical the use of extremely long TIs, allowing nulling of fluid signal on fluid-attenuated inversion recovery (FLAIR) images.

SINGLE-SHOT FAST SPIN ECHO (HASTE) TECHNIQUES

Generally, fast spin echo image quality is best if the echo train is not longer than necessary to fill the TE_{ef} with echoes, because longer echo trains tend to increase blurring and other artifacts. However, there are benefits that result when *all* echoes are obtained in one train.

Single-shot techniques can be used if acquisition time is minimized. Several concurrent strategies are used. Data sampling should be as fast as possible, which can be accomplished using high receiver bandwidth and rapid switching of gradients. Measures to reduce the amount of data needed for image reconstruction further decrease the duration of the echo train. These measures include partial sampling of each echo and half-Fourier reconstruction, which together involve acquisition of only slightly more than 25% of k-space and interpolation of the remainder.

Single-shot fast spin echo has infinite TR, since the excitation pulse is not repeated. This removes T1-weighting. Motion artifact is far less severe on single-shot images, which can often be acquired in less than half a second. Additional benefits include the lack of abrupt transitions in the filling of k-space and, therefore, the absence of certain edge and ghost artifacts that may be more conspicuous on multishot images. Another advantage of single-shot fast spin echo over multishot fast spin echo is reduced MT contrast, because only one image section is excited during any given period. The major limitations of single-shot fast spin echo are low SNR and blurring of tissues with short or intermediate T2. As with multishot fast spin echo, image contrast depends on the order of phase encoding. If the last echo is chosen to provide data for the center of k-space (i.e., the TE_{ef} is extremely long), images will consist entirely of signal from free fluid (Figs. 15–12 and 15–13).

ECHO PLANAR AND GRADIENT ECHO AND SPIN ECHO

Echo planar imaging was implemented initially as a single-shot technique. This form of

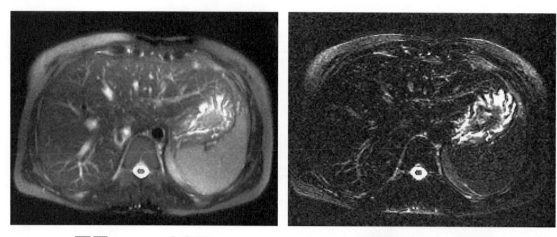

$\text{TE}_{\text{ef}} = 105$ $\text{TE}_{\text{ef}} = 458$

FIGURE 15–12. Axial single-shot fast spin echo images with TE_{ef} of 105 *(left)* and 458 *(right)* msec. With TE_{ef} of 458, only free fluid is visible.

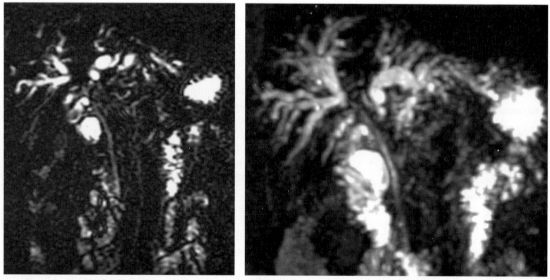

5 mm thick section   Maximum Intensity Projection

FIGURE 15–13. Single-shot fast spin echo technique with TE_{ef} greater than 500 msec. Fluid is depicted clearly. In this example, contiguous 5-mm thick coronal sections *(left)* were obtained during a single breath hold, forming a maximum intensity projection "MR cholangiogram" *(right)* in a patient with an obstructing cholangiocarcinoma at the confluence of the left and right bile ducts.

Single-Shot FSE

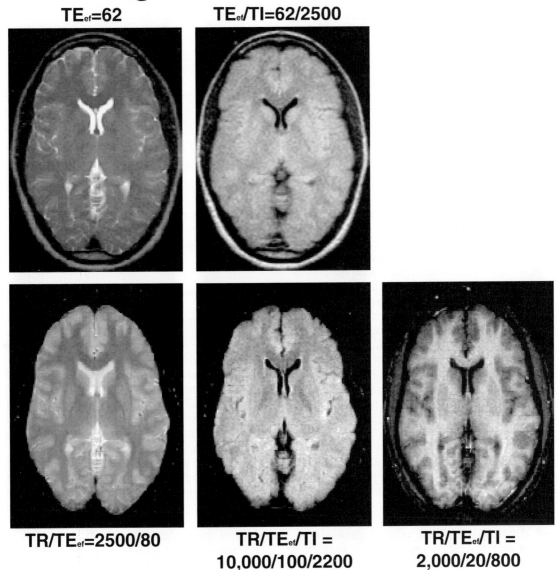

Multishot Echo Planar

FIGURE 15-14. Axial images of the brain using single-shot fast spin echo and multishot spin echo–echo planar techniques. At top, images with TE_{ef} of 62 msec are compared without *(left)* and with *(right)* the use of a single inversion pulse with TI of 2500 msec. With a TI of this length, fluid signal is nulled (fluid-attenuated inversion recovery [FLAIR]). At bottom, echo planar images are compared without an inversion pulse *(left)*, with a TI of 2200 msec (FLAIR) and with short TE_{ef} (20 msec) and TI of 800 msec, producing T1-weighted images. FSE, fast spin echo.

TABLE 15-1. COMPARISON OF T2-WEIGHTED PULSE SEQUENCES*

| Pulse Sequence | Attributes for T2-Weighting | | | |
	Contrast	*SNR*	*Efficiency*	*Artifact-Free*
Spin echo	+ + + +	+	−	+ +
Steady-state free precession	+	−	+ + +	−
Multishot fast spin echo	+ + +	+ + + +	+ + +	+ + +
Single-shot fast spin echo	+ +	−	+ + + +	+ + + +
Fast spin echo–STIR	+ + + +	+ +	+ + +	+ +
Gradient echo	+	+ +	+ + +	+
Spin echo–prepared gradient echo	+	−	+	−
Echo planar	+ + + +	+	+ + + + +	−
GRASE	+ + +	+	+ + + +	+

*Relative advantages of various T2-weighted pulse sequences regarding T2 contrast, SNR, efficiency, and freedom from artifacts. Due to inherent magnetization transfer contrast, soft tissue contrast may be suboptimal for fast spin echo techniques, although other attributes may be more desirable. Signal-to-noise ratio (SNR) is highest for three dimensional Fourier transform (3D-FT) and two dimensional (2D) multisection techniques, and lowest for single section techniques. Efficiency is greatest for echo planar techniques, and least for spin echo or magnetization-prepared techniques.

echo planar imaging is useful principally for maximizing temporal resolution, which is helpful for cardiac imaging and monitoring of other processes that exhibit rapid physiologic variation, such as those documented with functional neuroimaging. Single-shot echo planar T2-weighted techniques have the added advantage of having an "infinite" TR, which eliminates T1 contrast. They have the disadvantage of requiring an extremely long echo train, during which there is no RF refocusing except at the central echo. Artifacts can thus be far more intrusive than with single-shot fast spin echo.

Multishot echo planar techniques have a much shorter echo train length, which leads to less severe susceptibility artifacts than single-shot echo planar. Although multishot techniques do not have infinite TR, they can be obtained with TRs of more than 5000 msec, allowing for nearly complete recovery of longitudinal magnetization; however, susceptibility, eddy current, and chemical shift artifacts can still occur, and, as with other techniques acquired over several seconds or more, multishot echo planar images are very sensitive to motion.

Although long or infinite TR reduces or eliminates T1 contrast, T1-weighted images can be obtained with echo planar technique. By preceding each excitation pulse with an inversion pulse, inversion recovery images can be obtained, as they can with fast spin echo techniques (Fig. 15–14; Table 15–1).

Gradient echo and spin echo (GRASE) technique can be used to produce T2-weighted images with efficiency intermediate between that of fast spin echo and echo planar (see Chapter 13). However, artifacts may degrade the images. GRASE is currently not widely available, and its role in clinical imaging has not yet been defined.

ESSENTIAL POINTS TO REMEMBER

1. Although T2-weighted spin echo images may be diagnostically useful, their acquisition is very inefficient owing to substantial dead time during the long TE.
2. T2- or T2*-weighted gradient echo and steady-state free precession images tend to have significant artifacts from magnetic field heterogeneity.
3. Fast spin echo images have fewer artifacts than gradient echo and steady-state free precession images and can be acquired more efficiently than standard spin echo images.
4. Fast spin echo images tend to be blurrier than standard spin echo images and may have more artifacts. This can be compensated for by using higher acquisition matrices.
5. The high signal intensity of adipose tissue on fast spin echo images, if considered undesirable, can be reduced by using fat-saturation or inversion recovery techniques.
6. Fast spin echo images have more MT contrast than do standard spin echo images. This causes solid tissues to lose more signal intensity than fat or fluid, increasing

the conspicuousness of fluid but reducing some forms of tissue contrast.

7. Dual TE_{ef} fast spin echo techniques require more acquisition time than single TE_{ef} fast spin echo images.

8. With multishot fast spin echo, choice of TE_{ef} should be based on the desired tissue contrast. Echo train should be long enough to accommodate this TE_{ef} but otherwise should generally be as short as possible to reduce artifacts and blurring.

9. Once TE_{ef} and echo train are chosen, TR should generally be chosen to allow adequate anatomic coverage.

10. Echo planar and GRASE images can be acquired in less time than standard spin echo or fast spin echo images, but they may have more artifacts.

11. Single-shot echo planar images can show physiologic phenomena with greater temporal resolution than multishot techniques, but they usually have lower spatial resolution and more artifacts.

16 Intermediate-Weighted Pulse Sequences

Early clinical MRI protocols almost invariably included spin echo images with (1) short repetition time (TR) and short echo time (TE) (T1-weighted), (2) long TR and long TE (T2-weighted), and (3) long TR and short TE. The latter type of image is commonly referred to as being *proton density weighted*. In this chapter we discuss contrast on this image, and explain why, in fact, *intermediate-weighted* is a more appropriate description for such images. We then describe attributes of these images that lend them clinical importance and review the pulse sequences that can be used to obtain this type of contrast.

DEFINITION

T1 contrast is usually achieved by using a TR short enough so that the longitudinal magnetization of some tissues does not relax completely between excitations. T2 contrast is achieved by using a TE long enough so that substantial decay of transverse magnetization of some tissues occurs. In other words, both T1 contrast and T2 contrast depend on achieving lower signal intensity of some tissues than would occur solely from proton density. If the longitudinal magnetization of all tissues is allowed to relax completely between excitations (infinitely long TR and/or small flip angle), and if no transverse magnetization is allowed to decay (infinitely short TE), T1 contrast and T2 contrast could both be eliminated. Tissue contrast would thus be dominated by other contrast mechanisms, such as proton density, chemical shift, and magnetization transfer.

Full recovery of longitudinal magnetization of all tissues can be ensured by using a single-shot technique or if an extremely long TR is used (e.g., 10,000 msec). Decay of transverse

magnetization can be prevented if transverse magnetization is measured as soon as it is created, with TE of 0. Even though pulse sequences have been introduced clinically with TE less than 2 msec, there is some decay of transverse magnetization of some tissues, and therefore at least some T2 or T2* contrast.

The term *proton density weighting* suggests that proton density contrast is, in fact, the dominant contrast mechanism in the image; however, often this is not true. Many so-called proton density weighted images have TR that is too short, or TE that is too long, to completely eliminate T1 and T2 contrast. Tissue contrast on these images commonly includes a combination of T1 and T2 contrast, in addition to other effects such as chemical shift and magnetization transfer.

To indicate that T1 contrast and T2 contrast are present, images with long TR and short TE have been referred to as *balanced,* but this term is also misleading, because it suggests that the effect on tissue contrast of T1 differences is equal to that of T2 differences. There is no basis for this assumption, however, because, depending on the pulse sequence and pair of tissues, either T1 or T2 contrast may dominate.

One term that does not include any incorrect assumptions is *intermediate-weighted.* In all situations, contrast on an image that might be called *proton density weighted* is intermediate between that of a T1-weighted image and a T2-weighted one. Therefore, we recommend use of this term in place of more popular but less appropriate terms such as *proton density weighted.*

ATTRIBUTES FOR CLINICAL USE

Intermediate-weighted images usually have higher overall signal-to-noise ratio (SNR) than comparable T1-weighted or T2-weighted pulse sequences because longitudinal recovery is maximized and transverse decay minimized. Generally, intermediate-weighted images are particularly useful for depicting structures with low signal intensity, such as bone, fibrous tissue, or air, contrasted with a background of soft tissues or fluid with higher signal intensity. These often can be depicted best if intermediate-weighted images are acquired using high-resolution technique, taking advantage of their typically high SNR. Intermediate-weighted images are useful for imaging the brain, vertebral column, and musculoskeletal system. They provide a useful combination of mild T1 contrast and mild T2 contrast (Fig. 16–1).

SPIN ECHO TECHNIQUES

Spin echo technique is generally the best method for obtaining intermediate-weighted images. During the first decade of clinical MRI, intermediate-weighted images were routinely obtained as the first echo of a dual-echo spin echo technique. In this manner, intermediate-weighted and T2-weighted images are obtained simultaneously, in the acquisition time necessary for T2-weighted images alone. If spin echo technique is used to obtain T2-weighted images, obtaining a first echo with short TE is certainly the most efficient way to provide additional images with intermediate weighting.

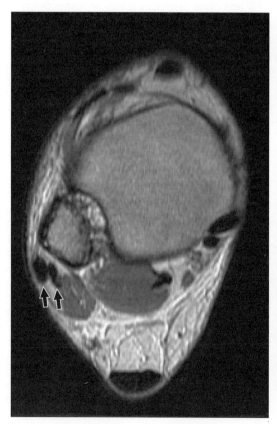

FSE 4433/40

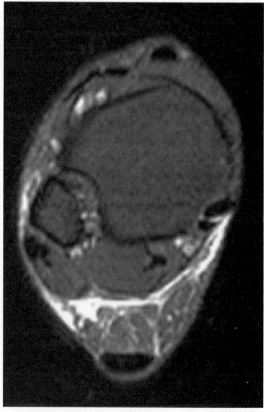

FatSat FSE 3817/72

FIGURE 16–1. Axial intermediate-weighted fast spin echo (FSE) 4433/40 image of the ankle *(left)*. TE_{ef} of 40 msec is long enough for tendons to be depicted as signal voids but short enough for muscle to have much higher signal intensity. A shorter echo train length (4), and a larger matrix (512 × 256) were used than for the fat-saturated T2-weighted FSE 3817/72 image at right. Separate acquisition of intermediate- and T2-weighted images allows separate optimization of parameters for each. Arrows in image at left indicate the peroneus longus and brevis tendons, which are depicted more clearly than at right; however, high-signal perimuscular edema is shown better at right.

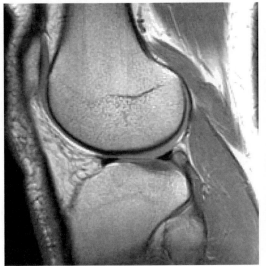
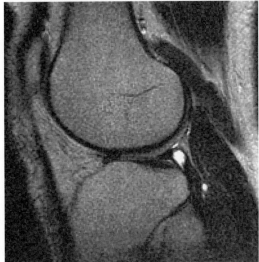

SE 2000/15   SE 2000/90

FIGURE 16-2. Double spin echo sagittal images of the knee. The intermediate-weighted image *(left)* depicts anatomic detail with high SNR and no additional time for acquisition than the T2-weighted image *(right)*, which is needed to depict fluid. TR, matrix, and other parameters are identical.

When intermediate images are acquired simultaneously with T2-weighted spin echo (SE) images, TR, acquisition matrix, section thickness, and many other parameters are identical for both images (Fig. 16-2).

FAST SPIN ECHO VERSUS SPIN ECHO TECHNIQUES

For most applications fast spin echo (FSE) is replacing spin echo as the preferred technique for acquiring T2-weighted images. With fast spin echo, acquisition of intermediate-weighted images in addition to T2-weighted images takes substantially longer than acquisition of T2-weighted images alone. Therefore, simultaneous acquisition of intermediate-weighted and T2-weighted images by dual-echo fast spin echo is not the only method that should be considered.

If intermediate-weighted and T2-weighted images are acquired together as part of a dual-echo pulse sequence, parameters such as TR, acquisition matrix, and number of signal averages, must be identical, even though the *optimal* parameters may not be identical for the two images. Acquisition of two independent

sets of images should be considered so that intermediate-weighted and T2-weighted images can be optimized separately. The two most attractive techniques for acquiring intermediate-weighted images are multishot fast spin echo and spin echo, so these techniques are compared next.

Blurring with fast spin echo is most severe when the effective TE (TE_{ef}) is short, because of the rapid changes in transverse magnetization between successive echoes that occur at short TE_{ef}. Since the high spatial resolution of intermediate-weighted images is one of their most important attributes, it is especially important to eliminate any source of blurring. For this reason, intermediate-weighted images should generally be acquired using standard spin echo technique (Fig. 16-3). Alternatively, intermediate-weighted fast spin echo images with mild T2-weighted and short echo train may be useful, particularly for musculoskeletal imaging.

The principal advantage of fast spin echo versus spin echo for acquiring images with long TE is that, with fast spin echo, the TE_{ef} is not dead time that decreases the efficiency of data acquisition. With short TE/TE_{ef} imaging, however, the efficiency of data acquisition is similar with fast spin echo and spin echo. Spin echo remains an attractive technique for acquiring intermediate images, even if it is no longer a

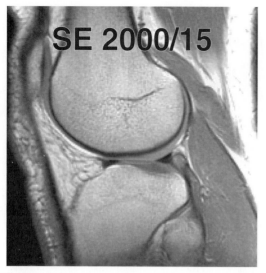 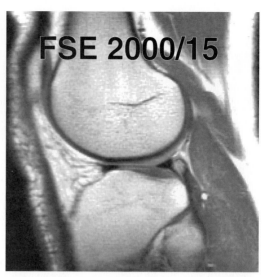

FIGURE 16–3. Image detail on sagittal 2000/15 images is slightly superior with spin echo technique *(left)* than with fast spin echo technique *(right)*.

"free lunch" associated with acquisition of T2-weighted images.

T2-weighted images require long TR to reduce contributions from T1 contrast. Additionally, because there are no data acquisitions during the long TEs used for T2-weighted spin echo acquisitions, long TR is often needed to ensure adequate anatomic coverage. Thus, dual spin echo techniques may require longer TR than is necessary to produce satisfactory intermediate-weighted images.

OPTIMIZING INDEPENDENT ACQUISITION OF INTERMEDIATE-WEIGHTED IMAGES

Intermediate-weighted pulse sequences are usually used to provide clear definition of high-contrast structures (e.g., bone, ligaments) rather than to depict subtle tissue contrast. Thus, a mild component of T1 contrast, resulting from incompletely recovered longitudinal magnetization of some tissues, may not substantially reduce the utility of intermediate-weighted pulse sequences. Because of the highly efficient data acquisition of pulse sequences with short TE, long TR may not be needed to provide adequate anatomic coverage with intermediate-weighted spin echo pulse sequences. For example, a TR of 3000 msec might be needed for adequate coverage with TE of 100 msec, whereas a TR of 1200 msec might

be sufficient if TE is 15 msec. Clarity of the desired lesions and anatomic structures is more important than using a TR as long as that used for T2-weighted images. The use of an "intermediate" TR such as this may allow depiction of the desired anatomy in shorter acquisition time (Figs. 16–4 and 16–5).

Other parameters may also be optimized separately when intermediate-weighted pulse images are acquired independently. Because of their high SNR, intermediate-weighted pulse sequences can often be obtained with smaller voxel size—and therefore with higher spatial resolution—than can T2-weighted images.

If other parameters are left unchanged, either the echo train length or the TR must be doubled to change from a single TE_{ef} to a dual-TE_{ef} multishot fast spin echo acquisition. Doubling the TR reduces contributions from T1 contrast, which is usually desirable with fast spin echo. Increasing the echo train length, however, generally increases blurring and the severity of artifacts.

If a dual-TE_{ef} multishot fast spin echo pulse sequence is changed to a single-TE_{ef} sequence, acquisition time of the T2-weighted pulse sequence can be decreased by approximately 50%. In most instances, the acquisition time is reduced by lowering TR. If this reduced TR introduces unwanted T1 contrast, image quality can deteriorate. (For example, sagittal coverage of the spine might be accomplished using a dual-TE_{ef} technique with TR of 2500 msec. Reducing TR to 1250 msec for a single–TE_{ef} acquisition is unlikely to yield satisfactory T2-

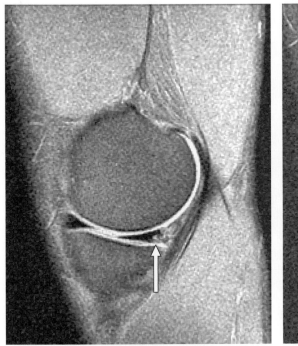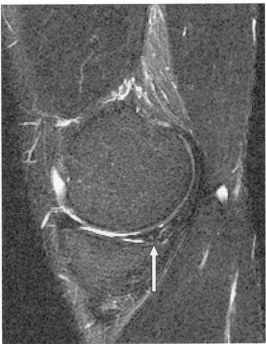

SE 1283/25   FSE 4733/100

FIGURE 16-4. Separate optimization of intermediate-weighted spin echo *(left)* and T2-weighted fast spin echo *(right)* images of the knee, both with fat suppression. For the intermediate-weighted images, a TR of 1283 msec was long enough for coverage of the entire knee. Arrows indicate a tear of the posterior horn of the medial meniscus.

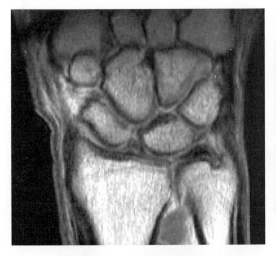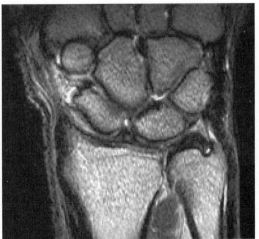

FSE 2000/29   FSE 4000/87

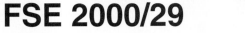

FIGURE 16-5. Separate optimization of intermediate-weighted *(left)* and T2-weighted *(right)* fast spin echo images of the wrist. With shorter TE_ef and short echo train, the intermediate-weighted image shows ligaments of the wrist more clearly. The shorter echo train allowed adequate coverage with a TR half that of the T2-weighted image.

weighted images.) One alternative is to double echo train length rather than reducing TR, possibly exacerbating blurring and artifacts. Alternatively, the best choice in this situation might be to use a dual-TE_{ef} multishot fast spin echo technique, even though the intermediate-weighted image may have poorer quality than a comparable image obtained with standard spin echo technique. Essentially, the choice here is whether to prioritize optimization of the T2-weighted or the intermediate-weighted images. The other set of images should then be tailored

to avoid unduly prolonging total examination time.

GRADIENT ECHO TECHNIQUES

Gradient echo technique can be used to obtain intermediate-weighted pulse sequences, although it is more difficult to remove T2* contrast or chemical shift effects. For these reasons, gradient echo technique is not often used to

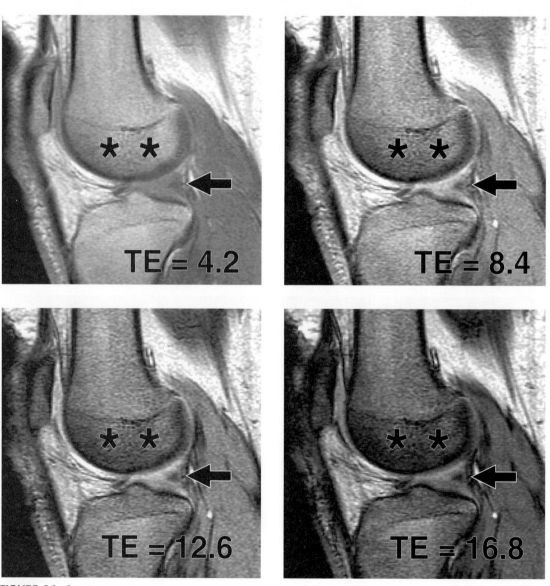

FIGURE 16–6. Effects of increasing echo time (TE) on clarity of fibrocartilage and trabecular bone. In-phase spoiled gradient echo images show the posterior horn of the lateral meniscus *(arrow)* with increasing clarity as TE increases. In addition, note decreasing signal intensity of the distal femoral epiphysis (**) owing to increasing susceptibility contrast from bone trabeculae.

TABLE 16–1. COMPARISON OF INTERMEDIATE-WEIGHTED PULSE SEQUENCES*

Pulse Sequence	Attributes			
	Contrast	*SNR*	*Efficiency*	*Artifact-Free*
Spin echo	+ + +	+ + + +	+ + +	+ + + +
Multishot fast spin echo	+ + +	+ + + +	+ + +	+ + +
Gradient echo	+ + +	+ + + +	+ + + +	+ + +

*Relative advantages of various intermediate-weighted pulse sequences regarding contrast, SNR, efficiency, and freedom from artifacts. All three techniques can generate high-quality images, although artifacts tend to be least with spin echo techniques. The gradient echo technique is most efficient.

obtain intermediate-weighted images, unless three-dimensional Fourier transform (3D-FT) images with intermediate weighting are desired.

To reduce T1 contrast, intermediate-weighted gradient echo images can be acquired using intermediate (e.g., less than 800 msec) or short (e.g., less than 50 msec) TR and reduced excitation flip angle. Reducing the excitation flip angle decreases the saturation resulting from each excitation radio pulse and thus reduces the time needed for complete recovery of longitudinal magnetization after excitation. The use of increasingly shorter TRs demands increasingly smaller flip angles, especially if T1 contrast is not desired.

To reduce the contribution of T2* contrast, TE must be minimized. This may be difficult if chemical shift effects are not desired. To eliminate chemical shift effects, the TE must be a multiple of the period with which methylene (CH₂) and water protons with respect to each other oscillate between in-phase and opposed-phase. The shortest TE that can be used to obtain such in-phase images is approximately 4.2 msec at 1.5 T, approximately 6.3 msec at 1.0 T, and 12.6 msec at 0.5 T. Maximally opposed-phase images with minimized TEs can be achieved at these field strengths, respectively, with TEs of 2.1, 3.15, and 6.3 msec. Shorter TEs than these have milder chemical shift effects.

For some applications, complete elimination of T2* contrast on intermediate-weighted images may not be desirable. For example, fibrocartilage and tendons are best depicted by en-

suring that they have low signal intensity. These structures may have too much signal intensity, and therefore be obscured, if the TE is too short (Fig. 16–6).

ESSENTIAL POINTS TO REMEMBER

1. Both T1 and T2 contrast can be reduced by using both long TR and short TE. Other contrast mechanisms, such as proton density, chemical shift, and magnetization transfer then become more conspicuous.
2. The term *proton density weighting* is misleading, because proton density is not necessarily the most important source of contrast on these images. A preferable expression is *intermediate weighting*.
3. Intermediate-weighted images tend to have high SNR and to show low-signal structures, such as bone and ligaments, with great anatomic detail.
4. Spin echo technique allows efficient acquisition of high-quality intermediate-weighted images, whether as a separate acquisition or along with T2-weighted images as part of a dual-TE technique.
5. Image quality of intermediate-weighted images is usually better with standard spin echo than with fast spin echo technique because they have less blurring and fewer artifacts.
6. Separate acquisition of T2-weighted images using fast spin echo technique and of intermediate-weighted images using standard spin echo technique allows parameters for each of these acquisitions to be optimized independently. This allows the use of shorter TR and higher resolution for the intermediate-weighted images.
7. Intermediate-weighted images can be obtained using gradient echo technique with small flip angle and short TE, but additional contrast from T2* and chemical shift differences is more difficult to eliminate than with spin echo technique.
8. With gradient echo technique, T1 contrast can be minimized, even with relatively short TR, if the excitation flip angle is reduced.

CHAPTER

17 Contrast Agents

Current clinical MRI techniques are based entirely on measuring signals from protons. The active components of most MRI contrast agents contain no protons and, thus, are not detected directly during the MR measurement process; however, the contrast agents act by shortening the relaxation time of water protons that are close to the contrast agent. Therefore, MRI contrast agents act by a mechanism different from that of contrast agents for all other modalities.

Most contrast agents reduce both T1 and T2 relaxation, but some affect one more than they do the other. The effect of contrast agents depends on their biodistribution as well as on pulse sequence parameters.

In this chapter, we consider a variety of contrast agents, classified principally by their biodistribution and tissue effects. Relevant compartments to consider include the intravascular space, which can be subdivided into (1) arterial-capillary and (2) venous spaces; the interstitial space; the reticuloendothelial system; and the parenchymal cells of various organs. Some contrast agents principally affect one of these compartments, while others are distributed to two or more of them. Figure 17–1 depicts the relevant compartments in hepatic parenchyma, as an example of the biodistribution of various MRI contrast agents. After considering current intravenous and oral agents, we will discuss their nomenclature.

EXTRACELLULAR PARAMAGNETIC AGENTS

3The extracellular space consists of the sum of the intravascular and interstitial spaces. Currently available chelates of gadolinium (e.g., gadopentetate dimeglumine, gadoteridol, gadoversetamide, and gadodiamide) are considered extracellular space agents. Materials such as these are distributed initially within the intravascular space and diffuse rapidly throughout the extracellular (vascular plus interstitial) space, much as water-soluble iodinated contrast agents do.

Although these agents have been described as "nonspecific," they can be quite specific and versatile if proper attention is directed toward choice of pulse sequence and timing of image acquisition relative to contrast agent administration. Immediately after intravenous injection, these agents first traverse the pulmonary circulation and are then distributed throughout systemic arteries, followed by distribution throughout the vascular space. Within seconds, substantial amounts of contrast material diffuse across capillaries into the interstitial space of tissues outside the central nervous system and across renal glomeruli into the urinary collecting system. One can consider three basic phases of vascular and tissue enhancement following administration of extracellular space agents—arterial, blood pool, and extracellular phases.

Arterial Phase

If the image data for the center of k-space are acquired during the first pass of contrast agent through the arterial system, arteriographic images can be obtained. Although two-dimensional Fourier transform (2D-FT) techniques may be used for these gadolinium-enhanced arteriograms, 3D-FT techniques are preferable for acquiring thin, contiguous sections that can be used to generate projection images via maximum intensity projection (MIP) (Fig. 17–2).

Images obtained during the arterial phase are also useful for depicting tissue perfusion. Only

213

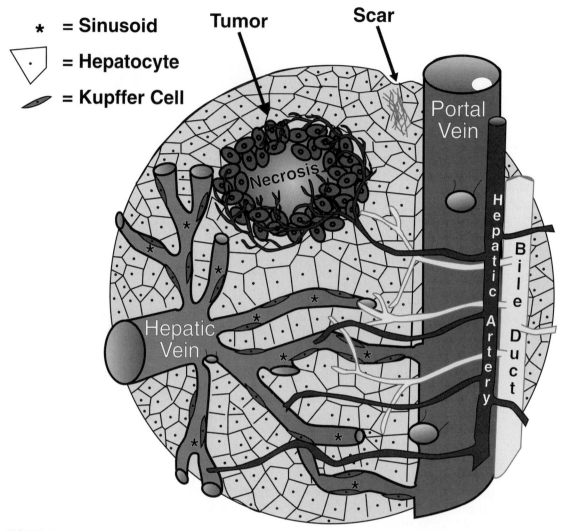

* = Sinusoid

= Hepatocyte

= Kupffer Cell

Tumor

Scar

Portal Vein

Hepatic Artery

Bile Duct

Hepatic Vein

Necrosis

FIGURE 17-1. Compartments within the liver serve as an example for biodistribution of various MRI contrast agents. The hepatic vascular supply comes principally via the portal vein, while the hepatic artery supplies about one third of its perfusion. These vessels drain into hepatic sinusoids, the abundance of which gives the liver a large blood volume. Kupffer cells are reticuloendothelial cells that line the walls of hepatic sinusoids. Tumors tend to have abundant arterial supply, while scars are hypovascular. Both tumors and scars have large interstitial spaces. Hepatocytes produce bile, which is excreted into bile ducts.

images captured during this phase can be used to judge a tissue's vascularity; images obtained at a later phase are affected by contrast agent in the venous and capillary systems and in tissue interstitium (Figs. 17–3 and 17–4).

Arterial phase images are best acquired using pulse sequences that allow completion of imaging within 30 seconds or less. Suitable techniques include single-section or multisection 2D-FT spoiled gradient echo images or 3D-FT spoiled gradient echo images with very short repetition time (TR). Preparation pulses, such as fat suppression or inversion recovery, can improve depiction of enhancing tissue, al-

though they increase acquisition time. The contrast agent must be injected rapidly (e.g., faster than 2 ml per second), either by hand or by machine. The contrast agent bolus should be followed by a rapid flush of approximately 10 to 20 ml of saline or other solution to clear the intravenous tubing and peripheral veins of contrast agent.

The arterial phase is the most technically difficult one to image. The window of opportunity for this phase—between initial arrival of contrast material in arteries and filling of veins—is usually no longer than 20 seconds. Signs of a successful acquisition of arterial-

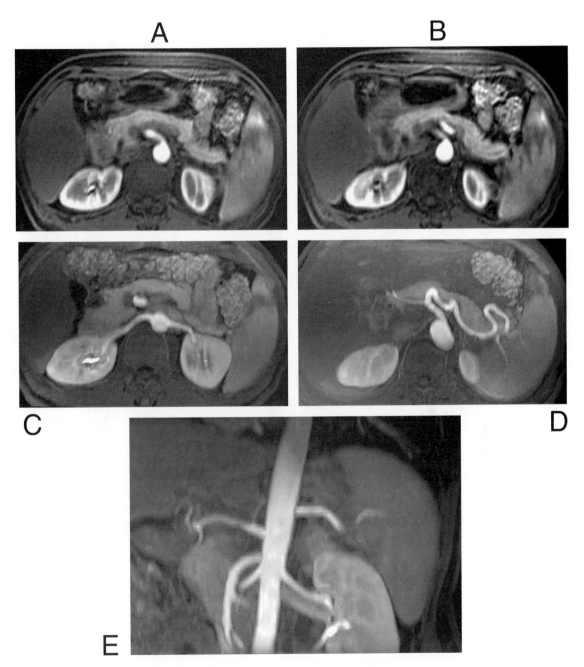

FIGURE 17–2. Arterial phase 3D gradient echo images used to generate MRA images. *(A)* and *(B)* Axial 5-mm sections obtained immediately after a bolus of 0.1 mmol/kg of gadolinium chelate. *C* and *D,* Axial MIP images at, respectively, the renal artery and celiac axis levels. *E,* Oblique coronal reconstruction shows these vessels.

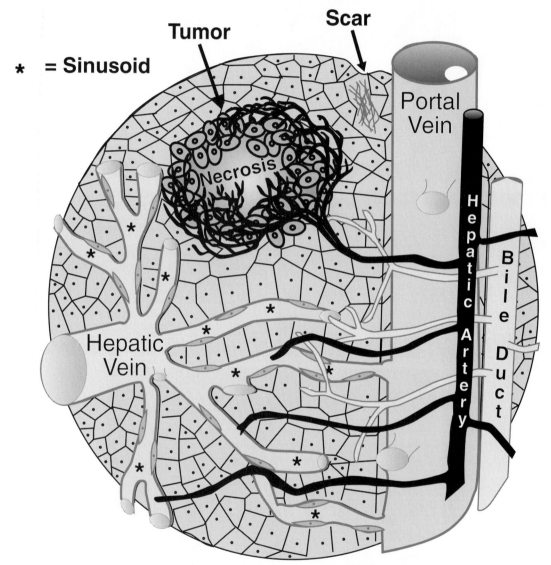

FIGURE 17–3. Early arterial phase of hepatic enhancement. Dark shades indicate arterial enhancement. There is no enhancement of portal veins, sinusoids (*), or hepatic veins. Intense enhancement of the tumor is due to its abundant arterial supply.

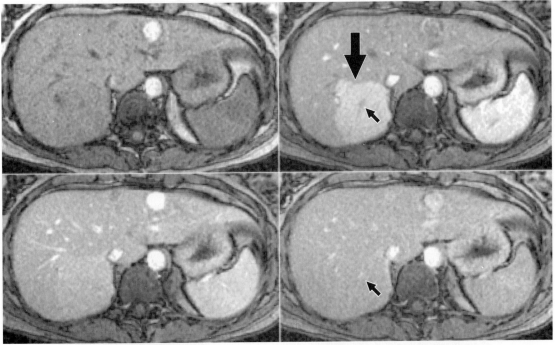

Unenhanced

Arterial

Blood Pool

Extracellular

FIGURE 17–4. Hypervascular hepatic focal nodular hyperplasia *(large arrow)*, depicted best on T1-weighted spoiled gradient echo 122/2.3/90° images during the arterial phase after injection of gadolinium chelate. The mass is subtle during later phases, because the size of its blood pool and extracellular space are similar to those of the liver. Small arrow indicates a central scar that is hyperintense only during the extracellular phase, because it has a larger extracellular space than the rest of the tumor, even though it is less vascular.

phase images include intense enhancement of arteries and little or no enhancement of veins. In the abdomen, arterial phase images are characterized by intense and approximately equivalent enhancement of pancreas, spleen, and renal cortex; marked heterogeneity of the spleen; near absence of renal medullary enhancement; and minimal enhancement of liver parenchyma. Although contrast material is usually visible in major portal vein branches on good capillary phase images of the liver, there is little if any contrast material in microscopic portal branches and in hepatic sinusoids, and none in the hepatic veins (except for the major central hepatic veins in some patients with tricuspid regurgitation) (Figs. 17–5 and 17–6).

Blood Pool Phase

Less than a minute after intravenous injection, contrast material typically is distributed throughout the body's blood vessels. At this time the distribution of extracellular space contrast agents most closely approximates the blood pool, although some diffusion into the interstitial space and renal tubules has occurred. Throughout much of the body, tumors are depicted best during this phase, owing to the small blood pool of skeletal muscle (Fig. 17–7).

In the abdomen, the blood pool phase is usually referred to as the *portal venous phase,* although arteries and parenchymal tissues are enhanced prominently during this phase as well. Although hypervascular tissues such as the pancreas enhance maximally during the arterial phase, the blood pool phase is the phase of maximal hepatic enhancement (see Fig. 17–6); approximately two thirds of blood flow to normal livers is supplied by the portal circulation, which arrives 20 to 30 seconds after hepatic arterial flow (Fig. 17–8). Because of the large volume of blood in hepatic sinusoids, even many moderately hypervascular malignancies

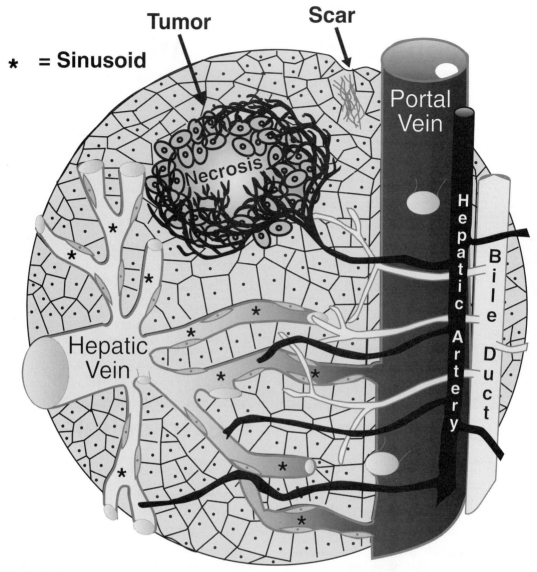

FIGURE 17-5. Late arterial phase. Although there is some enhancement of the portal vein and its major branches, the sinusoids (*) and hepatic veins are not yet enhanced.

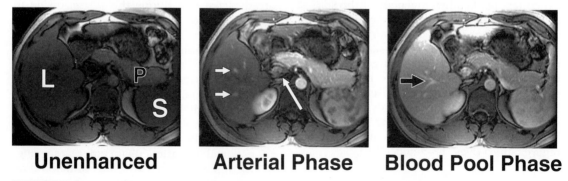

FIGURE 17-6. Axial images of the abdomen obtained before *(left)* and during the arterial *(center)* and blood pool *(right)* phases after bolus injection of gadolinium chelate. The liver (L) enhances little during the arterial phase, while the pancreas (P) and spleen (S) enhance intensely. There is some contrast material in the main portal vein *(long white arrow)* and its major branches *(short white arrows)*. During the blood pool phase, contrast material has filled hepatic sinusoids, causing the liver to become isointense with pancreas and spleen. Black arrow indicates enhanced hepatic vein.

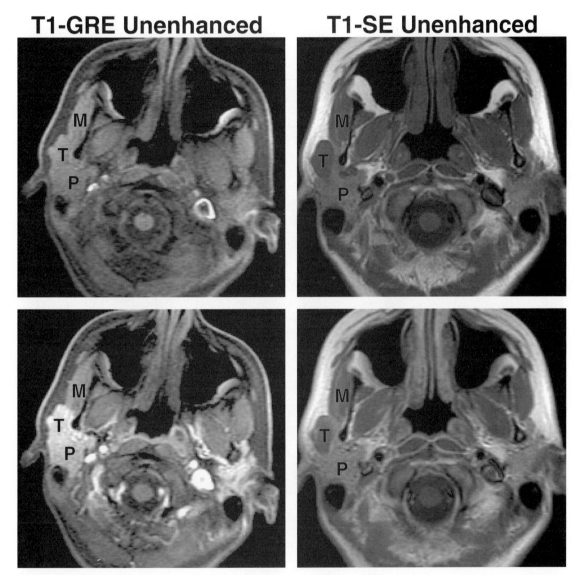

FIGURE 17–7. Hypervascular parotid tumor (T) at the anterior edge of the parotid gland (P) is isointense with skeletal muscle (M) on unenhanced images *(top left, top right)* and during the extracellular phase *(bottom right)*. Contrast with muscle is greatest during the vascular phase *(bottom left)*. The parotid gland is hyperintense compared with tumor on T1-spin echo images before and after contrast agent administration, owing to fat content; fat is suppressed on the gradient echo images.

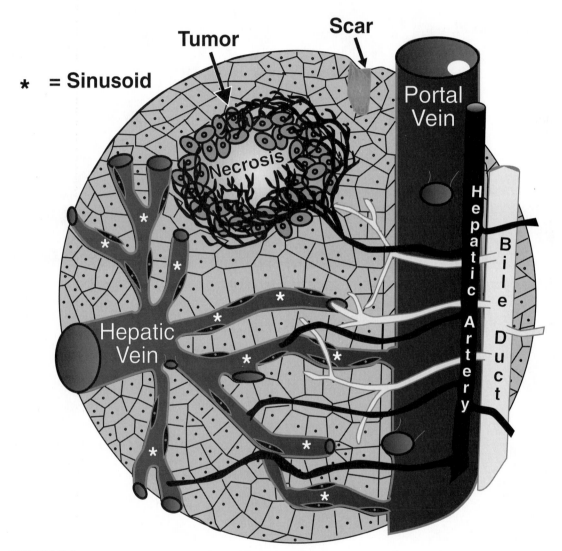

FIGURE 17–8. Blood pool (portal venous) phase. All blood vessels, including arteries, veins, and hepatic sinusoids (*), are filled with contrast material. Necrotic tumor and scar have small blood pools and, thus, are relatively unenhanced.

are less intense than liver on these images. Contrast between liver and hypovascular lesions is maximal on blood pool phase images (Fig. 17-9). Hypervascular lesions may be obscured on these images, however, because their blood pool may be similar to or greater than that of hepatic parenchyma (Fig. 17-10).

Extracellular Phase

Extracellular phase images are acquired at least 2 minutes after injection of contrast material. By this time, contrast material has diffused widely across capillary walls into the interstitium of most tissues, although there is still substantial contrast agent in the vessels (Fig. 17-

11). Capillaries in the central nervous system and the testes are not permeable to contrast agents, unlike capillaries throughout the rest of the body. Interstitial contrast enhancement is particularly prominent in edematous tissues such as neoplasms and areas of inflammation. Fibrous tissue typically has a large interstitial space. Therefore, fibrous tissue is much enhanced on extracellular phase images, although it is usually extremely hypovascular. Many metastases have large interstitial spaces and are therefore hyperintense on extracellular phase images (Fig. 17-12).

In addition to diffusing across tissue capillary walls, extracellular space contrast agents diffuse across glomerular walls into renal tubules, within which they are concentrated as water is

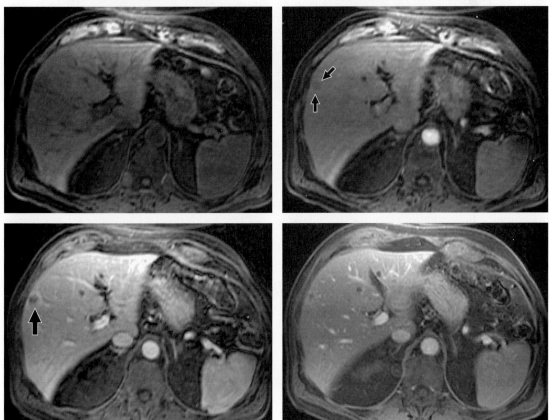

Unenhanced   **Arterial Phase**

Blood Pool Phase   **Extracellular Phase**

FIGURE 17–9. Hypovascular hepatic metastasis from colonic carcinoma depicted best on blood pool (portal venous) phase images (T1-weighted gradient echo images with fat saturation). The lesion is subtle on unenhanced image *(top left)*. During the arterial phase *(top right)*, there is subtle rim enhancement *(small arrows)*. The lesion is best seen during the blood pool phase *(arrow; bottom left)* and is subtle during the extracelluar phase.

Unenhanced   Arterial

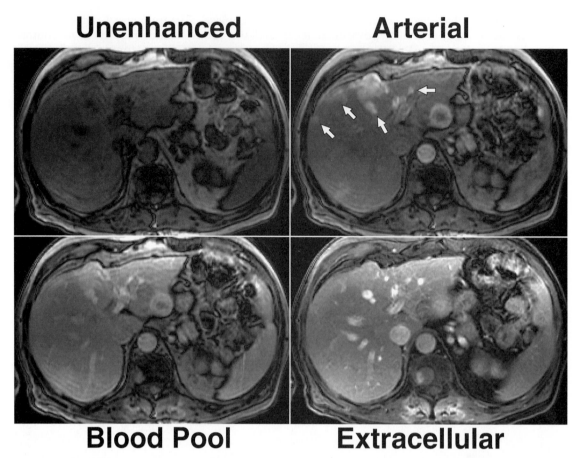

Blood Pool   Extracellular

FIGURE 17-10. Hypervascular metastases *(arrows)* are best depicted during the arterial phase, after injection of gadolinium chelate. On later phases, the lesions are subtle or obscured.

reabsorbed. Elimination of current extracellular space MRI contrast agents occurs entirely by renal excretion. Owing to the concentration of extracellular space agents in the renal parenchyma and collecting system, these agents are highly effective for enhancing renal MRI.

Since the extracellular phase of enhancement changes little over several minutes, fast scanning techniques are less important than they are for acquiring arterial or blood pool phase images. Frequently, extracellular phase images are obtained with suppression of lipid signal intensity via frequency-selective saturation. On these images, interstitial enhancement is particularly conspicuous. Note that, if fat is nulled via inversion recovery with short inversion time (STIR), enhancing tissue is also nulled because of its short T1 relaxation time. Therefore, STIR technique is not recommended after administration of T1-shortening contrast agents.

Brain and testicular capillaries are not permeable to gadolinium chelates. This is the basis for most clinical use of contrast agents for imaging the central nervous system (Fig. 17-13). Enhancement of the brain is minimal, owing entirely to enhancement of the blood pool. Tumors and injured brain parenchyma enhance much more, because of the enhancement of their interstitial spaces. Depiction on postcontrast images of brain lesions as high-signal intensity entities is best if at least a few minutes elapse after injection of contrast agent. This interval allows contrast agent to diffuse into the interstitium of diseased tissue while the blood pool contrast agent concentration decreases. Extracellular phase images are helpful for documenting enhancement of solid masses, allowing them to be distinguished from cysts. Careful comparison to adjacent tissues, either visually or quantitatively, may be necessary (Fig. 17-14).

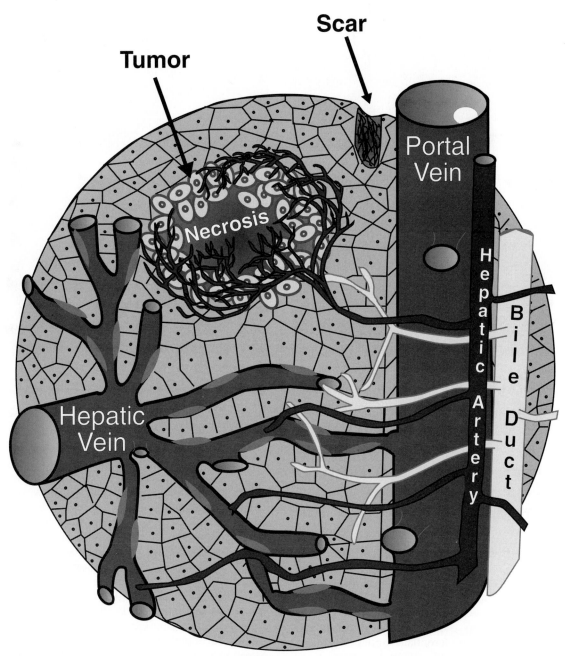

FIGURE 17-11. Extracellular phase. The entire extracellular space, including the vascular and interstitial compartments, is enhanced. Many tumors and scars have a large interstitial space and thus are hyperintense during this phase.

Unenhanced

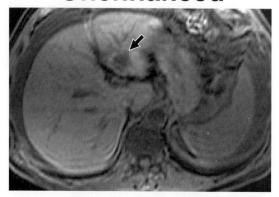

Arterial Phase

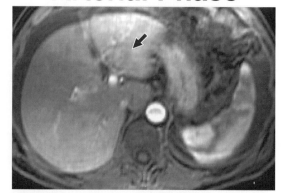

Blood Pool Phase

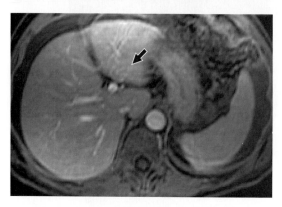

Extracellular Phase

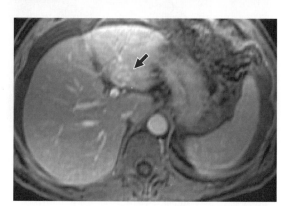

FIGURE 17–12. Hypervascular liver lesion *(arrows)*, obscured on arterial and on blood pool (portal venous) phase images, is depicted as hyperintense during the extracellular phase because of its large interstitial space.

TISSUE-DIRECTED PARAMAGNETIC AGENTS

Gadolinium Chelates

Attachment of a suitable structure to an extracellular gadolinium chelate may allow it to be transported across cell membranes. Compounds such as these have been developed most often for preferentially enhancing hepatocytes (Fig. 17-15). Hepatocyte-directed paramagnetic agents that have been tested in humans include gadobenate dimeglumine (formerly Gd-BOPTA) and gadoxetic acid, disodium (formerly Gd-EOB-DTPA).

Like other gadolinium chelates, these tissue-directed chelates diffuse across non–central nervous system capillaries and renal glomeruli,

accumulating in interstitial spaces and in urine. Unlike extracellular space chelates, however, tissue-directed gadolinium chelates have dual excretory pathways, being eliminated by both renal and hepatobiliary routes. In this respect, the biodistribution of these agents resembles that of iodinated radiographic contrast agents more than that of extracellular space gadolinium chelates, because iodinated agents also have a dual excretory pathway. However, both gadobenate dimeglumine and gadoxetic acid disodium have higher ratios of biliary to renal excretion than do iodinated radiographic contrast agents.

The proportion of renal versus hepatobiliary elimination depends on the particular contrast agent, and on the patient's relative renal and hepatobiliary function. Five or ten minutes after intravenous administration, substantial contrast agent has been distributed throughout the vas-

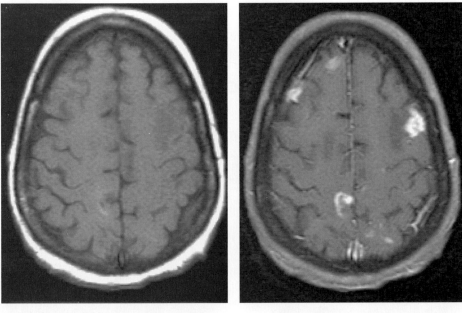

Unenhanced   **Enhanced**

FIGURE 17–13. Enhancement of intracranial metastases. After administration of gadolinium chelate *(right)*, there is little enhancement of brain parenchyma owing to the blood-brain barrier. Contrast material had diffused into the interstitium of the metastases, causing intense enhancement of them.

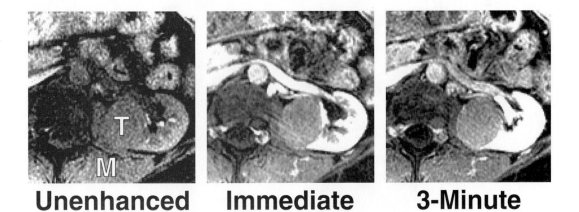

Unenhanced   Immediate   3-Minute

FIGURE 17–14. Hypovascular renal carcinoid tumor (T) with subtle enhancement. The tumor is slightly less intense than skeletal muscle (M) before administration of contrast agent *(left)*; isointense during the vascular phase *(center)*; and slightly hyperintense during the extracellular phase *(right)*. A cyst would be less intense than skeletal muscle during these phases, owing to greater enhancement of skeletal muscle relative to that of the cyst.

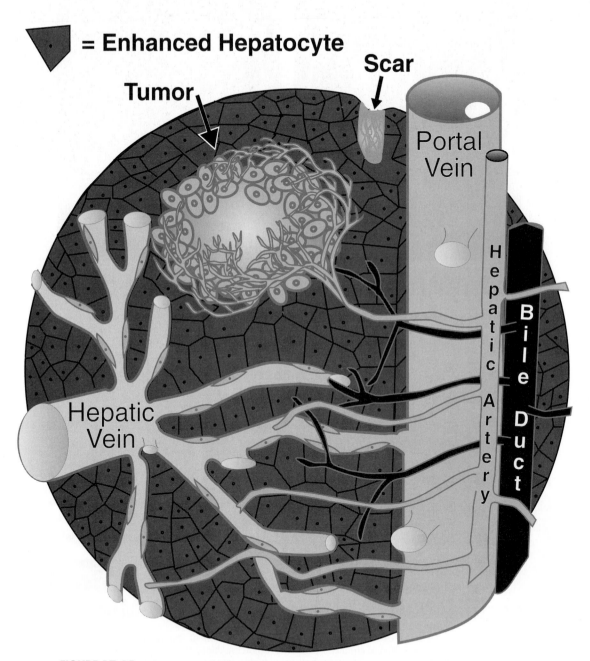

FIGURE 17–15. Enhancement of hepatocytes and bile ducts by hepatocyte-directed contrast material.

Unenhanced   1 Minute

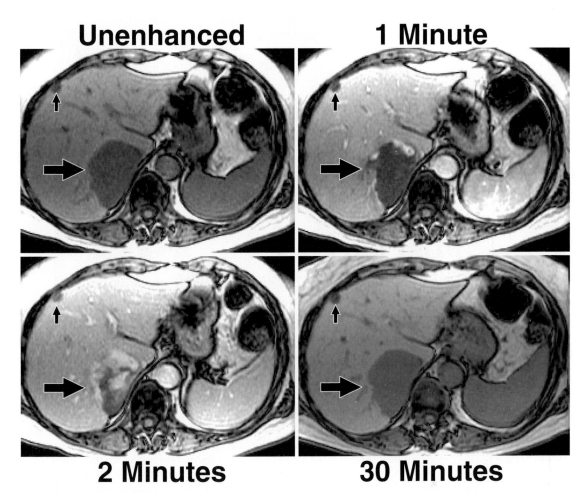

2 Minutes   30 Minutes

FIGURE 17–16. Unenhanced, 1-minute, 2-minute, and 30-minute T1-weighted gradient echo images following injection of gadobenate dimeglumine. The 1-minute and 2-minute images show typical progressive enhancement of a cavernous hemangioma *(large arrow)* and no enhancement of a cyst *(small arrow)*. By 30 minutes, contrast agent has been cleared from the blood pool but remains within hepatocytes.

cular and interstitial spaces, and in hepatocytes. On later images (i.e., after 30 minutes or more), contrast agent is cleared from the extracellular space and is then present principally in hepatocytes, bile ducts, and proximal small bowel, owing to its biliary excretion (Fig. 17–16).

Manganese-Based Compounds

Manganese (Mn^{++}), like gadolinium (Gd^{+++}), is strongly paramagnetic. Although manganese is an important component of a normal human diet and plays an important role in several cellular functions, free manganese is toxic if injected directly into the bloodstream. Manganese is tolerated better if it is complexed to a molecule that facilitates binding to plasma

proteins. Protein binding occurs after oral ingestion of manganese, and after in vivo decomplexation of some manganese chelates. In the body, manganese is located principally within mitochondria, where it is involved in cell respiration. Manganese is eliminated by biliary and intestinal secretion.

Thus far, the only parenteral manganese compound tested in humans is mangafodipir trisodium (formerly Mn-DPDP). Although mangafodipir trisodium was designed to be extracted primarily by hepatocytes, manganese appears to be delivered to several tissues with active aerobic metabolism, including pancreas, renal cortex, gastrointestinal mucosa, myocardium, and the adrenal glands (Fig. 17–17). Thus, mangafodipir trisodium appears to be more of a metabolic contrast agent than are other current

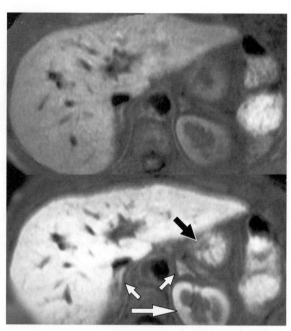

Unenhanced

Post Mn

FIGURE 17–17. Fat-suppressed T1-weighted spin echo images before *(top)* and after *(bottom)* intravenous injection of mangafodipir trisodium. In addition to the liver, there is prominent enhancement of the renal cortex *(large white arrow)*, adrenal glands *(small white arrows)*, and gastric wall *(black arrow)*.

contrast agents; however, clinical testing in humans has thus far been restricted to diagnosis of liver lesions.

PARTICULATE AGENTS

Polysaccharide-coated superparamagnetic iron oxide particles, often referred to as *SPIO,* can be designed to have various properties. These particles contain a crystalline core composed of ferrous (Fe^{2+}), ferric (Fe^{3+}), and oxygen, coated with dextran or some other polysaccharide. Most of these particles measure between 4 and 10 nm, but their biologic behavior is altered by their polysaccharide coating.

The blood half-life and distribution to different organs of the reticuloendothelial system change with effective particle or cluster size. One particulate iron oxide agent, ferumoxides (also referred to as Feridex® or AMI-25), has a thin, incomplete dextran coating that causes individual particles to form polycrystalline aggregates. These aggregates behave in solution or within cells as larger particles. A different agent, ferumoxtran (also referred to as Combidex® or AMI 227), contains a thicker, more

complete coating, which causes these particles to remain as separate monocrystals in solution. Large particles or aggregates accumulate rapidly within reticuloendothelial cells of the liver and spleen (Fig. 17–18), while smaller particles remain in circulation longer and are taken up more avidly by lymph nodes.

Iron oxide polycrystalline aggregates with an average diameter of approximately 50 to 200 nm are phagocytosed rapidly by reticuloendothelial cells and are cleared from the blood in an hour or less. Iron oxide particles such as these are far more effective for T2 and T2* enhancement than for T1 enhancement. Therefore, the major use of SPIO is for reducing the signal intensity of targeted tissues on T2-weighted or T2*-weighted images (Fig. 17–19).

Reticuloendothelial contrast agents can also be created by incorporating a paramagnetic or superparamagnetic material to hollow structures with surrounding lipid bilayers (i.e., liposomes).

Blood Pool Agents

As effective particle size decreases, the efficiency of phagocytosis by macrophages and re-

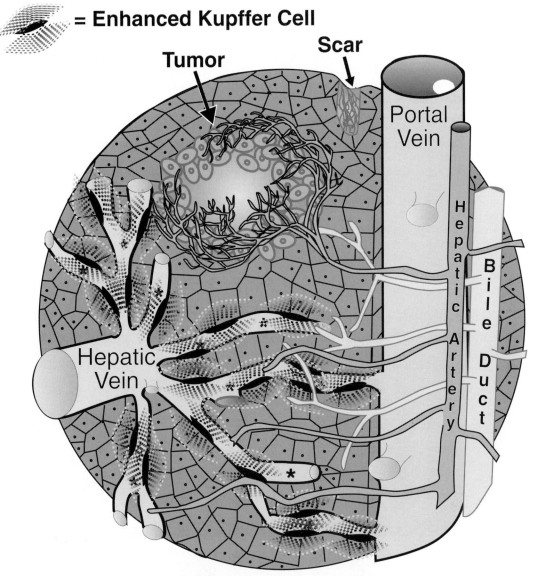

FIGURE 17–18. Enhancement by iron oxide particles of Kupffer cells of the liver. The powerful effect of the superparamagnetic particles extends far beyond the Kupffer cells themselves.

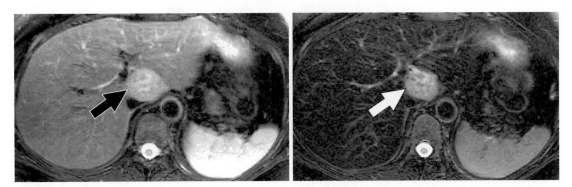

FIGURE 17–19. T2-weighted fast spin echo 3000/96 images before *(left)* and 10 minutes after *(right)* intravenous administration of iron oxide particles (Ferrixan) show greater conspicuousness of a colonic metastasis *(arrows)* owing to decreased signal intensity of the liver. The spleen also has slightly decreased signal intensity.

ticuloendothelial cells is reduced. Therefore, smaller particles remain longer in the blood. Eventually, these particles either degrade or are phagocytosed at a slow rate by macrophages, particularly by those within lymph nodes (Fig. 17-20). These ultrasmall superparamagnetic iron oxide agents are sometimes referred to as *USPIO.*

Small iron oxide monocrystals such as ferumoxtran facilitate T2 relaxation less efficiently than do large particles. These particles reduce both T1 and T2 substantially, and by comparable magnitudes, increasing signal intensity on T1-weighted images and decreasing it on T2-weighted images (Fig. 17-21).

T1 enhancement of vascular spaces by larger iron oxide particles can also be depicted using appropriate pulse sequences (Fig. 17-22). T1 enhancement by iron oxide particles of the blood pool often increases during the first several minutes. This is because particulate agents usually contain particles of a variety of sizes. Particles larger than desired are filtered and discarded during production of the product. Among the spectrum of particles sizes remaining, the largest particles are taken up most rapidly by reticuloendothelial cells and thus are cleared from the blood pool. Smaller particles, with greater T1 relaxivity and less T2* relaxivity than large particles exhibit, predominate on later images and therefore increase the signal intensity of the blood pool on images with sufficiently short TE.

Paramagnetic blood pool contrast agents

FSE 4000/96 Unenhanced

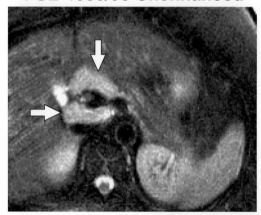

FSE 4000/96 24H Post USPIO

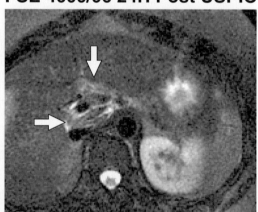

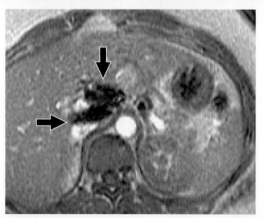

GRE 120/4.2/90° 24H Post USPIO

FIGURE 17-20. Concentration of ultrasmall iron oxide particles within hyperplastic inflammatory lymph nodes *(arrows),* 24-hour postdose on T2-weighted fast spin echo (FSE) 4000/96 *(top right)* and gradient echo (GRE) 120/4.2/90° *(bottom)* images.

GRE 44/2.3/90° Pre

FSE 3416/102 Pre

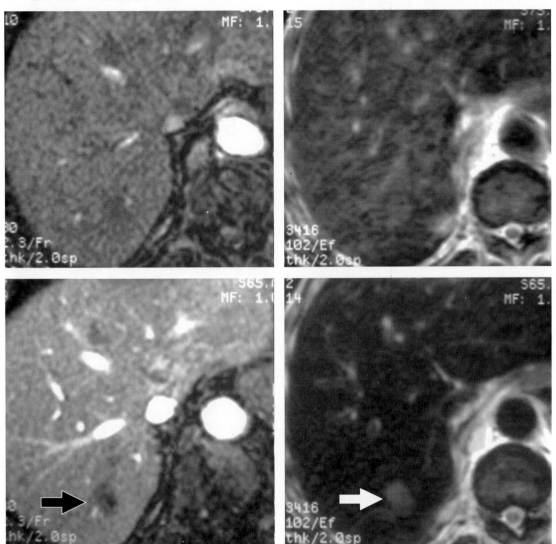

GRE 44/2.3/90° Post

FSE 3416/102 Post

FIGURE 17–21. Blood pool effects of USPIO (ferumoxtran) increasing signal intensity on T1-weighted images *(left)* and decreasing signal intensity on T2-weighted images *(right)*. On T1-weighted images *(bottom left)*, hepatic parenchyma and vessels both have increased signal intensity, increasing visibility of a metastasis *(arrow)*. On T2-weighted images *(bottom right)*, hepatic parenchyma and vessels both have decreased signal intensity, again increasing visibility of the metastasis *(arrow)*.

have also been created by attaching paramagnetic material such as gadolinium diethylenetriamine pentaacetic acid (Gd-DTPA) to larger molecules, such as albumen or polylysine.

Blood pool contrast agents are effective for enhancing blood vessels, for demonstrating perfusion dynamics on rapid sequential images, and for enhancing organs with large blood spaces such as the liver and spleen. In fact, the success of the portal phase for hepatic imaging after administration of extracellular agents such as iodinated contrast material for computed tomography and gadolinium chelates for MRI is based on blood pool principles. In other words, the reason the liver enhances more than most tumors during the portal phase is that its blood pool is larger than that of most tumors. In fact, the portal phase after administration of

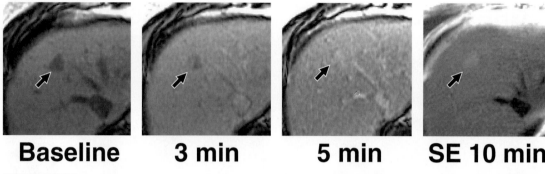

FIGURE 17-22. T1-enhancing effects of iron oxide particules (Ferrixan) increasing the intensity of a cavernous hemangioma *(arrow)* and hepatic vessels relative to the hepatic parenchyma. Enhancement of blood vessels and the hemangioma is more apparent at 5 minutes than at 3 minutes, because larger particles have been cleared from the blood pool by this time.

extracellular space agents is contaminated somewhat by leakage of the contrast material into the interstitial space of tumors. It must be emphasized that the use of a blood pool agent results in enhancement that is much different from that which results from the extracellular phase after administration of an extracellular space agent, owing to interstitial enhancement by the latter.

ORAL AGENTS

A variety of oral contrast agents have been investigated for improved delineation of bowel. These can be divided into ones that have (1) low signal intensity on all pulse sequences (proton displacement or T2 shortening), (2) high signal intensity on all pulse sequence (T1 shortening), (3) high signal intensity on T1-weighted and low signal intensity on T2-weighted images (T1 and T2 shortening), and (4) low signal intensity on T1-weighted images and high signal intensity on T2-weighted images (water based).

Low-Low Intensity

The principal advantage of reducing the signal intensity of bowel on all pulse sequences is that artifacts from moving bowel can be eliminated. This may be particularly desirable on T2-weighted images, where artifact from bowel motion can be particularly pronounced. Additionally, distinction between bowel and high–signal intensity masses or fluid collections can be accentuated if bowel signal intensity is reduced. On T1-weighted images, however, masses and fluid collections might be difficult to distinguish from low–signal intensity bowel.

The signal intensity within bowel can be reduced by displacing bowel contents with a material that contains no protons, such as air. Air can be administered by intubation of the small bowel or rectum. This method has not found widespread acceptance, principally because of patient discomfort. Additionally, susceptibility artifacts from air degrade T2*-weighted gradient echo images and echo planar images.

Bowel contents can also be displaced with perfluorocarbons. Perfluorocarbons do not contain protons, but they have the same susceptibility as water and thus do not cause artifacts. The first oral MRI contrast agent approved for clinical use was a perfluorocarbon formulation, perflubron (Imagent®), but it was prohibitively expensive and was withdrawn from the market.

The signal intensity of bowel can be reduced on all pulse sequences by administering superparamagnetic iron oxide particles (SPIO). A high enough concentration of these agents can shorten T2 and T2* enough to eliminate signal from bowel even on so-called T1-weighted images. The major disadvantage of SPIO as a bowel agent is the resulting distortion of the local magnetic field, which can exacerbate artifacts. Fat-suppression techniques are particularly vulnerable to magnetic field distortions.

Clays, such as kaolin and attapulgite (both used in formulations of Kaopectate®) and bentonite, restrict the motion of water, shortening T1 and T2 relaxation times. The T2-shortening is profound enough to eliminate signal from bowel on standard SE images with TE 20 msec or more. Therefore, clay agents have been described as reducing signal intensity on all pulse sequences; however, T1-weighted gradient echo images with TE less than 3 msec have little T2 contrast and therefore depict clay in bowel contents as high signal intensity owing to their short T1 (Fig. 17-23).

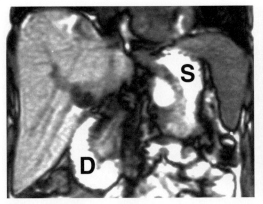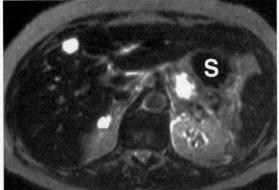

FIGURE 17–23. Intraluminal clay in Kaopectate causes high signal intensity on coronal T1-weighted gradient echo 101/2.3/90° image *(left)* and low intensity on T2-weighted spin echo 2500/100 image *(right)*. A hemorrhagic pancreatic pseudocyst medial to the stomach has high signal intensity on both images. S, stomach; D, duodenum.

High-High Intensity

Paramagnetic materials can reduce T1 relaxation time and therefore increase the signal intensity of bowel contents on T1-weighted images. If the concentration of paramagnetic material is low enough, the effects on T2 relaxation time are minimal, and the signal intensity of bowel contents remains high on T2-weighted images.

Many nutritional supplements or foods have been used as oral contrast agents owing to their high fat content or inclusion of paramagnetic materials such as manganese. Contrast agents that produce high signal intensity of bowel may be useful for depicting the low signal intensity of the bowel wall, but the images are rendered more sensitive to degradation by motion.

High-Low Intensity

Some materials shorten both T1 and T2 relaxation times enough so that bowel contents have high signal intensity on T1-weighted images and low signal intensity on T2-weighted images. Examples of this type of agent include clay, gadolinium chelates in high concentrations, and compounds of manganese (Fig. 17–24). Manganese is present in high concentrations in some foods, such as bananas and blueberries.

The major appeal of a high-low agent is that the resulting signal intensity of bowel is different on all pulse sequences from those of fluid collections and tumors, which tend to have low signal intensity on T1-weighted images and high signal intensity on T2-weighted images. However, some T2-weighted pulse sequences (e.g., fast spin echo) may depict bowel more clearly if its contents have high signal intensity, so this form of contrast is not necessarily desirable for every application. While reduction of bowel signal intensity may improve depiction of biliary and pancreatic ducts on magnetic resonance cholangiopancreatograms (MRCPs), the location of the duodenum on these images may be obscured.

Low-High Intensity

The least expensive, most widely available, and best understood oral contrast agent used for MRI is water. It can be used to mark bowel as low signal intensity on T1-weighted images and high signal intensity on T2-weighted images. Compounds that contain water such as barium sulfate have been used to produce similar effects.

Low-high agents are useful for delineating the pancreas, which has relatively high signal intensity on T1-weighted images and intermediate signal intensity on T2-weighted images. However, bowel may be difficult to distinguish from fluid collections and tumors, and high bowel signal intensity can intensify motion artifacts.

CONTRAST AGENT NOMENCLATURE

The most precise term for a contrast agent, or for any other chemical substance, is its name as established by the International Union of Pure and Applied Chemistry (IUPAC). The sys-

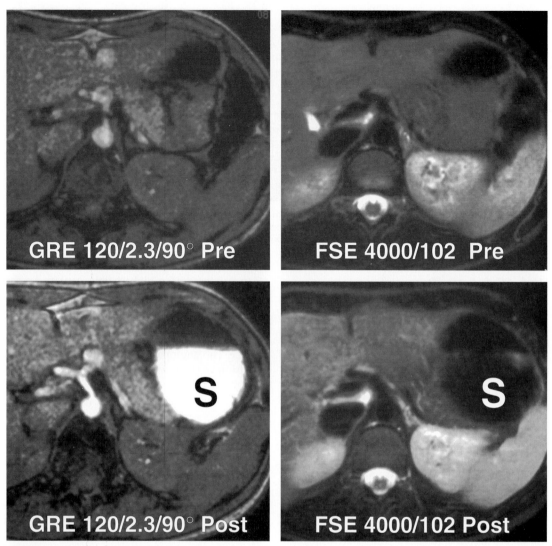

FIGURE 17–24. Manganese-based oral contrast agent that enhances T1 and T2. Axial T1-weighted gradient echo (GRE) *(left)* and T2-weighted fast spin echo (FSE) *(right)* images before *(top)* and after *(bottom)* oral administration of LumenHance®. Contrast agent in the stomach (S) has high signal intensity on T1-weighted images *(bottom left)* and low signal intensity on T2-weighted images *(bottom right)*.

tematic chemical name indicates unambiguously the exact structure of the contrast agent; however, such names often consume several lines of text and are virtually unpronounceable. For these reasons, the systematic chemical name is rarely used in clinical practice and generally appears in the radiology literature only during the early stages of contrast agent development. For example, the first gadolinium chelate approved for human use has the chemical name of 1-deoxy-1-(methylamino)-D-glucitol dihydrogen [N,N-bis[2-[bis(carboxymethyl)amino]ethyl]-glycinato-(5-)]gadolinate (2-)(2:1).

To facilitate dissemination of information, a pharmaceutical company usually derives an ab-

breviated name or company code name for a new contrast agent. Thus, 1-deoxy-1-(methylamino)-D-glucitol dihydrogen [N,N-bis[2-[bis(carboxymethyl)amino]ethyl]-glycinato-(5-)]gadolinate (2-)(2:1) has been referred to as gadolinium–diethylenetriamine pentaacetic acid, or, still shorter Gd-DTPA. This term, although now obsolete, is still commonly used.

During early investigation of a contrast agent in humans, an official U.S. Adopted Name (USAN) is assigned to a contrast agent. The USAN is an agent's official generic name. Once this occurs, the abbreviated name introduced by the pharmaceutical company should no longer be used. Thus, the agent formerly known

TABLE 17–1. NAMES AND VENDORS* OF CONTRAST AGENTS, BY CLASSIFICATION

Generic (IUP) Name	Commercial Name	Vendor	Other Terms
Gadolinium Chelates—Extracellular			
Gadopentetate dimeglumine	Magnevist®	Berlex Laboratories, Wayne, NJ	Gadolinium diethylenetriaminepentaacetic acid dimeglumine (Gd-DTPA)
Gadoterate meglumine	Dotarem®	Laboratoire Guerbet, Aulnay-sous-Bois, France	Gadolinium tetraazacyclododecanetetraacetic acid meglumine (Gd-DOTA)
Gadoteridol	ProHance®	Bracco Diagnostics, Milan, Italy	Gd-HP-DO3A
Gadodiamide	Omniscan®	Nycomed AS, Oslo, Norway	Gadolinium diethylenetriaminepentaacetic acid bis (methylamide) (Gd-DTPA-BMA)
Gadobutrol	Gadovist™	Berlex Laboratories, Wayne, NJ	Gd-DO3A-butantriol
Gadoversetamide	Optimark®	Mallinckrodt Medical, Inc., St. Louis, MO	MP-1177/10
Gadolinium Chelates—Biliary Excretion			
Gadoxetic acid disodium	Eovist®	Berlex Laboratories, Wayne, NJ	Gadolinium ethoxybenzyl diethylenetriaminepentaacetic acid (Gd-EOB-DTPA)
Gadobenate dimeglumine	MultiHance®	Bracco Diagnostics, Milan, Italy	Gadolinium benzyloxypropionictetraacetate (Gd-BOPTA/Dimeg)
Manganese Agents			
Mangafodipir trisodium		Nycomed AS, Oslo, Norway	Manganese dipyridoxyl diphosphate (Mn-DPDP)
Iron Oxide Particles (Intravenous)			
Ferumoxides*	Feridex I.V.®	Berlex Laboratories, Wayne, NJ	AMI-25
Ferrixan*	Resovist™	Schering AG, Berlin, Germany	SH U 555 A
Ferumoxtran*	Combidex™	Advanced Magnetics, Inc., Cambridge, MA	Code 7227; BMS 180549; AMI-227
Oral Agents			
Ferric ammonium citrate	FerriSelz	Otsuka Pharmaceuticals, Tokyo, Japan	Oral magnetic resonance (OMR)
Ferumoxsil oral suspension*	GastroMARK®	Mallinckrodt Medical, Inc, St. Louis, MO	AMI-121
Gadopentetate dimeglumine	Magnevist® Enteral	Schering AG, Berlin, Germany	Gd-DTPA (gadolinium diethylenetriaminepentaacetic acid dimeglumine)
Perflubron	Imagent® GI	Alliance Pharmaceutical Corp, San Diego, CA	Perfluoro-octylbromide (PFOB)
Manganese chloride	LumenHance®	Bracco Diagnostics, Milan, Italy	
Gadolinium zeolite	Gadolite™ 60 Oral Suspension	Pharmacyclics, Sunnyvale, CA	

*For iron oxide agents marketed or tested in the United States and, by a different name, in other nations, only the United States vendor is listed.
From Mitchell DG: MR imaging contrast agents—what's in a name? JMRI 1997;7:1–7.

as Gd-DTPA should now be referred to as *gadopentetate dimeglumine.*

As development of an agent continues, a pharmaceutical company creates a brand name for marketing. While applying to the United States Patent and Trademark Office for an official trademark, the symbol "™" is applied (e.g., Magnevist™). Once the brand name is officially registered, the symbol changes to "®" (e.g., Magnevist®). Table 17–1 lists the generic and commercial names of several currently used MRI contrast agents.

ESSENTIAL POINTS TO REMEMBER

1. Current chelates of gadolinium are extracellular space agents. They are distributed throughout the vascular space and diffuse

across capillary walls into the interstitial space, except in the central nervous system and testes.

2. Extracellular space MRI contrast agents are eliminated entirely by renal excretion.

3. Images for which the center of k-space is acquired within approximately 30 seconds after injection of MRI contrast agent depict arterial anatomy and vascularity.

4. Images acquired approximately 1 minute after injection of MRI contrast agent depict the blood pool. In the abdomen, these images are often referred to as portal venous phase images.

5. Images acquired more than 3 minutes after injection of extracellular space agent depict enhancement of the entire extracellular (vascular plus interstitial) space. This includes enhancement of fibrous tissue, edema, and partial necrosis.

6. Gadolinium chelates can be attached to a structure that causes them to be transported across cell (e.g., hepatocyte) membranes. Hepatocyte-directed gadolinium chelates are excreted by both renal and biliary mechanisms.

7. Mangafodipir trisodium (Mn-DPDP) is rapidly decomplexed. The released manganese is transported to mitochondria within aerobically active tissues throughout the body (e.g., pancreas, renal cortex, adrenal glands, gastrointestinal mucosa). Excretion is entirely biliary and intestinal.

8. Iron oxide particules are taken up by reticuloendothelial cells. Large particles (i.e., 50 to 200 nm) are taken up rapidly. These agents preferentially enhance T2 and T2*, reducing signal intensity on T2-weighted and T2*-weighted images.

9. Small iron oxide particles, which are taken up more slowly, have a much longer blood half-life and are concentrated within lymph nodes. These agents enhance T1, T2, and T2*, causing high signal intensity on T1-weighted images and low signal intensity on T2-weighted images.

10. Oral agents that displace protons or have a very short T2 have low signal intensity on all pulse sequences.

11. Oral agents that have strong T1 enhancement and mild T2 enhancement have high signal intensity on most pulse sequences.

12. Oral agents with strong T1 and T2 enhancement have high signal intensity on T1-weighted images and low signal intensity on T2-weighted ones.

13. Contrast agents initially are given an abbreviated chemical name or a company code name. When an official generic name is given, it should be used in place of the older name. For example, the agents formerly known as Gd-DTPA and Mn-DPDP are now called, respectively, *gadopentetate dimeglumine* and *mangafodipir trisodium*.

CHAPTER

18 Vascular Techniques

If blood were not moving, its magnetic resonance (MR) signal intensity would result directly from its proton density, T1 and T2. Blood has more free water than almost any tissue in the body, only somewhat less than cerebrospinal fluid and urine. Therefore, its proton density is higher than that of most other tissues.

The high iron content of blood has the potential to affect its signal intensity. Deoxyhemoglobin within deoxygenated red blood cells is weakly paramagnetic, which can lead to reduced T2 if it is unevenly distributed, as within subacute hemorrhage. Within circulating blood, the effect on signal intensity of deoxyhemoglobin is weaker. Heavily T2*-weighted images are needed to distinguish oxygenated from deoxygenated flowing blood. This phenomenon is used to evaluate brain perfusion via blood oxygen level dependent (BOLD) techniques.

Since circulating blood has relatively long T1 and long T2, if it were not moving it would have low signal intensity on T1-weighted images and high signal intensity on T2-weighted images.

The signal intensity of blood can be altered by many techniques, allowing many strategies for magnetic resonance angiography (MRA). Vessels can be depicted effectively by MRI using either "dark blood" or "bright blood" techniques. First, we will consider mechanisms that can produce low signal intensity of blood. These can be used to create images that depict vessel and myocardial walls, and intraluminal thrombus or tissue. Then, we will consider three basic methods of producing bright blood images, all of which include strategies for avoiding dark blood mechanisms. Finally, we will discuss methods for showing perfusion and diffusion that do not involve depicting blood vessels.

DARK BLOOD MECHANISMS

Because of the long T2 of blood, dark blood images are difficult to produce with T2-weighted techniques. However, the long T1 of blood provides one strategy for reducing its signal intensity. In the absence of mechanisms that increase its signal intensity, blood will be dark on T1-weighted images. The T1 of blood can also be used to null its signal throughout an image by applying an inversion recovery preparation pulse with an inversion time (TI) long enough to null blood signal.

With single-section acquisitions, blood flowing into an image section between excitation pulses often has high signal intensity because it has not been affected by previous excitation pulses. With multisection acquisitions, blood is often bright on *entry sections*, that is, on sections at the edge of the imaged volume that flowing blood encounters first. The signal intensity of flowing blood is progressively lower on sections farther from the entry section, owing to increased saturation as the blood flows through more sections. One strategy for producing dark blood, therefore, is to use a multisection technique, so that each excitation pulse saturates blood as it moves into adjacent image sections. Intravascular signal intensity can be reduced further by applying spatial saturation pulses, so that flowing blood is saturated before it enters an image section. This is discussed in greater detail in Chapters 10 and 12.

Conventional spin echo and fast spin echo images are usually more effective than gradient echo images for depicting blood vessels as having low–signal intensity lumens. For blood to generate signal intensity on spin echo images it must be exposed to both the excitation and refocusing pulses. If blood is excited but flows out of the image section before the refocusing pulse, the rephasing lobe of the frequency-encoding gradient (Gf) will cause further dephasing, rather than rephasing. Therefore, blood that leaves an image section before the refocusing pulse generates no signal on spin echo images.

237

237

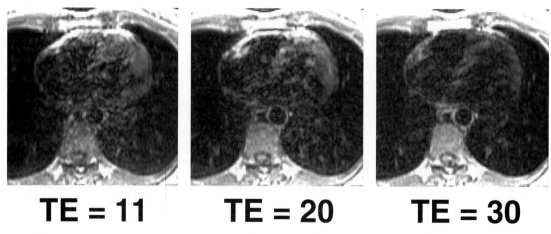

TE = 11   TE = 20   TE = 30

FIGURE 18–1. Effect of echo time (TE) on intravascular signal intensity on cardiac gated axial SE images with repetition time (TR) of 861 msec. With TE of 11 msec *(left)*, intravascular signal and artifact are prominent. These decrease with progressive increases in TE to 20 *(center)* and 30 *(right)* msec. However, myocardial signal intensity also decreases with increasing TE.

On conventional spin echo images, increasing echo time (TE) is a mechanism for reducing the signal intensity of blood (Fig. 18-1). At some centers, for example, gated spin echo images of the heart are obtained with a TE of 20 to 30 msec rather than the minimum TE, to decrease intraluminal signal intensity. This is only partially effective, however, because increased TE also reduces the signal intensity of background tissue, which usually has shorter T2 than blood, and allows increased motion artifacts.

Loss of coherent phase within a voxel is probably the most important mechanism for signal intensity reduction of flowing blood. As discussed in Chapter 10, motion during the application of imaging gradients causes dephasing, which is not corrected by the rephasing gradient unless gradient moment nulling is used. If dark blood imaging is desired, gradient moment nulling is not used, and additional gradients may even be applied to further dephase moving spins. Even in the absence of gradient moment nulling, intravascular dephasing is minimal if TE is very short (e.g., less than 3 msec). Strategies for reducing the signal intensity of blood, and their underlying mechanisms, are summarized in Table 18-1.

PARAMAGNETIC ENHANCEMENT

The signal intensity of blood can be increased by intravenous injection of a paramagnetic agent. With a sufficient dose, blood has higher signal intensity than other tissues on T1-weighted images, as long as mechanisms that reduce the signal intensity of flowing blood are avoided. If the concentration of paramagnetic agent is sufficiently high, longitudinal magnetization recovers fast enough to minimize saturation by previous excitation pulses. Therefore, three-dimensional Fourier transform (3D-FT) gradient echo techniques with extremely short repetition times (TRs) can be used. The use of the shortest possible TE maximizes phase coherence and allows efficient image acquisition.

High-quality paramagnetic contrast-enhanced bright blood images can be obtained using 2D-FT spoiled multisection gradient echo images, but 3D-FT techniques are usually preferred for this (Fig. 18-2). The use of 3D-FT ensures high

TABLE 18–1. STRATEGIES AND MECHANISMS FOR REDUCING SIGNAL INTENSITY OF BLOOD

Dark Blood Strategy	Mechanism
Short TR	Blood is saturated owing to long T1
Moderate TE	Allows motion-induced intravoxel dephasing
Inversion recovery	Nulls blood signal based on its T1
Spatial saturation	Saturates blood before entering region of interest
90°/180° washout	Blood leaves image section between 90° and 180° pulses
Gradient dephasing	Increases motion-induced intravoxel dephasing

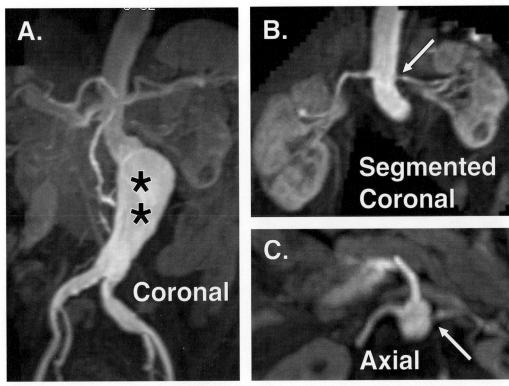

FIGURE 18–2. Maximum intensity projection (MIP) projections based on a coronal three-dimensional gradient echo (3D-GRE) 7/2.2/50° acquisition during the first-pass arterial phase of a 30-mL injection of gadolinium chelate. *(A)* Coronal projection shows an aortic aneurysm *(asterisks)*. The renal arteries are obscured by overlying vessels. *(B)* Segmented coronal projection based on a limited portion of the data, excluding the anterior tissues and vessels that obscured the renal arteries in *(A)*. *(C)* Axial projection. Arrows in *(B)* and *(C)* indicate left renal artery stenosis.

signal-to-noise ratio (SNR) and contiguous image sections. TR and TE should be as short as possible. Flip angle should be high enough so that background tissue remains sufficiently saturated, causing low signal intensity. The optimal flip angle for contrast-enhanced 3D-FT MRA is usually between 30° and 60°.

Contrast agent should be administered so that the bolus is maximally present within the vessels of interest during acquisition of the weakest phase-encoded views (the center of k-space). For a full-Fourier sequential acquisition (where the high negative views are acquired first and the high positive views last), the center of k-space is acquired during the midpoint of the acquisition, when intravascular paramagnetic concentration should be maximal. For centric or half-Fourier acquisitions, where the center of k-space is acquired at or near the beginning of the acquisition, paramagnetic concentration should be maximal at the beginning of the acquisition. If the center of k-space is acquired before intravascular paramagnetic concentration is high enough, high signal intensity may be restricted to the edges of the vessel,

corresponding to enhancement of edge detail only (Fig. 18–3).

TIME-OF-FLIGHT TECHNIQUES

All time-of-flight (TOF) techniques are based on the same basic principle: blood flowing into an image section has higher magnetization than the partially saturated stationary tissue within the section. The *time* it takes for the *flight* of blood into an image section is the mechanism for vascular enhancement. This is a simple principle that does not require contrast agents, dedicated hardware, signal processing, or sophisticated software beyond that needed for a simple gradient echo pulse sequence. In fact, current two-dimensional TOF (2D-TOF) techniques are merely refinements of gradient echo pulse sequences introduced and used clinically more than a decade ago.

Two-Dimensional Time of Flight

The basis of a 2D-TOF pulse sequence is slice by slice generation of individual images on

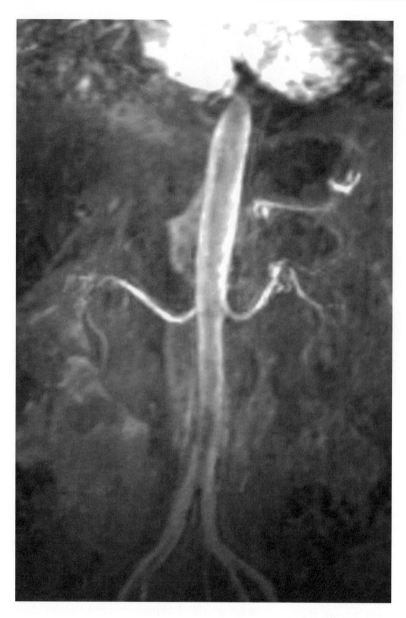

FIGURE 18-3. Coronal MIP projection of a coronal 3D-GRE 11/2.3/60° set of images acquired too early relative to the bolus of gadolinium chelate. Enhancement peaked after the central views of k-space were obtained, so signal magnitude was greater for the peripheral views. This caused higher signal intensity of fine detail, resulting in greater signal intensity of the edges of the aorta and of the renal arteries than of the aortic lumen.

which blood is white and other tissues are dark or intermediate shades of gray. Stationary tissue within each image section is exposed to repeated excitation pulses, causing it to be partially saturated. Between each excitation pulse, fresh unexcited blood flows into the image section, replacing blood that had been exposed to the previous excitation pulse. Because it is less saturated than background tissue, flowing blood has higher signal intensity. The signal intensity of background tissue can be reduced further by the use of magnetization transfer (MT) saturation, which reduces the signal intensity of tissue without affecting blood. Projection MRA images can be created by combining the data from multiple 2D-TOF sections (Fig. 18-4). Time-of-flight techniques are sensitive only to flow perpendicular to the image plane, although sufficiently thin sections usually depict this component of flow even within vessels nearly parallel to the image (Fig. 18-5).

There are three basic requirements for successful 2D-TOF imaging:

1. Background tissue must be kept relatively saturated. This requires a short TR and intermediate or high flip angle.

2. Enough blood must flow into the imaging section or volume between excitations to increase signal intensity beyond that of nearby

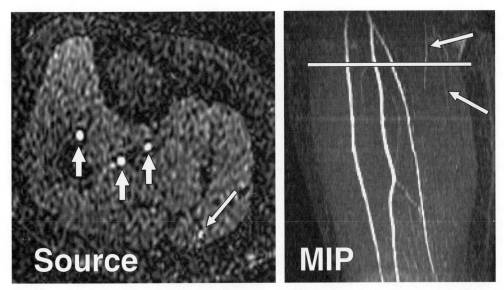

FIGURE 18-4. Axial source two-dimensional time of flight (2D-TOF) 37/7/60° image of the calf *(left)* shows anterior tibial, peroneal, and posterior tibial arteries *(thick arrows)* as high signal intensity relative to the partially saturated background tissue. Thin arrow indicates a small muscular branch vessel. Venous signal was suppressed by using inferior spatial saturation pulses. Coronal maximal intensity projection (MIP) image *(right)* depicts the patent arteries. Arrows indicate small muscular branches. The horizontal white line indicates the plane of the source image.

stationary tissue. This requires a sufficiently long TR and thin sections.

3. The phase of blood signals must remain coherent. This is accomplished by using the shortest possible TE, gradient moment nulling, or cardiac compensation or gating.

With these three basic principles in mind, the following parameters will be addressed individually. The effects of many of these parameters are illustrated in Chapter 10.

Repetition Time. TR should be long enough to allow sufficient inflow of unsaturated spins between repetitions and short enough to maintain saturation of stationary tissue. An additional benefit of shorter TR is less variation in the signal intensity of blood between successive echoes, which reduces artifacts from pulsatile flow. Most successful implementations of 2D-TOF techniques use TRs between 20 and 50 msec.

Flip Angle. As flip angle is increased, more transverse magnetization is created. Therefore, the transverse magnetization of unsaturated blood flowing into an image section increases. Increased flip angle will also result in greater saturation of stationary tissue in the image section, decreasing the resultant transverse magnetization. Thus, increased flip angle increases the signal intensity of flowing blood and decreases the signal intensity of stationary tissue, increasing the contrast between flowing blood and background tissue.

However, the use of a high flip angle reduces the signal intensity of slowly flowing blood, which is not completely replaced during the time between repetitions. During diastole, there is little forward flow in many vessels; higher flip angles reduce the signal intensity of blood during diastole. Since systolic signal intensity increases (greater transverse magnetization created) and diastolic signal intensity decreases (greater saturation) with higher flip angle, view-to-view intensity changes and the resulting phase artifacts from pulsation are exacerbated as flip angle increases. In most instances, a flip angle between 30° and 60° yields satisfactory images, the lower angle reserved for minimizing artifacts from highly pulsatile flow.

Section Thickness. Sections should be thin enough to allow sufficient replacement of blood protons from inflow between repetitions but thick enough to ensure adequate SNR and anatomic coverage. Section thickness of 5 to 8 mm can provide a rapid "road map" of major vessels. Thinner sections are especially important for imaging slow flow and flow within small in-plane vessels and for depicting details of vascular anatomy such as stenoses (Fig. 18-6). The use of 2D-TOF for detecting arterial stenosis requires section thickness of 2 mm or less for most applications. The use of thin sections also improves the quality of 3D-maximum intensity projection (MIP) reconstructed images.

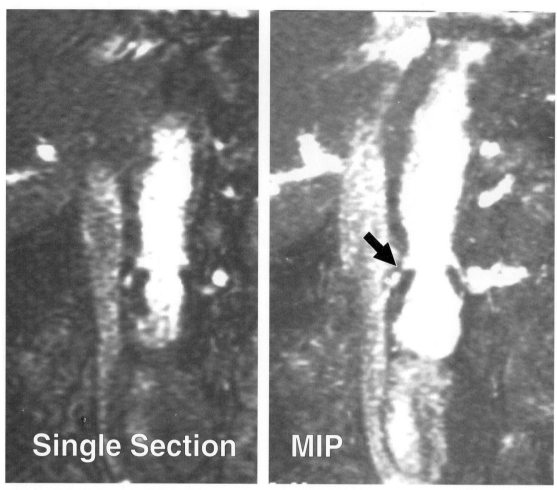

FIGURE 18–5. Coronal 2D-TOF image *(left)* and MIP projection *(right)* showing left renal artery stenosis *(arrow)*. Even though the aorta and renal arteries are parallel to the imaging plane, the image sections are thin enough so that through-plane flow is adequate for their depiction.

Echo Time. Generally, TE should be as short as possible within the limitations of the system hardware. Several user-selected parameters affect TE, and the choice of these parameters involves a series of tradeoffs. Desirable features of 2D-TOF implementations include thin sections to increase sensitivity to slow flow, gradient moment nulling to decrease loss of vascular signal intensity from phase differences within each voxel, and sufficiently low sampling bandwidth to ensure adequate SNR. All of these measures increase TE somewhat, but these tradeoffs are usually acceptable or unavoidable.

Motion Compensation Techniques. Most current implementations of 2D-TOF use gradient moment nulling to compensate for phase incoherence resulting from the first order of motion, constant velocity. During the short interval of echo sampling (usually less than 10 msec) constant velocity is a close enough approximation to compensate for phase errors resulting from even pulsatile flow. Higher orders of motion (e.g., acceleration and jerk) have little effect on the phase coherence of each individual echo. In fact, higher orders of gradient moment nulling are counterproductive, since the resulting increase in TE leads to additional degradation of vascular signal intensity.

Artifacts from pulsatile flow result primarily from variations in vascular magnetization between echoes, rather than from phase differences within each echo. Therefore, artifacts from pulsatile flow are best reduced by decreasing magnetization differences between systole and diastole. These differences can be reduced by decreasing TR and/or flip angle (see above) or by using cardiac gating or triggering.

Signal Averaging. Pulsation artifacts often

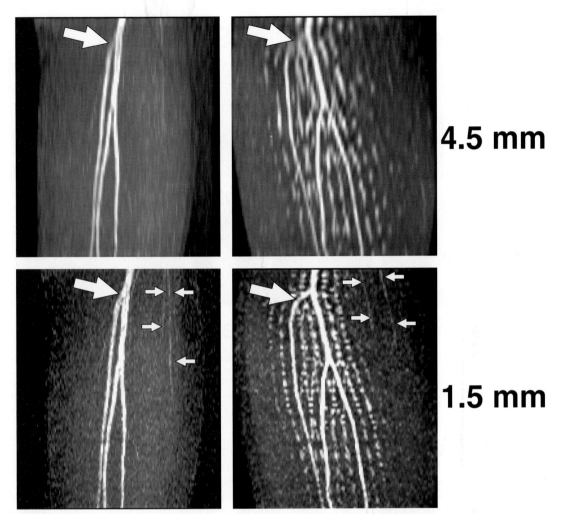

FIGURE 18-6. Effect of section thickness on 2D-TOF images of the calf, acquired using axial 33/5/45° source images. The phase axis of the source images was left-to-right; the ghost artifacts from pulsatile flow are therefore depicted on the coronal projections *(right)* but not on the sagittal projections *(left)*. Although signal-to-noise (SNR) is higher with 4.5-mm section thickness *(top)*, partially in-plane flow at the origin of the anterior tibial artery *(large arrows)* is depicted with greater clarity with 1.5-mm section thickness *(bottom)*, as are small peripheral vessels *(small arrows)*.

increase with signal averaging, unlike spin echo images, where increased signal averaging reduces the conspicuousness of motion artifact. Motion artifacts on breath holding images decrease when the central views of k-space, which determine tissue contrast, are acquired during a single cardiac cycle. Signal averaging requires sampling each point of k-space more than once, thereby increasing the time needed for sampling k-space. This usually splits the central views into two or more different cardiac cycles, increasing the distance between ghost artifacts and the conspicuousness of ghosts and decreasing edge sharpness.

Decreasing the time required for sampling the center of k-space decreases pulsation artifacts. This can be accomplished by using one

or fewer signal averages, decreasing TR, or minimizing the field of view (FOV) in the phase-encoding axis by using rectangular FOV.

Saturation Pulses. Pulsation artifacts and signal from overlapping arteries or veins can be reduced by judicious use of saturation bands. For example, axial images of carotid artery flow can be clarified by saturation bands placed immediately cephalad to each image section, to reduce the signal intensity of blood within caudad-flowing veins. Similarly, jugular veins can be imaged without overlying arteries by inferiorly placed saturation bands.

For longitudinally oriented vessels such as those in the neck and extremities, the location of the saturation band can be changed for each image section, to saturate blood optimally im-

Floating Superior Saturation

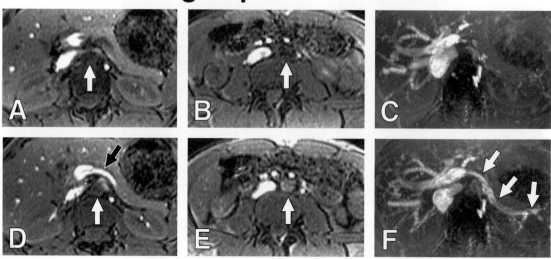

Fixed Superior Saturation

FIGURE 18-7. Effects of floating *(A–C)* versus fixed *(D–F)* superior saturation pulses on axial 2D-TOF images of the abdomen. *(A)* and *(D)* are at the level of the splenic vein *(black arrow in D)*, *(B)* and *(E)* are at an inferior level, and *(C)* and *(F)* are axial MIP images covering the splenic vein *(arrows in F)*. With floating saturation pulses, signal intensity of inferiorly flowing blood in the aorta *(arrows in A, B, D, E)* is more completely suppressed. However, the splenic vein is seen only if the superior saturation pulse has a fixed location superior to that of this vein *(arrows in D, F)*.

mediately before it enters the image section. Saturation bands that change their location with each image section are sometimes referred to as *floating saturation pulses*. For some applications, such as imaging peripheral arteries, these saturation bands should not be immediately adjacent to the image section but should be separated by at least a few millimeters. This ensures that reversed blood flow during diastole will not be inadvertently saturated by a pulse too close to the image section; inadvertent saturation of reversed diastolic flow would decrease arterial signal intensity.

It must be remembered that 2D-TOF "MR arteriograms" and "MR venograms" do not necessarily depict only arteries or only veins. Rather, they depict inferiorly flowing or superiorly flowing blood. For example, retrograde arterial flow within collateral vessels is not depicted on a typical TOF MR arteriogram.

Floating saturation pulses can cause inadvertent saturation of desired blood vessels in body parts with complex vascular anatomy, such as the abdomen. For example, renal arteries commonly curve so that their distal portions are angled cephalad. Images obtained with floating inferior saturation pulses therefore show the aorta and proximal (inferiorly oriented) renal

arteries but fail to depict any portion of the artery with upward angulation. Similarly, saturating blood immediately above each image section eliminates signal intensity from a patent splenic vein (Fig. 18–7), which usually courses inferiorly toward the confluence with the superior mesenteric vein. Portal vein flow voids may result. If used at all in body parts such as these, saturation pulses should have a fixed location that does not overlap any portion of the vessel of interest.

If a 2D-TOF technique is optimized, administration of gadolinium chelates does not improve depiction of vessels. The high signal intensity of unsaturated blood flowing into an image section does not depend on its T1 relaxation time; since unsaturated blood has not experienced an excitation pulse, time for recovery of longitudinal magnetization is not necessary. Therefore, shortening the relaxation time of blood via contrast agents is not beneficial for optimized 2D-TOF techniques. The signal intensity of background tissue, however, increases after administration of contrast agents, potentially obscuring vessels. If in fact administration of current gadolinium chelates improves 2D-TOF images, the 2D-TOF technique itself was not optimized for depiction of slow or in-plane flow. However, if thick image sections are used to increase SNR and reduce acquisition time, gadolinium chelates increase intravascular signal from slow or in-plane flow.

Paradoxically, the severity of ghost artifact may actually decrease after administration of gadolinium chelate, because the intensity of flowing blood will become more uniform throughout the cardiac cycle. During systole, blood magnetization is high because blood entering an image section has not been exposed to an excitation pulse. Reducing its T1, therefore, does not affect its signal intensity; however, blood may remain within an image section during diastole, so it *is* affected by the prior excitation pulse. Its magnetization recovers faster from the resulting saturation when a contrast agent has been administered. The resulting signal intensity of blood during diastole is thus closer to that during systole after contrast agent administration, reducing artifacts from view-to-view intensity changes.

TOF images can be very sensitive to slow flow but sometimes do not completely depict complex flow within aneurysms or distal to stenoses. Contrast-enhanced MRA techniques generally depict vascular lumens with greater accuracy in these situations (Fig. 18–8).

Three-Dimensional Time of Flight

Three-dimensional-TOF techniques consist of a gradient echo acquisition of a volume into which blood is flowing. The advantage of 3D-TOF over 2D-TOF is generally higher spatial resolution in the section direction and a greater SNR. The 3D-TOF techniques have been most useful for imaging rapid flow like that in the carotid arteries and circle of Willis (Fig. 18–9); however, 3D-TOF techniques are usually suboptimal for imaging slow flow like that in the abdominal vessels. It is also more difficult to adapt 3D-TOF technique to allow suspended respiration.

Unlike optimized 2D-TOF techniques, 3D-TOF techniques can benefit from the administration of contrast agents to shorten the T1 relaxation time of blood. This is because blood within the imaged volume is partially saturated with 3D-TOF techniques; longitudinal magnetization recovers more rapidly after contrast agent administration, increasing vascular signal intensity. In fact, some so-called contrast-enhanced 3D-TOF techniques are not really TOF techniques at all, since they depict blood vessels based on the short T1 of enhanced blood rather than the actual TOF principle.

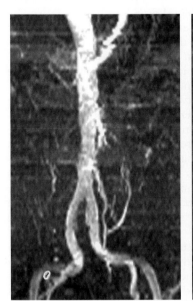 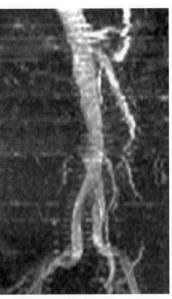 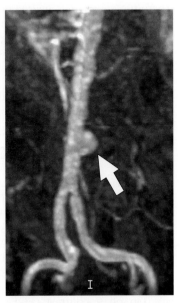

Time-of-Flight   Gadolinium

FIGURE 18–8. Coronal and oblique 2D-TOF MIP images acquired from 2-mm thick axial source 37/6.5/50° images *(left and center)* show aortic and iliac ectasia, but no aneurysm. The gadolinium-enhanced 3D 11.2/2.3/60° MIP image *(right)* clearly depicts a saccular aneurysm *(arrow)*.

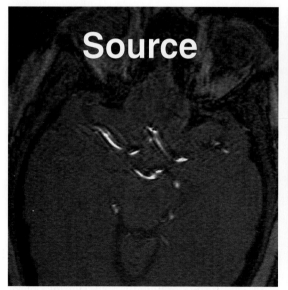
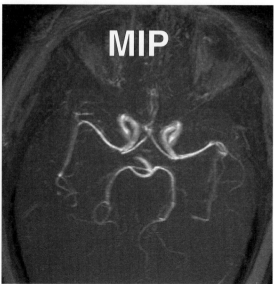

FIGURE 18–9. Three-dimensional-TOF axial source *(left)* and MIP *(right)* images using TR/TE/flip angle of 59/6.9/30°. Background signal has been partially suppressed using magnetization transfer saturation. The 3D-FT acquisition has resulted in high SNR.

One method of increasing the sensitivity of 3D-TOF techniques to moderate velocity flow is to use multiple overlapping thin slab acquisitions (MOTSA). MOTSA can be thought of as a compromise between 2D-TOF and 3D-TOF. By decreasing the slab thickness, sensitivity to slow and moderate flow velocities is increased. Anatomic coverage is maintained by using multiple acquisitions. Smooth transitions between slabs is ensured by overlapping the slabs. Compared to 2D-TOF, MOTSA has a higher SNR but less sensitivity to slow flow (Fig. 18–10). Compared to 3D-TOF, MOTSA has lower SNR but greater sensitivity to slow flow.

PHASE-CONTRAST TECHNIQUE

One disadvantage of all pulse sequences discussed thus far for depicting flowing blood is the possibility of ambiguous signal. On dark blood images (e.g., those with spatial saturation pulses), air, bone, and other substances also have low signal intensity. On bright blood images based either on TOF or contrast enhancement, other tissues may have high signal intensity. On phase-contrast (PC) pulse sequences, the phase changes from motion itself are used to depict flowing blood. The principal advantages of PC sequences are better suppression of background tissue and greater potential for measuring blood flow.

In Chapter 10 we discussed how phase changes that result from motion can create artifacts in phase encoding. We have also mentioned how these effects can be reduced by altering the gradient waveforms through gradient moment nulling. The same principles provide the basis for using phase changes to depict and measure blood flow.

PC images are reconstructed from two or more separate data sets, usually acquired simultaneously in an interleaved manner. These two data sets are identical except for the phase changes from motion along one particular axis. For example, two data sets may differ because gradient moment nulling is applied in the frequency-encoding axis in one set but not in the other. The difference between these two data sets is the phase shifts along the frequency-encoding axis. Subtraction of these data sets produces an image of motion along this axis. Images of flow along the phase-encoding and section-select axes can be similarly created (Fig. 18–11).

The amount of phase change that arises from motion of a given velocity can be varied by altering the gradient waveform. This flow-sensitive gradient adjustment is often referred to as the *velocity-encoding variable* (v_{enc}), which is the value that produces a phase shift of 180°. The v_{enc} represents the practical upper limit of velocities that can be depicted unambiguously. Flow velocity higher than the v_{enc} may be misrepresented owing to velocity aliasing, depicted

2D-TOF

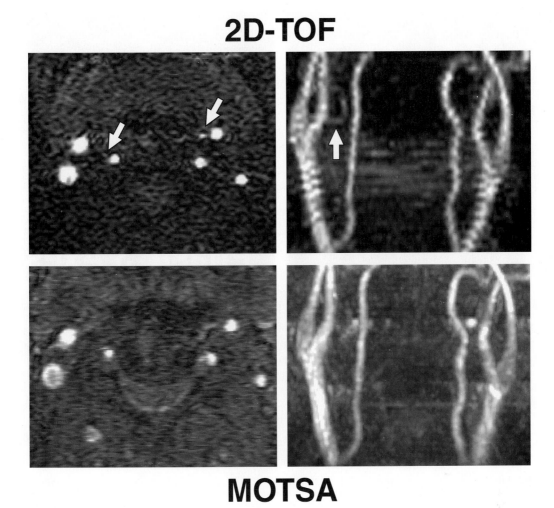

MOTSA

FIGURE 18–10. Two-dimensional-TOF 38/8.6/60° *(top)* and multiple overlapping thin slab acquisitions (MOTSA) 57/6.9/30° *(bottom)* images of the neck. Axial source images are at left and coronal MIP images at right. Patient motion and vascular pulsations during acquisition has resulted in a stair-step pattern in the 2D-TOF MIP. The MOTSA images have higher SNR but greater background signal. Arrows indicate small vessels that are depicted better by 2D-TOF owing to its greater sensitivity to slow flow.

as if it were flow in the opposite direction (Fig. 18-12). Slow flow is depicted more sensitively with lower v_{enc}.

Signal intensity on PC images is proportional to the velocity of motion in the encoded axis. The accuracy of the data, however, depends on the strength of the signal—that is, on SNR. Therefore, gradient echo techniques are usually used for PC, because flowing blood has higher signal intensity on these images. Paramagnetic contrast agents can also increase the signal intensity of flowing blood, thus increasing the sensitivity and accuracy of PC images.

One disadvantage of PC images as compared to other pulse sequences is their generally longer acquisition time. To encode motion or flow along one axis, two data sets must be compared. To encode flow in three orthogonal directions, four data sets must be acquired, consisting of one motion-compensated set and three sets with flow encoded in each of the three axes.

Two-Dimensional Phase Contrast

Two-dimensional PC (2D-PC) is useful for obtaining images during suspended respiration or during different phases of the cardiac cycle. On these images, background stationary tissue is usually gray; flow in one direction is light, and flow in the other direction is dark. The shade

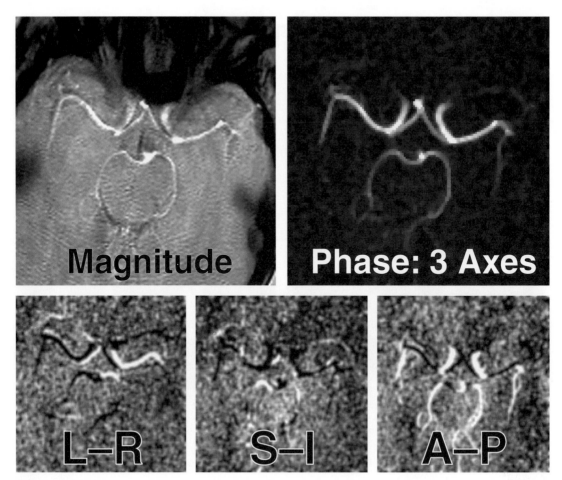

FIGURE 18–11. Two-dimensional phase contrast (2D-PC) 28/7.4/20° acquisition of a single 1.5-cm thick section at the circle of Willis (same patient as in Fig. 18–18). The received magnitude (amplitude) of the MR signals is used to construct the image at top left. Separate phase images are depicted at bottom, sensitive to flow directions of left to right *(left)*, superior to inferior *(center)*, and anterior to posterior *(right)*. Flow in one direction is white, flow in the other black, and static tissue is represented as neutral gray noise. The reconstructed phase image, sensitive to flow in all three axes, is depicted at top right without directional sensitivity, showing flow in any direction as white and nonmoving tissue as black.

of gray depends on the velocity of flow; rapid flow is depicted as white or black. These images are analogous to the color portion of color Doppler ultrasound images. In fact, PC images can be encoded in color and superimposed on gray-scale magnitude images, as with color Doppler imaging.

Two-dimensional PC images are useful for measuring the velocity and volume of blood flow. Velocity is directly proportional to the phase shift, whereas the volume of flow depends in addition on the cross-sectional area of the blood vessel.

Imaging and measurement of pulsatile flow is usually most accurate if cardiac gating techniques are used to produce 2D-PC images at different phases of the cardiac cycle. These techniques are often referred to as *cine phase contrast.*

Three-Dimensional Phase Contrast

Three-dimensional PC (3D-PC) images are useful for depicting flow with high SNR, high spatial resolution, and high background suppression. The major disadvantage of 3D-PC is the long acquisition time required for encoding motion along three orthogonal axes. Additionally, complex flow often results in heterogeneous phase changes within a voxel, reducing vascular flow signal. This can exaggerate the severity of vascular abnormalities or give false-positive results. However, this property of 3D-PC can be useful for confirming disturbed flow distal to a stenosis, implying hemodynamic significance (Fig. 18–13). If a vessel is not depicted on 3D-PC images distal to a stenosis, hemodynamic significance is likely.

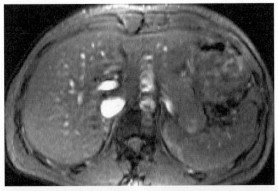

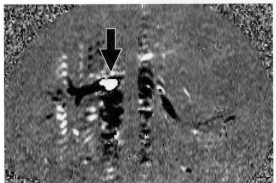 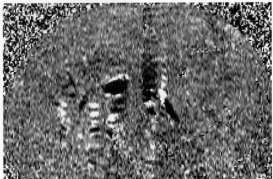

VENC = 20 cm/sec VENC = 80 cm/sec

FIGURE 18–12. Effect of different velocity-encoding value (v_{enc}) on 2D-PC 18/9/20° images sensitive to flow in the superior-inferior axis. Magnitude image is at top. With a low v_{enc} of 20 cm/sec *(bottom left)*, the velocity of flow in the portal vein is above the limit for unambiguous encoding of direction, causing aliasing in the portal vein *(arrow)*. With a higher v_{enc} of 80 cm/sec *(bottom right)*, flow in the portal vein is encoded unambiguously. Fewer small intrahepatic vessels are depicted, however, owing to less sensitivity to slow flow.

PERFUSION AND DIFFUSION TECHNIQUES

The previous sections of this chapter have focused on anatomic depiction of blood vessels. Vascular pathology and physiology can also be investigated with methods that rely on depiction of perfusion or diffusion rather than vascular anatomy. Many of these methods follow directly from principles introduced earlier in this book, including contrast agents, signal loss from motion or susceptibility, and the use of magnetization preparation pulses. Techniques for depicting perfusion and diffusion are discussed in the remainder of this chapter.

Perfusion

Dynamic bolus techniques are described in Chapter 17 and earlier in this chapter. Refine-ments of these techniques can be used to depict or measure tissue perfusion.

Perfusion of a tissue can be studied with any contrast agent that can be administered in a short, rapid bolus. Contrast agents that diffuse across capillary walls, such as most gadolinium chelates, can be used for perfusion techniques if images are acquired only during the first pass of the contrast agent through the tissue. The interval until arrival of the contrast agent to the tissue, the tissue's rate of enhancement, or the time required for the contrast agent to pass through the tissue, is measured and depicted. Ideal bolus administration for perfusion studies should be nearly instantaneous. The use of prolonged boluses leads to decreased precision of results.

Fast T1-weighted gradient echo techniques can be used to depict perfusion as increased signal intensity after bolus administration of gadolinium chelate. Alternatively, T2*-weighted gradient echo or echo planar images can be

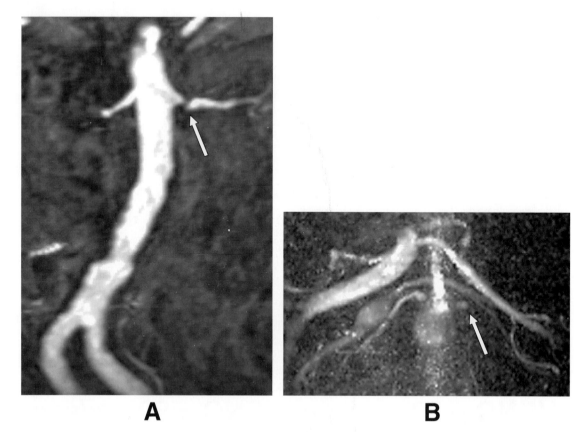

FIGURE 18–13. High-grade stenosis *(arrow)* depicted by gadolinium-enhanced 3D-GRE 7.5/2.2/50° MIP *(A)*, exaggerated by 3D-PC 33/7.7/20° technique *(B)* owing to dephasing of complex flow distal to the stenosis *(arrow)*.

used to depict perfusion as decreased signal intensity.

Principles related to magnetic susceptibility were discussed in Chapters 2 and 4. Paramagnetic materials in a magnetic field increase its strength in their immediate vicinity, causing local magnetic field heterogeneity. This decreases T2* relaxation time, decreasing signal intensity on certain pulse sequences. Pulse sequences that are sensitive to susceptibility-induced signal loss are referred to as T2*-weighted. Sensitivity to T2* contrast can be minimized by refocusing transverse magnetization via a 180° refocusing pulse transmitted at one half the TE or effective TE (TE$_{ef}$). Conversely, T2* contrast can be *increased* by omitting 180° refocusing pulses and by using long TEs or TE$_{ef}$. Particularly fast and efficient T2*-weighted images can be obtained using echo planar techniques.

The susceptibility effect of uneven distribution of contrast agent extends farther than the more local paramagnetic effect of T1 reduction. Heterogeneous susceptibility causes signal loss extending beyond the boundaries of the vessels into the surrounding tissue, whereas increased signal intensity due to paramagnetic substances affects only water protons in the blood vessels themselves (Fig. 18-14).

While small doses of superparamagnetic contrast agent (e.g., iron oxide particles or dysprosium chelates) may be used, these are not currently approved for rapid bolus administration in clinical practice. Fortunately, currently available gadolinium chelates produce sufficient T2* shortening when they are unevenly distributed in tissue, as when present only within capillaries during initial arrival to a tissue (Fig. 18-15). Echo planar techniques are ideal for perfusion imaging because of their rapidity and sensitivity to T2* enhancement.

Dilution of the contrast agent during the passage from peripheral vein to the tissue of interest produces unavoidable broadening of the effective bolus. A tighter bolus, for more precise depiction of tissue perfusion, could be obtained by direct intraarterial injection just proximal to the tissue of interest; however, invasive techniques are necessary for this. An alternative approach is to tag the blood magnetically. This can be accomplished with a spatial saturation

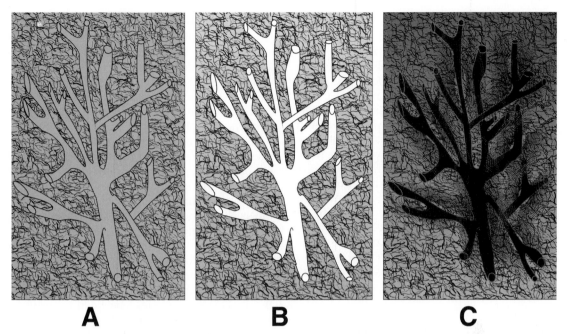

A   **B**   **C**

FIGURE 18-14. Effects of gadolinium chelates on brain parenchymal signal intensity using T1-weighted and T2*-weighted pulse sequences. *(A)* Baseline illustration. *(B)* On T1-weighted images, signal intensity increases markedly within vessels, but effect on parenchyma is minimal. *(C)* Susceptibility effects of gadolinium chelate extend beyond the vessel walls, decreasing parenchymal signal intensity on T2*-weighted images.

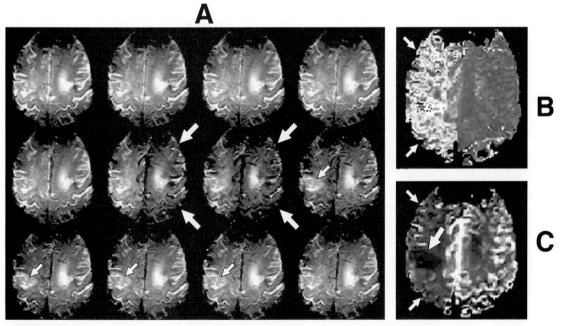

FIGURE 18-15. Acute cerebral infarction depicted by echo planar perfusion imaging following a bolus of 0.1 mmol/kg gadolinium chelate. *(A)* Twelve T2*-weighted images at the same location, each of which was acquired as part of a multiplanar whole-brain set of images at 40 different phases after contrast agent injection. These 12 images were acquired during an interval of 42 seconds. Upon arrival of the contrast agent, signal intensity of the normally perfused left hemisphere decreases *(large arrows)*; perfusion to the right hemisphere is delayed. Within the right hemisphere, the actual infarct is not perfused *(small arrows)*. *(B)* Mean transit time map depicts slow transit through the right hemisphere secondary to ischemia *(arrows)*. *(C)* Regional cerebral blood volume (rCBV) map, depicting decreased blood volume of the ischemic region *(small arrows)*, and nonperfusion of the infarct *(large arrow)*. (Courtesy of M. Moseley, M. Marks, D. Tong and G. Albert; Department of Radiology and Stanford Stroke Center.)

pulse, so that blood flowing into an image section or volume is more saturated. The effects of saturation pulses are most apparent on large vessels, but there are more subtle effects on tissue signal intensity. These effects are somewhat greater if 180° selective inversion pulses are used. Even so, the change in parenchymal signal intensity produced by such inversion pulses can be as small as 2%; depiction of these small changes requires postprocessing techniques such as image subtraction. If two images of the same site, one acquired with a preceding inversion pulse and one without, are subtracted from each other, the difference image will reflect tissue perfusion. One successful implementation of selective inversion recovery perfusion imaging has been referred to as *echo planar imaging signal targeting with alternating radiofrequency* (EPISTAR).

Blood Oxygen Level–Dependent Techniques

In the preceding section we discussed the use of T2*-weighted gradient echo or echo planar images, obtained following a bolus of para-magnetic contrast agent, for depicting perfusion. Disadvantages to the use of contrast agents include the added time, effort, and invasiveness of injections and the direct cost of the contrast agent. Additionally, it may be necessary to wait several minutes or hours before repeating the observation. However, intravascular deoxyhemoglobin may be used as an endogenous contrast agent for obtaining repetitive images depicting changes in perfusion after a variety of physiologic provocations.

Deoxyhemoglobin has four unpaired electrons, rendering it paramagnetic. Oxyhemoglobin is diamagnetic and has little effect on MR images. On heavily T2*-weighted pulse sequences, signal intensity is inversely related to deoxyhemoglobin concentration. Pulse sequences that are sensitive to concentrations of deoxyhemoglobin are commonly referred to as BOLD. These techniques have been successfully applied to depict changes in brain oxygen levels after various physiologic stimuli. With increased stimulation, blood flow to activated brain areas increases to deliver more oxygen, but tissue extraction of oxygen from the blood changes little. The increased blood flow to activated brain results in delivery of more fully oxygen-

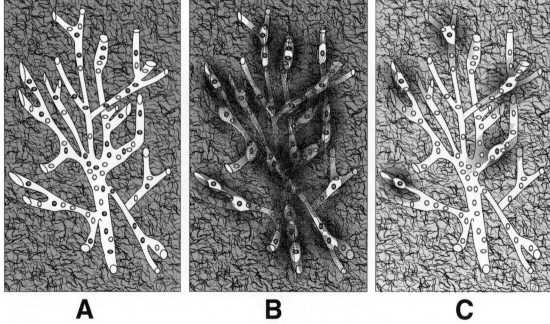

A   **B**   **C**

FIGURE 18–16. Principles of blood oxygen level dependent (BOLD) technique. *(A)* Light and dark ovals represent, respectively, oxygenated and deoxygenated red blood cells within microvasculature. *(B)* The paramagnetism of deoxyhemoglobin within deoxygenated red blood cells induces a higher local magnetic field, creating local field heterogeneities that extend beyond the blood vessels, decreasing parenchymal signal intensity on T2*-weighted images. *(C)* With increased flow, more oxygenated blood cells are delivered to the tissue, decreasing the concentration of deoxyhemoglobin and thus increasing signal intensity.

ated blood, decreasing the concentration of deoxyhemoglobin and increasing the signal intensity of activated brain on $T2^*$-weighted images (Fig. 18-16). The increased signal intensity caused by increased brain oxygen levels is 10% or less, so unambiguous depiction depends on postprocessing techniques such as subtraction (Fig. 18-17). Care must be taken to determine whether the observed increased signal intensity from increased blood oxygenation is within brain parenchyma or within cortical veins.

Diffusion

In Chapter 10 we discussed the loss of signal intensity caused by intravoxel phase dispersion; uncompensated motion during the interval between excitation and signal measurement can reduce the amplitude of the resultant echo. This principle can be applied to generate images in which loss of signal intensity results from random microscopic motion of water in relatively unstructured tissues such as fluid collections. This random motion is referred to as *diffusion*. Water diffuses randomly in tissue capillaries and the interstitium between cells, and it diffuses continually across cell membranes and between the various tissue compartments. Pure water at 37°C diffuses at a rate of approximately 0.003 mm^2/sec; this value is called the *diffusion coefficient* (D) of water. The diffusion of water in tissue is restricted and less random, so an apparent diffusion coefficient (ADC, or D^*) is used. ADC is smaller than the unrestricted value of D, and it continues to decrease as the time of its measurement (the diffusion time, T_d) increases. T_d can be increased to reduce the contribution from restricted diffusion, rendering the pulse sequence more specific for unrestricted diffusion.

Diffusion imaging is accomplished by incorporating into a pulse sequence pulsed gradients that increase sensitivity to diffusion. These dif-

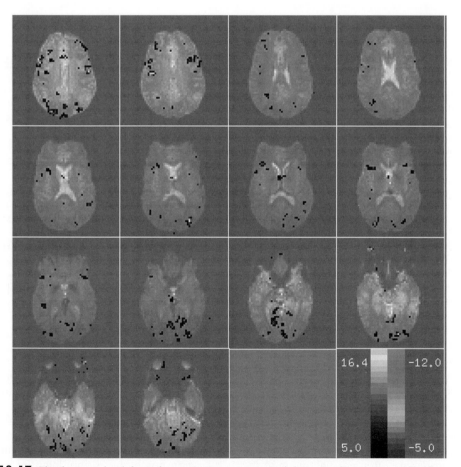

FIGURE 18-17. Blood oxygen level dependent activation map acquired during reading sentences. Baseline nonactivated areas are indicated in pale shades; activated areas are darker. Typically, overlays such as this use color to depict activated areas of parenchyma. (Courtesy of Keith R. Thulborn, M.D., Ph.D., University of Pittsburgh.)

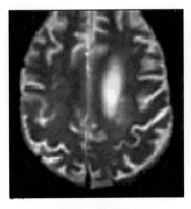 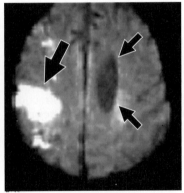

T2WI   DWI

FIGURE 18–18. Depiction of an acute cerebral infarction by diffusion-weighted images (same patient as in Fig. 18–11). The T2-weighted echo planar image *(left)* shows no abnormality owing to the relative lack of edema in this acute infarct. On the diffusion-weighted image with b = 1000 sec/mm² *(right)* there is markedly decreased signal intensity in the left lateral ventricle *(small arrows)* owing to the high apparent diffusion within free fluid. There is moderate apparent diffusion within brain parenchyma, but little within the infarct *(large arrow).* (Courtesy of M. Moseley, M. Marks, D. Tong and G. Albert; Department of Radiology and Stanford Stroke Center.)

fusion-sensitizing dephasing gradients are analogous to the flow-sensitizing dephasing gradients used for PC MRA techniques. The sensitivity of these pulse sequences can be altered by adjusting strength and timing of the diffusion-sensitive gradients, expressed by the diffusion sensitization parameter b. Generally, b values of 500 to 1500 sec/mm² are used. As the b value increases, TE (typically about 100 to 200 msec) must increase as well.

Diffusion-weighted images tend to resemble the inverse of T2-weighted images, because both are generally sensitive to free water, which is depicted as low signal intensity on diffusion-weighted images and as high signal intensity on T2-weighted images. However, diffusion-weighted images depict certain abnormalities better than T2-weighted images do. In particular, acute cerebral infarction involves decreased axonal cytoplasmic streaming owing to interruption of the sodium-potassium-ATPase pump, which results in decreased diffusion in the superoinferior plane. Additionally, the resulting cell swelling causes decreased interstitial and intravascular volume. These changes are depicted as markedly reduced diffusion in the section-select direction on axial diffusion-weighted images. At this early stage, T2-weighted images are often normal owing to the absence of edema (Fig. 18–18).

ESSENTIAL POINTS TO REMEMBER

1. Stationary oxygenated blood has low signal intensity on T1-weighted images and high signal intensity on T2-weighted images.
2. Saturation pulses can be applied to reduce the signal intensity of blood before it flows into an image section.
3. The flow of blood out of an image section between the excitation and refocusing pulses causes decreased intravascular signal.
4. Loss of phase coherence secondary to different flow velocities within a voxel causes decreased intravascular signal intensity.
5. Administration of gadolinium chelate reduces the T1 of blood, increasing its signal intensity.
6. Gadolinium-enhanced bright blood arteriographic images are best obtained using 3D-FT techniques, timed so that the weak phase-encoded views are acquired during the first pass of contrast agent through the vessels of interest.
7. TOF techniques depend on saturating background tissue with rapid repeated excitations. Blood flowing into the image section has higher signal intensity because it has not been saturated.

8. Two-dimensional TOF techniques are very sensitive to slow flow, owing to the short distance that blood must flow to leave the image section between excitations.

9. Three-dimensional TOF techniques have higher SNR and lower sensitivity to slow flow than do 2D-TOF techniques.

10. MOTSA is one method of increasing the sensitivity to slow flow of 3D-TOF techniques, at the expense of lower SNR.

11. PC techniques use phase changes from motion itself to encode flow. They allow measurement of flow velocity and usually have high background suppression, but acquisition time is longer than for most other vascular imaging techniques.

12. Perfusion can be depicted on a series of images acquired immediately after rapid bolus injection of contrast agent.

13. For depicting perfusion, T2*-weighted images are useful because intravascular contrast agent causes heterogeneous susceptibility and heterogeneous magnetic field that extend across vessel walls into the parenchyma.

14. For perfusion imaging, T2*-weighted images can be obtained after a bolus of either a particulate agent (e.g., iron oxide) or gadolinium chelate.

15. Perfusion imaging can be accomplished by magnetically tagging blood, using a saturation or inversion preparatory pulse, before its entry into a region of interest.

16. Deoxyhemoglobin is paramagnetic and is distributed heterogeneously, since it is present only within blood vessels. Thus, deoxyhemoglobin within blood vessels causes heterogeneous susceptibility and decreased signal intensity on T2*-weighted images.

17. Stimulated by activity, cerebral blood flow increases—and, thus, the delivery of fully oxygenated blood. This decreases the concentration of deoxyhemoglobin, increasing brain parenchymal signal intensity.

18. Parenchymal effects of perfusion and BOLD on images may be subtle. Thus, image subtraction is often used, subtracting baseline from, respectively, enhanced or stimulated images.

19. Diffusion of water molecules in blood vessels or interstitial fluid causes intravoxel phase dispersion, which decreases signal intensity on sensitive images. Sensitivity to diffusion can be increased by applying additional pulsed gradients.

CHAPTER

19 Artifacts

During the course of our discussion of magnetic resonance imaging (MRI) principles we have explained the basics of several artifacts. Now, we will review several common artifacts and methods by which they can be avoided.

WRAP-AROUND

As discussed in Chapters 5 and 8, spatial resolution of an image can be improved by decreasing its field of view (FOV). Often, the FOV is smaller than the body part being imaged. These situations can lead to wrap-around artifacts, in which image data outside the FOV are "wrapped around" and represented on the opposite side of the image. Wrap-around artifact can occur in both axes of an image section and in the section-encoding axis of a three-dimensional Fourier transform (3D-FT) acquisition.

In the frequency-encoded axis, image data is represented according to the frequency of received MR signals. The range of frequencies sampled is defined by the sampling bandwidth, which is synonymous with the sampling rate. The highest frequency that can be sampled unambiguously, also referred to as the *Nyquist frequency*, is half of the sampling bandwidth. Frequencies outside the range of ± the Nyquist frequency (i.e., the sampling bandwidth) cannot be distinguished from frequencies within the range. Figure 19–1 illustrates how a wave with a frequency higher than that of the sampling rate might be sampled so that its frequency appears to be lower.

In older imaging systems, frequencies just above the sampled range would be encoded as if they were at the low end of the range, producing wrap-around in the frequency-encoded axis. On these imaging systems, wrap-around in

the frequency-encoded axis can be avoided by using a sufficiently large FOV or by obtaining more frequency samples than are needed. For example, 512 samples can be obtained, even though the frequency-encoded resolution is only 256. The drawback of this technique is that sampling time is lengthened. On modern equipment, wrap-around in the frequency axis is avoided by using digital filters, which eliminate signals with frequencies outside the desired range.

Wrap-around in the phase-encoded axis is more difficult to prevent. Typically, an image is encoded for 360° of phase. A phase change of slightly more than 360° is identical to a small phase change. For example, a phase of 405° is the same as a phase of 45° (Fig. 19–2).

Wrap-around artifact can produce a distinctive "zebra stripe" moiré fringe artifact on gradient echo images of large body parts (Fig. 19–3). Magnetic field heterogeneities outside the FOV produce artifacts that overlap the primary image. Stripes are caused by the resulting phase interference.

The only way to avoid ambiguous measurement of phase is to use a large enough FOV in the phase-encoded axis, so that the range of phases sampled is not more than 360°. It is not necessary, however, to use this data to create an image with an FOV larger than that desired. After the Fourier transform, only the pixel data that correspond to the region of interest are represented.

Although the pixel data from the unwanted region is discarded, acquisition of the views (echoes) that allowed the creation of this pixel data was not a wasted effort. It must be remembered that for 2D-FT techniques, *every view contains information, and thus contributes to signal-to-noise ratio (SNR), for every pixel within the image section*. For 3D-FT techniques, every view contains information for ev-

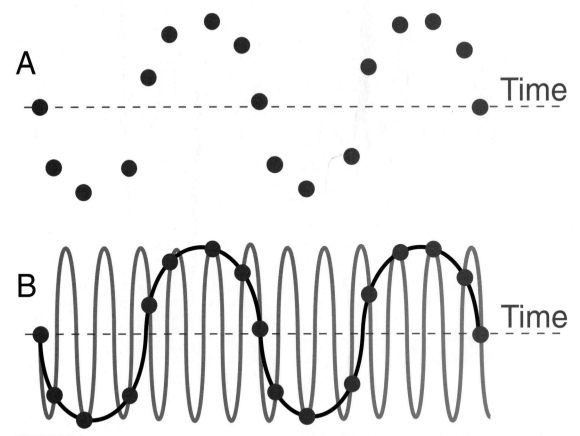

FIGURE 19-1. Frequency ambiguity results because waves of high and low frequency can both fit a given set of data samples. *(A)* A finite set of data samples is shown as points that fit the low-frequency waveform shown as a dark line in *B*. To unambiguously determine the high frequency shown with the lighter line, a faster sampling rate would have been needed.

ery pixel in the image volume. This principle allows some vendors to eliminate phase wrap in a way that is nearly transparent to clinical users; choosing a "no phase wrap" option eliminates phase wrap-around artifact without producing any apparent effects on the image or slowing acquisition time.

Consider an image with a 256 by 256 matrix, a 20-cm² FOV, and number of signals averaged (NSA) of 2. The number of views obtained is therefore 256 × 2 = 512. Spatial resolution is determined by the pixel size. Phase wrap can be eliminated by doubling the FOV in the phase-encoded axis from 20 to 40 cm. If the pixel size is not changed, it is necessary to double the number of phase-encoding views from 256 to 512. The matrix is now 256 by 512, and the FOV is 20 by 40 cm. If NSA is decreased from two to one, the total number of views obtained remains the same: 512. Because pixel size and the number of views have not changed, spatial resolution and SNR do not change (Fig. 19-4). Vendors may choose to label this image as having increased FOV and

matrix and decreased NSA or may choose simply to display image annotation as if nothing had changed, because, indeed, spatial resolution, SNR, and apparent FOV have not changed.

The principal disadvantage of phase axis oversampling is increased acquisition time for pulse sequences without signal averaging. If the minimum number of signal averages is already being used, phase axis oversampling cannot be accomplished without increasing the total number of views obtained. For applications such as high-resolution dynamic imaging after a bolus of contrast material, other approaches are needed. Phase axis wrap-around can often be avoided by judicious choice of FOV and phase-encoding axis. When wrap-around occurs, careful viewing of images is essential so that wrap-around artifact is not mistaken for disease (Fig. 19-5).

For 2D-FT techniques, section thickness is determined by selectively exciting, along the section select gradient, protons of a desired range of frequencies. Protons with frequencies outside this range are not excited, so wrap-

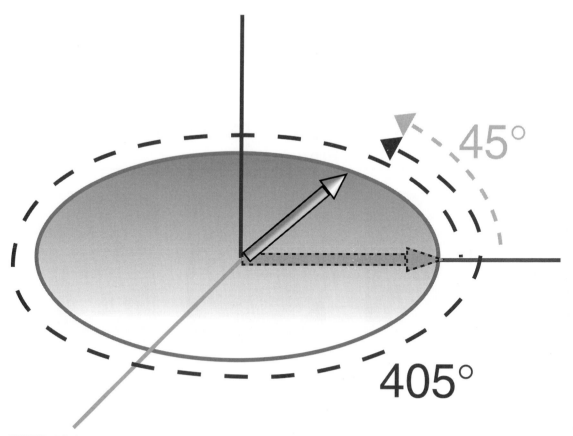

FIGURE 19-2. Phase ambiguity. Rotations of 45° and 405° produce the same phase, resulting in ambiguous phase encoding, which is depicted as aliasing.

FIGURE 19-3. Zebra stripe artifact *(arrows)* at the periphery of a gradient echo 11/2.2/30° image, results from phase interference between tissue in the image and aliased artifact from magnetic field heterogeneity outside the field of view.

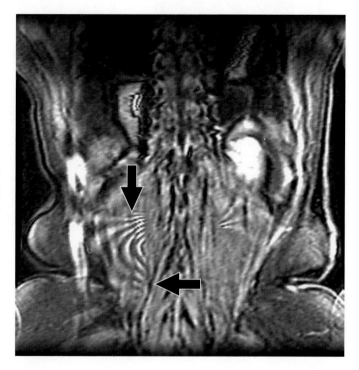

Phase Axis Wrap-Around

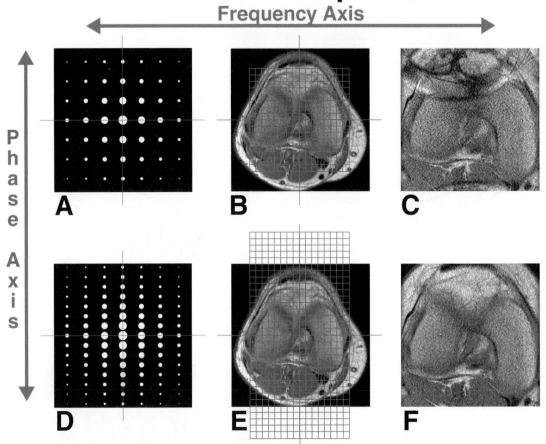

Increased Phase Axis Field-of-View

FIGURE 19–4. Phase axis wrap-around results from a body part extending beyond the field of view (FOV) in the phase axis *(top)*. *(A)* The map of k-space for the small FOV is depicted by the grid in *(B)*. The part of the knee that extends outside the acquired FOV is depicted ambiguously as wrap-around artifact in *(C)*. This artifact is eliminated if the acquisition FOV in the phase axis is increased, even if the reconstructed FOV is not changed *(bottom)*. *(D)* The map of k-space for the increased FOV depicted by the grid in *(E)*. There are twice as many points in k-space. Two signal averages of the top scenario and one signal average of the bottom scenario have the same total number of views, so signal-to-noise ratio (SNR) is unchanged. Pixel size is unchanged, so *(F)* has the same spatial resolution as *(C)*, but without wrap-around artifact. Wrap-around in the frequency axis is eliminated by digital filters.

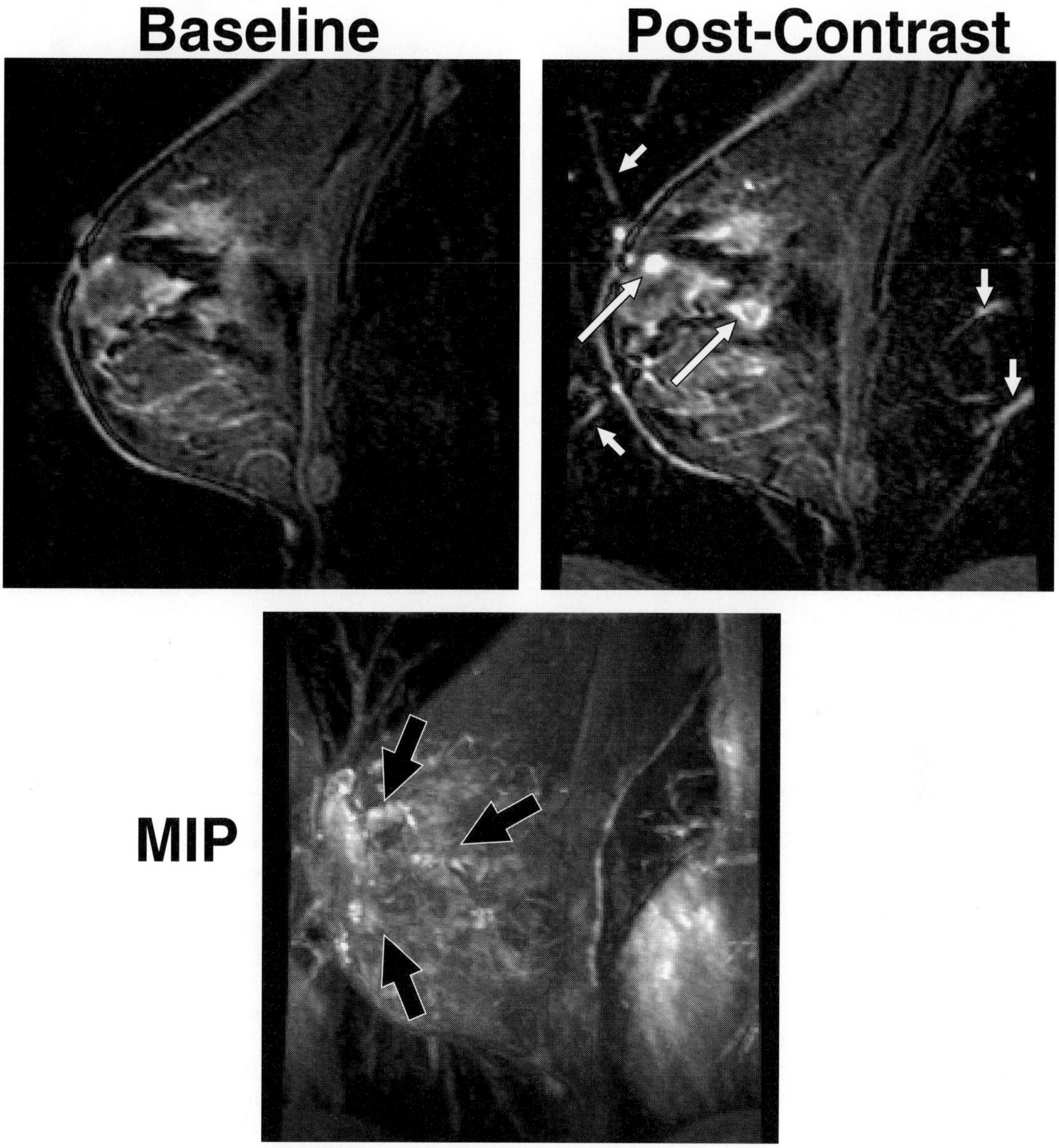

Baseline

Post-Contrast

MIP

FIGURE 19–5. Pseudonodules on sagittal images of the breast result from aliased pulmonary and hilar vessels. The phase axis is anteroposterior. Baseline image *(top left)* shows no breast lesions. On the post-contrast image, two round, enhancing structures *(large arrows)* project over the breast. Small arrows indicate pulmonary vessels. At bottom, the maximum-intensity projection (MIP) image shows the hilar structures *(black arrows)* overlying the breast, accounting for the enhancing pseudonodules.

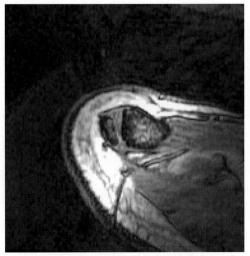 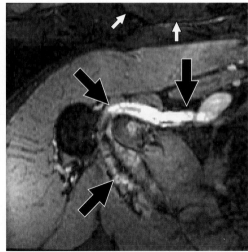

Top Section   Bottom Section

FIGURE 19–6. Wrap-around artifact in the section-encoded direction in axial three-dimensional Fourier transform (3D-FT) images of the shoulder. At right, a ghost of the top of the shoulder *(black arrows)* is projected onto the bottom section. White arrows indicate wrap-around artifact in the phase axis.

around artifact does not occur in the section-select axis. With 3D-FT techniques, however, sections are phase *encoded*, so phase wrap can occur in the section-encoded direction (Fig. 19–6). Wrap-around in the section-encoded direction can be avoided by encoding additional sections beyond the region of interest. Acquisition of the data for these sections contributes to the SNR of all other sections, whether or not these sections are reconstructed; each echo measured contributes information to all voxels throughout the volume of a 3D-FT acquisition.

EDGE ARTIFACTS

Detail of an image can be reduced by a variety of edge artifacts, even if voxel size is small and ghost artifacts are avoided. Many edge artifacts occur as a result of the FT processing of the image data.

Partial-Volume Artifacts

Partial-volume artifacts are intrinsic to all imaging, owing to finite limits of image resolution. In MRI and other digital techniques, image resolution is limited by the size of image voxels. The signals of different tissues or structures within a voxel are averaged so that they are not resolved. Thus, the interface between two objects with different signal intensities may be depicted as intermediate signal intensity (Fig. 19–7).

Chemical Shift Edge Artifacts

The difference between the resonant frequencies of water, lipid, and silicone protons produces chemical shift artifacts. Chemical shift *misregistration* artifact is erroneous mapping of protons with different chemical shifts (see Chapter 5). High signal bands result when protons with different chemical shifts are mapped as if they were in the same pixel, causing summation of their signals. Signal voids result when protons with different chemical shifts are mapped more distant from each other than their true separation. Chemical shift misregistration artifact is most visible on MR images when the magnetizations of different chemical shifts are *in phase* with respect to each other so that summation bands may be observed.

The amount of displacement of lipid relative to water depends on the magnetic field strength and the bandwidth per pixel. In an image with a frequency-encoding axis resolution of 256 and a sampling bandwidth of 32 kHz, the bandwidth per pixel is 125 Hz (32,000 ÷ 32 = 125). The chemical shift between lipid and water protons, about 3.5 parts/million, increases with magnetic field strength. With this bandwidth, at 1.5 T, the shift is about 220 Hz, slightly less than the bandwidth of two pixels. Thus, the displacement of lipid relative to water is slightly less than two pixels.

The frequency shift between lipid and water depends on the magnetic field and thus cannot be changed by the MR operator. The amount of physical distance that corresponds to this chemical shift, however, can be decreased by increasing the frequency-encoding resolution, so that a given number of pixels corresponds to a smaller physical distance. The misregistration is also reduced by increasing the sampling bandwidth, so that the chemical shift corre-

sponds to a smaller number of pixels. For the example above, if the bandwidth is doubled to 250 Hz per pixel, the chemical shift displacement would be reduced to less than 1 pixel.

Chemical shift *cancellation* artifact occurs when the magnetization of different chemical shifts are *out of phase* with respect to each other. For example, opposed phases of lipid and water proton magnetizations reduce signal intensity, because the effect is signal cancellation rather than signal summation. Edge artifacts result from chemical shift differences when water and lipid protons occupy the same voxel, owing to partial volume artifact. Phase cancellation results from destructive interfer-

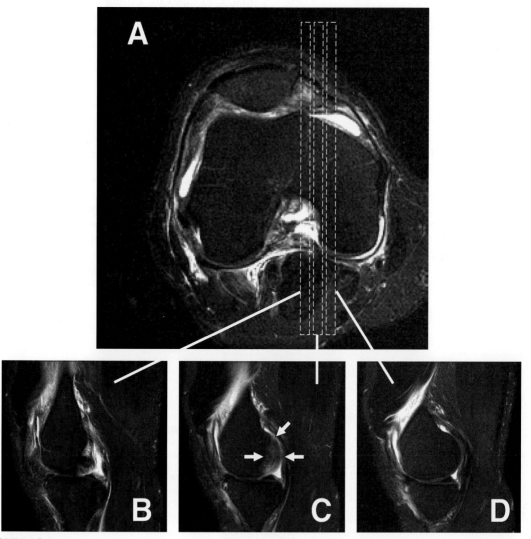

FIGURE 19–7. Partial volume artifact on fat-suppressed T2-weighted sagittal fast spin echo (FSE) images of the knee. The image sections for *(B)*, *(C)*, *(D)* are indicated by white-dotted rectangles on the axial fat-suppressed T2-weighted FSE image in *(A)*. *(C)* Arrows indicate moderately high signal intensity mimicking bone marrow edema caused by partial volume artifact between the high signal intensity of synovial fluid in *(B)* and the low signal intensity of bone and marrow in *(D)*.

ence between these signals and their discrepant phases. Chemical shift cancellation artifacts are eliminated by obtaining standard spin echo or fast spin echo images, in which the refocusing pulses correct for chemical shift differences. On gradient echo images, chemical shift cancellation artifacts are eliminated by choosing the echo time (TE) so that magnetizations of lipid and water protons are in phase. The conspicuousness of both types of chemical shift artifacts can be minimized by suppressing the signal of lipid, using either chemical shift fat-suppression or inversion recovery fat-nulling techniques.

Truncation Artifacts

MR signals are waves. They are mapped spatially according to their frequency and phase. In an attempt to create from a complex set of analog signals an image with a finite number of pixels, the data are truncated. This produces artifacts. The image is an approximation of the region of interest, spatial resolution being limited by the size of the voxels.

FT analysis involves expressing structure within an image as a complex combination of waves. Abrupt changes in signal intensity at the interface between high- and low–signal intensity structures can produce a "ring-down" artifact consisting of alternating bright and dark bands whose intensity decreases with distance from the high-contrast interface (Fig. 19–8).

The conspicuousness of truncation artifacts can be reduced by increasing the spatial resolution of the image or by decreasing the contrast of the interface. For example, truncation artifact adjacent to adipose tissue on a T1-weighted image can be reduced by suppressing the signal from fat.

Relaxation Artifacts

Edge artifacts result from any process that changes signal amplitude during image acquisition. For example, fast spin echo techniques rely on obtaining echoes with several different TEs. Signal decay increases with longer TE, owing to T2 relaxation. Thus, the signals from echoes with long TE are weaker than the signals from echoes with short TE. These edge artifacts are minimized in modern implementations of fast spin echo by careful design of the order of phase-encoding gradient strengths and by minimizing the time between echoes, so that signal intensity changes between successive echoes are small.

GHOST ARTIFACTS

Patient motion is a major cause of ghost artifacts. These artifacts, and ways of preventing them, are discussed in Chapter 10. These measures include spatial presaturation, gradient moment nulling, averaging, cardiac or respiratory monitoring, and decreased repetition time (TR) (Fig. 19–9). Ghost artifacts can also result from severe changes of signal intensity during image acquisition, such as in fast spin echo with incorrect phase-encoding order or with long echo spacing.

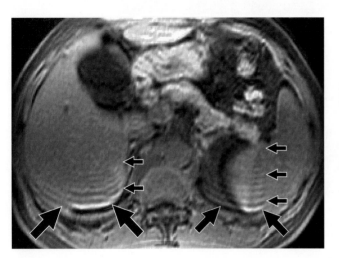

FIGURE 19–8. Truncation artifacts on an axial 3D gradient echo 7/2.2/20° image of the abdomen with 256 (left to right) by 128 (anteroposterior) matrix. The low anteroposterior spatial resolution has resulted in truncation artifact in this axis, which is manifested as a ring-down artifact *(small arrows)* originating from the high-contrast borders posteriorly *(large arrows)*.

TR = 120 msec

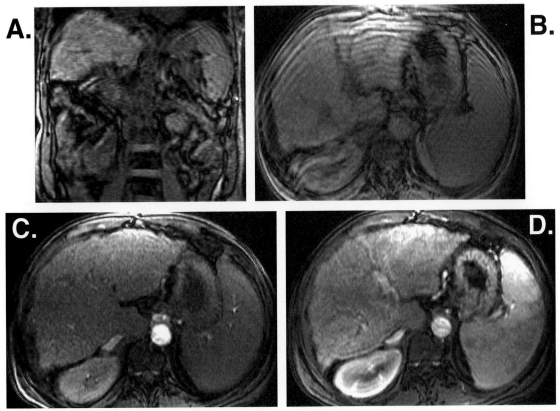

TR = 34 msec

FIGURE 19–9. Reduction of respiration-induced ghost artifacts by reducing repetition time (TR) in a patient who could not suspend respiration during imaging. Within-view errors are minimal owing to the short echo time (TE) of 2.2 msec for all images. Coronal *(A)* and axial *(B)* images with TR of 120 msec show pronounced artifact. When TR was reduced to 34 msec, unenhanced *(C)* and gadolinium-enhanced *(D)* images show less artifact. With shorter TR, there is less variability between views, so artifact is generally less pronounced.

STRIPES

Zipper Artifacts

Zipper artifacts consist of a stripe, often at the center of the frequency-encoding or phase-encoding axes. Alternating black and white spots produce a zipper appearance. At zero phase, a zipper parallel to the frequency-encoding axis can be caused by unwanted residual transverse magnetization before a radio pulse. This unwanted transverse magnetization can come from a nondecayed free induction decay (FID) or from stimulated echoes.

If side lobes of 180° refocusing pulses overlap the FID signal before it decays, zipper artifact

along the frequency-encoding axis at zero phase can result. The FID is the signal emitted immediately after creation of transverse magnetization by the excitation pulse. Normally, this signal decays rapidly, and later an echo is formed by the rephasing lobe of the frequency-encoding gradient. If the TE of a spin echo pulse sequence is short enough, the refocusing pulse may occur before the FID has fully decayed. A zipper results at the midpoint of the phase-encoding axis. This can be corrected by increasing the TE, which allows complete decay of the FID before the 180° refocusing pulse.

Zipper artifact at zero phase can also result if stimulated echoes are not adequately spoiled. Stimulated echoes are formed by imperfect radio pulses. For example, imperfect 180° pulses not only can refocus transverse magnetization, but can affect recovered longitudinal magnetization, to create new transverse magnetization. Because stimulated echoes are not phase encoded, they appear in the central line along the frequency-encoded axis, corresponding to zero phase encoding. This artifact can be eliminated by more complete spoiling.

A similar zipper artifact along the *phase-encoding* axis, at the point of zero frequency encoding, can be caused by radiofrequency (RF) feedthrough, which occurs when the excitation RF pulse is detected directly by the receiver coil. It is located in the center of the frequency-encoding axis because it matches the frequency of the excitation pulse, which corresponds to the central frequency of the sampled bandwidth (Fig. 19–10). RF feedthrough artifact can be eliminated by alternating the polarity of the excitation pulses, if more than one excitation are averaged. The positive and negative feedthroughs are averaged, producing zero artifact. If there is no signal averaging, RF feedthrough zipper artifacts can be eliminated by omitting the data that correspond to this central frequency and replacing it with data interpolated from adjacent points.

Zipper artifacts along the phase-encoding axis, away from the point of zero frequency encoding, can result from extraneous radio noise, which is collected along with sampled MR signals (Fig. 19–11). There are numerous sources of electronic noise, such as radio and television signals, fluorescent lighting, and electric equipment. The unwanted signals are mapped at the specific locations along the frequency-encoding axis that correspond to their frequencies.

Data Errors

Occasionally, mistakes in the filling of k-space lead to bad data points. These can result from static electricity in the magnetic bore, which can be caused by blankets or patients' clothing. The data errors are visible in maps of k-space as points of increased amplitude, and they produce a corduroy appearance on the resulting image. Fast imaging techniques that rely on interpolation based on the symmetry of k-space, such as partial echo sampling or partial Fourier techniques, are particularly prone to these artifacts, since the data errors are duplicated in the other half of k-space. The artifacts are less common and less severe when all of k-space is sampled at least once. The artifact can be reduced or eliminated if the causative data point is eliminated or if the image acquisition is repeated. Usually, only one image, or a few, in a multisection acquisition are affected (Fig. 19–12).

ALTERED SIGNAL INTENSITY

Susceptibility Artifacts

Magnetic susceptibility was discussed in Chapter 4. As with chemical shift artifact, image

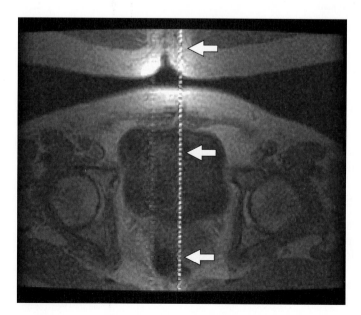

FIGURE 19–10. Radiofrequency feedthrough artifact *(arrows)* along the phase axis, at the point of zero frequency encoding. Note also phase axis wrap-around artifact, projecting the posterior tissues anteriorly.

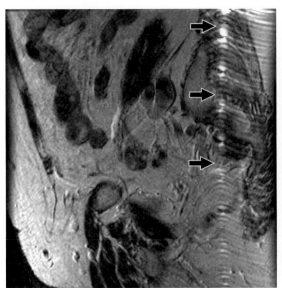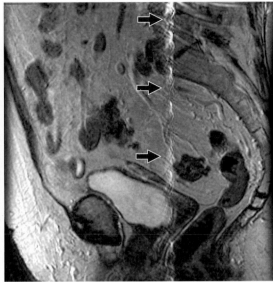

FIGURE 19-11. Zipper artifact from extraneous radio noise on two different image sections from the same acquisition.

distortion results from incorrect frequency encoding. Heterogeneous susceptibility causes magnetic field heterogeneity, which, in turn, alters the frequency of protons. Protons exposed to a higher magnetic field spin with increased frequency. These protons are thus mapped at a location that corresponds to a higher position along the frequency-encoding gradient and produce a signal void in the image where they should have been represented. A white band is commonly noted at the edge of this void; this reflects overlapping signals of the mismapped protons.

Susceptibility artifact can be minimized by using spin echo technique with the shortest possible TE, or fast spin echo technique with the shortest possible echo spacing. Susceptibility artifact is generally more pronounced with gradient echo techniques, although it can be reduced by using the shortest possible TE (Fig. 19-13). Sampling bandwidth should be as high as possible, and image gradients should have maximum strength; gradient strength can usually be maximized by using small FOV and thin image sections.

Cross-Talk

Radio pulses targeted to one section of a multisection acquisition may affect adjacent sections (see Chapter 7). This produces more saturation effects than would be expected from a given TR, because some saturation occurs during the TR. The result is equivalent to a

decrease in the "effective" TR. Thus, a given pulse sequence may have lower SNR and may appear more T1 weighted and less T2 weighted.

Heterogeneous Fat Suppression

Fat suppression via chemical shift saturation techniques involves exciting lipid protons by a radio pulse that matches their resonant frequency. If all lipid protons in the region of interest are precessing at the same frequency, they can be excited by a single radio pulse; however, if the main magnetic field is heterogeneous, or if the radio pulse is not transmitted uniformly throughout this region, excitation of lipid protons will not be uniform. Heterogeneous fat suppression is one of the most common artifacts, because the chemical shift between water and lipid protons is only about 3.5 parts per million. Slight variation of the main magnetic field causes lipid protons to precess at a different frequency from that of the narrowly focused chemical shift saturation pulse.

The homogeneity of even a perfect main magnetic field is disturbed once a patient lies within it. The most common cause of patient-induced magnetic field heterogeneity is air-tissue interfaces, whether within the patient or at the skin surface. Air and water have different magnetic susceptibilities, and this results in different local magnetic fields. Bone and water also have different susceptibilities, but the dis-

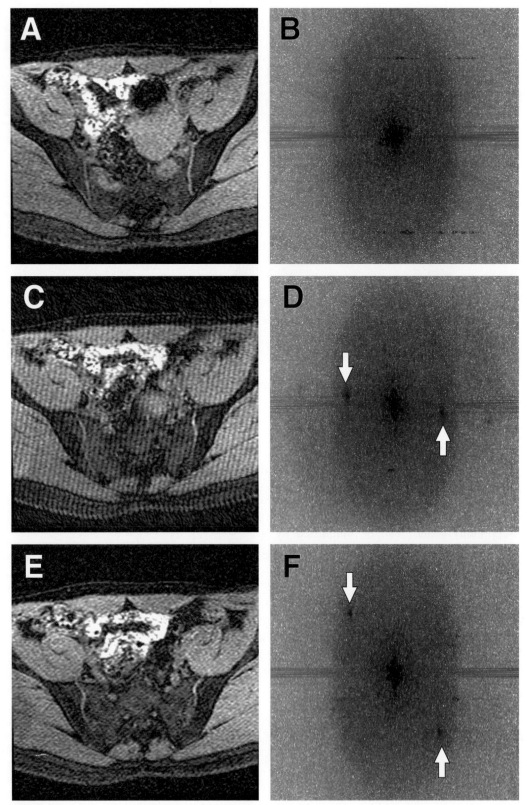

FIGURE 19–12. Artifact on fat-suppressed two-dimensional gradient echo (2D-GRE) 120/2.6/90° images from bad data points in k-space. The image in *(A)*, corresponding to the k-space map in *(B)*, shows no significant artifact. A prominent striped pattern overlies the adjacent image in *(C)*. This is caused by bad data points *(arrows)* in the k-space map in *(D)*. The striped artifact in *E* is more subtle, because the bad data points in *(F) (arrows)* are farther from the center of k-space.

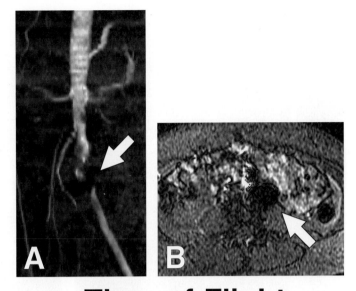

Time-of-Flight

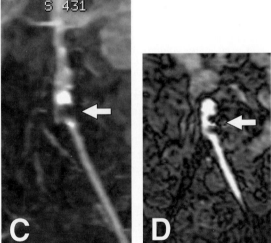

Gadolinium

FIGURE 19–13. Signal void *(arrows)* due to metallic surgical clips: effect of echo time (TE) on severity. *(A)* There is a large void in the coronal MIP, constructed from axial 37/6.5/60° two-dimensional time of flight (2D-TOF) source images *(B)*. *(C)* The signal void is much smaller in the coronal MIP image constructed from coronal gadolinium-enhanced three-dimensional gradient echo (3D-GRE) 11/2.2/60° source images *(D)*, owing to the shorter TE.

turbance of magnetic field homogeneity for these tissues is less pronounced.

With severe magnetic field heterogeneity, as in the presence of metal objects, most fat-suppression techniques should be avoided (Fig. 19-14). Generally, fat nulling by short inversion time recovery (STIR) is less affected than are fat-suppression techniques (Fig. 19-15). In some instances, magnetic field heterogeneity may cause the frequency of water protons in some portions of the image to correspond to the frequency of a fat-suppression pulse. This will result in unintended water saturation (Fig. 19-16).

Magic-Angle Effects

The decay of transverse magnetization is facilitated by nonrandom structure, particularly by a structure including oriented parallel components. Examples include tendons and ligaments, which contain parallel fibrous bands. For these

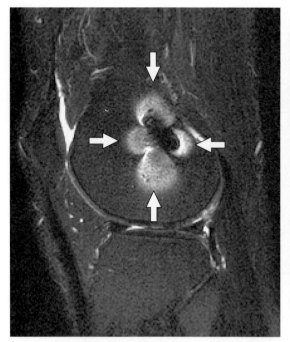 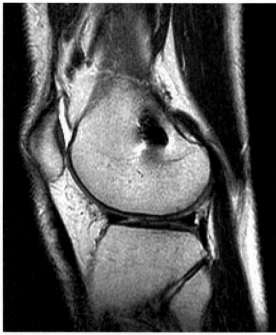

FSE FatSat   FSE

FIGURE 19–14. Pronounced artifact on fat-suppressed fast spin echo (FSE) 4500/100 image *(left)* from uneven fat suppression due to metal implant. Distortion is less on comparable FSE image without fat suppression *(right)*.

tissues T2 is thus particularly short, leading to low signal intensity on most MR images. However, if these parallel bands are oriented at 55° relative to the main magnetic field, the T2 facilitation is decreased, leading to increased signal intensity. For this reason, focal areas of increased signal intensity in tendons and ligaments are common on images with short or moderate TE (i.e., less than 25 msec). The location of the increased signal varies with position and angle of the fibers relative to the main magnetic field (Fig. 19–17).

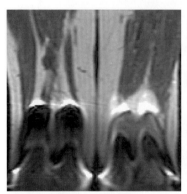 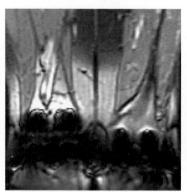 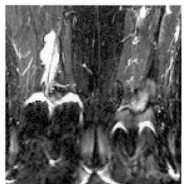

T1-SE   T1-FatSat   STIR

FIGURE 19–15. Susceptibility artifact from metallic prosthesis is exacerbated by uneven fat suppression. The local distortion and signal voids are comparable for the T1-weighted spin echo (T1-SE) 417/8 image *(left)*, T1-weighted fat-suppressed (T1-FatSat) gradient echo 250/1.6/90° image *(center)*, and fast spin echo-short inversion time inversion recovery (STIR) 6250/60/150 image *(right)*. Image degradation is exacerbated on the T1-weighted fat saturation image *(center)* due to heterogeneous fat suppression. Fat nulling is more homogeneous on the STIR image *(right)*.

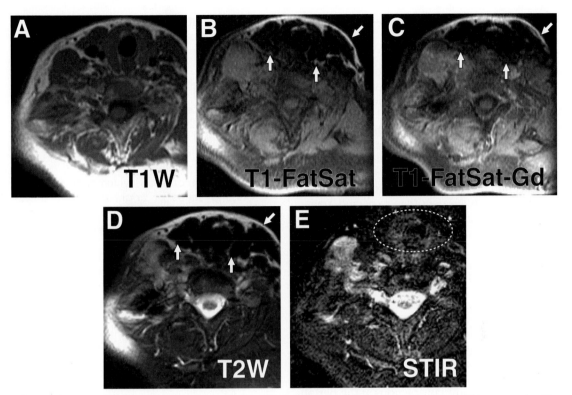

FIGURE 19–16. Artifactual water suppression *(arrows)* on fat-suppressed images (from magnetic field heterogeneity. The T1-weighted spin echo 467/8 image *(A)* shows increased signal intensity posteriorly, owing to a nonuniform profile of the local receiver coil. The T1-weighted, fat-suppressed gradient echo 250/1.6 image *(B)* shows water suppression of the anterior tissues of the neck. Following administration of gadolinium chelate (Gd) *(C)*, it is not possible to determine whether any tissue in this region is enhanced, as water signal is suppressed. Anterior water signal is also suppressed on the T2-weighted fat suppressed FSE 6100/98 image *(D)*. These tissues are depicted *(dotted circle)* on the FSE-STIR 8571/75/150 image *(E)*.

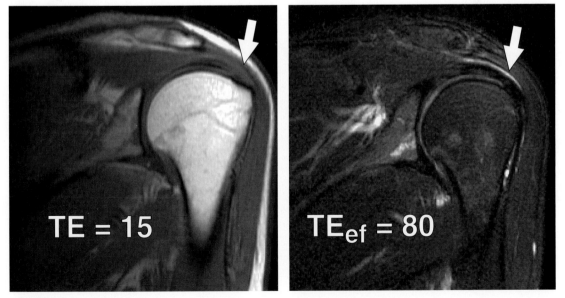

FIGURE 19–17. Magic angle effect produces an area of increased signal intensity *(arrow)* of the supraspinatus tendon on spin echo 600/15 image *(left)*. On FSE 3000/80 image *(right)*, the tendon has uniformly low signal intensity, owing to the longer effective echo time (TE$_{ef}$).

IMAGE DISTORTION

Imaging gradients are used for spatial location of MR signals. The depiction of structure on MR images depends on a linear correspondence between true anatomy and the phase and frequency changes caused by these gradients. Image distortion usually results from a nonlinear response to imaging gradients. This can be particularly pronounced near large differences in susceptibility, as near metallic objects. The magnetic field is stronger than expected, owing to the strength of the imaging gradient itself, so image distortion and signal loss occur.

Eddy Currents

Eddy currents are small electric currents that are caused by rapidly switching the gradients on and off. These currents produce persistent undesirable magnetic gradients that result in faster dephasing of transverse magnetization. Affected images show areas of reduced signal intensity that is most conspicuous at the periphery, where gradient profiles are often less adequate. Ghost artifacts in the phase axis, indistinguishable from motion artifact, can also occur.

ESSENTIAL POINTS TO REMEMBER

1. Wrap-around artifact, or aliasing, involves representation of a body part on the opposite side of an image when it extends beyond the acquired FOV.
2. Wrap-around artifact in the phase axis can be prevented by acquiring data for a larger FOV. If pixel size and the total number of echoes sampled do not change, SNR and spatial resolution are not affected.
3. With 3D-FT techniques, image sections are phase encoded, so wrap-around can occur in the section-encoding axis.
4. Partial volume artifact results when two different structures are included in the same voxel.

5. Chemical shift misregistration artifact is most conspicuous on images in which fat and water magnetizations are in phase and both have moderate or high signal intensity.
6. Chemical shift misregistration artifact can be reduced by increasing the sampling bandwidth.
7. Chemical shift cancellation artifact occurs when fat and water magnetizations have opposed phases.
8. Truncation artifacts, which appear as alternating series of bright and dark bands, occur because the FT reconstruction cannot accurately depict abrupt high-contrast borders.
9. The conspicuousness of truncation artifact can be reduced by increasing spatial resolution or by decreasing the contrast of the border, as by fat suppression.
10. Any cause of changing echo amplitude during acquisition, such as variable TEs within an echo train, can cause ghost artifacts.
11. Zipper artifacts can be caused by a variety of pulse sequence deficiencies or by extraneous radio signals that are detected by the MRI receiving coil.
12. A corduroy-like banding pattern can result from a single bad data point in k-space, which in turn can arise from static electricity as from a patient's clothing or blankets.
13. Heterogeneous susceptibility can be caused by air or metal, causing areas of signal loss and image distortion. Spin echo images with short TE and fast spin echo images with short echo spacing are least affected.
14. A nonhomogeneous magnetic field results in nonhomogeneous fat suppression, because the resulting various lipid frequencies cannot be matched by the single frequency of the fat-suppression pulse.
15. The T2 of tissues with oriented fibers is highest when these fibers are aligned at $55°$ (the magic angle) relative to the main magnetic field. Homogeneous low signal intensity of these tissues can be achieved by using a sufficiently long TE.

INDEX

Page numbers in *italics* refer to illustrations; page numbers followed by t refer to tables.